THE MOST COMPLETE GUIDE
TO NATURAL HEALING AND
HEALTH WITH TRADITIONAL
AYURVEDIC HERBALISM

the way of

AYURVEDIC HERBS

Ayurvedic herbs have reached the mainstream of American health care. Now two experts teach you about the earth's oldest healing system.

Karta Purkh Singh Khalsa
& Michael Tierra

LOTUS PRESS

P.O. BOX 325
TWIN LAKES, WI 53181 USA

DISCLAIMER

This book is not intended to treat, diagnose or prescribe. The information contained herein is in no way to be considered as a substitute for your own inner guidance or consultation with a duly licensed health-care professional. We wish the best of health and welfare to all.

First Edition 2008

Reprinted 2012, 2024

Printed in the United States of America

ISBN 978-0-9409-8598-8

Library of Congress Catalog Number 2007935723

LOTUS PRESS

Published by:
Lotus Press, P.O. Box 325, Twin Lakes, WI 53181 USA
web: www.lotuspress.com
Email: lotuspress@lotuspress.com
800.824.6396

CONTENTS

Author's Foreword to the Series ix
Introduction xi
1 The People's Medicine 1
2 The Five Elements and the Basis of Ayurveda 7
3 The Three Doshas 11
4 The Way of Health and Disease in Ayurveda 17
5 The Way of Ayurvedic Diagnosis 25
The Healer in Ayurveda 26
Constitution 27
Determining your body type 27
Personal Constitution Test 30
Constitutional Questionnaire 32
Making the best of your constitution 34
Mental Constitution 34
Symptoms 38
6 Food and Diet in Ayurveda 41
Fasting and Detoxification 45
Signs of the need for detoxification 46
Getting it Out 47
Milk Products 50
Ghee and Butter 52
Honey 54
Lemon 54
Salt 55
Protein 55
Beans 58
Mung Beans and Kicharee 58
Kanji 59
Karela 59
Eggplant 60
Onion 60
7 The Way of Ayurvedic Treatments 63
Ayurveda Treatment Categories 65
Massage Therapy in Ayurveda 66
Panchakarma 68

Herbs for the Mind 70
Nasal Rinsing- Spring Cleaning for your Nose 72

8 Ayurvedic Materia Medica 75
Temperature 75
Taste 76
Ayurvedic Dose and Preparations 82
Ajwain 86
Aloe 87
Amla 89
Angelica 91
Arjuna 92
Asafoetida 94
Asana 96
Ashwaganda 97
Bala 99
Barberry 100
Betel 101
Bhumy amalaki 102
Bibitaki 103
Bilwa 104
Black Pepper 105
Black tea 106
Brahmi 109
Bringraj 111
Calamus 112
Camphor 114
Cardamom 115
Castor 116
Chiretta 119
Chrysanthemum 120
Cinnamon 120
Clove 123
Coleus 124
Coriander 125
Cumin 126
Dandelion 127
Fennel 129
Fenugreek 130
Flaxseed 132
Garlic 133
Gentian 135
Ginger 136
Gokshura 138

Guduchi 139
Guggul 141
Gurmar 142
Haritaki 144
Hibiscus 145
Jambul 146
Juniper 147
Kalmegh 148
Kapi Kachu 149
Kokum 150
Kutaj 152
Kutki 152
Licorice 153
Lotus 155
Mandukaparni 156
Manjishta 158
Mugwort 159
Musta 160
Mustard 160
Myrrh 161
Neem 162
Nigella 163
Nutmeg 164
Peppermint 168
Pipali 169
Pomegranate 170
Poppy 171
Punarnava 172
Psyllium 173
Rauwolfia 174
Rhubarb 174
Rose 175
Safed Musali 176
Saffron 177
Salai Guggul 178
Sandalwood 178
Sarsaparilla 180
Senna 181
Sesame 182
Shankpushpi 183
Shatavari 184
Shigru 185
Spearmint 186

Tulsi 187
Turmeric 189
Valerian 196
Vamsha Rochana 198

9 Non-Herbal and Mineral Medicines 199
Bhasma 199
Shilajit 204
Sulfur Preparations 205
Medicated Ghee preparations 206

10 Ayurvedic Formulas 207
Agnitundi Vati 207
Ajmodali Churna 208
Arjunarisht 208
Avipattikar Churna 208
Chyavanprash 208
Dashmula 209
Hingvastak 210
Guggul Formulas 210
Kumariasava 211
Mahasudarshan 211
Narayan Oil 212
Sanjeevani Vati 213
Saptamrita Lauha 213
Saraswat Churna 213
Sitopladi Churna 213
Talisadi Churna 214
Trikatu 214
Triphala 214

11 Ayurvedic Home Remedies 219

12 Specific Diseases and Treatments 223
Acne and Dermatitis 225
Allergy 226
Anxiety 227
Amavata 228
Arthritis 227
Amavata 228
Asthma 230
Athlete's Foot 231
Bad Breath 233
Benign Prostatic Hyperplasia 233
Canker sores 236
Cardiovascular Conditions 236

Cataract 238
Cold and flu 241
Constipation 242
Depression 242
Detoxification 243
Diabetes 244
Fibromyalgia 248
Gallstones 248
Gastritis, Heartburn and Ulcer 250
Glaucoma 251
Hair 252
Hay Fever 254
Headache 254
Herpes and cold sores 254
Impotence and Erectile Dysfunction 255
Insomnia 258
Irritable Bowel Syndrome 261
Macular Degeneration 262
Memory 263
Menstrual cramps, PMS, Menopause 263
Premature Ejaculation 265
Skin Cancer 266
Weight Loss 268
13 Integrating Ayurvedic Herbs and Foods into Daily Life .. 273
How to live it day to day 280
Personalize Your Lifestyle with Ayurveda 282
14 Ayurveda, Kundalini and Yoga 291
15 Conclusion 297
Appendix Synopsis of Therapy 301
Appendix Vegetable Juices to for a Gentle Detox 303
Appendix of Selected Ayurvedic Recipes 305
Main Dishes and Soups 305
Vegetables 309
Drinks 311
Snacks and Desserts 313
Glossary 315
Bibliography 323
Recommended Reading 327
Ayurveda and Herbal Resources 329
Ayurveda Education 331
For More Information 333

TABLE OF FIGURES

Figure 1The Five Elements 9
Figure 2 Dosha Characteristics 12
Figure 3 Subdoshas 13
Figure 4 The 13 Agnis 21
Figure 5 The Three Malas 23
Figure 6 Constitutional Overview 29
Figure 7 Constitution (Short Form) 32
Figure 8 Mental Constitution Test 34
Figure 9 Diagnosis 37
Figure 10 Dietetic Factors 42
Figure 11 Foods for the Doshas 44
Figure 12 Melon Fast 50
Figure 13 Detoxifying Foods 50
Figure 14 Meat Properties 57
Figure 15 Ayurveda Branches 63
Figure 16 Ayurveda Treatment Categories 65
Figure 17 Therapeutic Settings 67
Figure 18 Panchakarma 69
Figure 19 Herbal Neti 73
Figure 20 The Six Tastes and Their Properties 78
Figure 21 Gurvadi Gunas 80
Figure 22 Special Potency 82
Figure 23 Ayurvedic Preparation Methods 84
Figure 24 Bhasma Preparations 201
Figure 25 Ten Lifestyle Tips for Erectile Dysfunction 257
Figure 26 Sleep Symptoms 260
Figure 27 Conquering Sleep 261
Figure 28 Dosha Cycles 274
Figure 29 Daily Routine 280

AUTHOR'S FOREWORD TO THE SERIES

Ayurveda, the traditional medicine of India, shares the distinction with Traditional Chinese Medicine (TCM) and Middle Eastern Unani Tibb Medicine as one of the three oldest surviving comprehensive herbal medicine systems on the planet. These are distinct insofar as, unlike local or native herbal medical systems, they evolved over a diverse cultural and geographical area to enable them to treat the most diverse variety of human diseases.

Even a cursory examination of the three systems will reveal a number of fundamental similarities, including the energetic classification of diseases and herbs, such as the use of cosmological theories with descriptive energetic medical terms, such as "hot," "cold," "damp," "dry" and "wind." Also, each is based on a similar "elemental" system, which was also the foundation of early Greco-Roman medicine.

In fact, there seems to be a common thread that forms the basis of the three great healing systems of the world, with similar approaches to healing, among apparently widespread and disparate cultures, ranging from India, China, to the Mediterranean and even extending to native cultures of the Americas, partially as a result of colonizing and pre-colonizing influences.

Could it be that there is a common wellspring of wisdom to all these healing systems? If so, much of it utilized a circular logic to represent our interconnection with all aspects of inner and outer nature. And just as early Asian and European systems used theories of four or five elements to represent an interdependent relationship with all aspects of being, so did Native North American Medicine use the Sacred Medicine Wheel, representing the four directions, north, south, east and west, and classified herbs as being heating cooling, moistening or drying, corresponding with their general effects on the sympathetic and parasympathetic nervous system.

Having evolved mostly as a self taught herbalist, with periods of intense study in all of these traditional healing methods, I was never satisfied to exclusively align myself to any single one of them. This inspired me to form the concept of *Planetary Herbology* that subsequently led to the publication of my book with the same title by Lotus Press. In it, I offer the possibility of a synthesis of essential elements from each of the primary three medical systems, Indian Ayurvedic, Traditional Chinese Medicine and Western herbalism, applying their medical classifications to the use of herbs from around the world.

This book is the third in *"The Way"* series beginning with *The Way of Herbs* and followed by *The Way of Chinese Herbs* (both published by Pocket books). While these were written based on my dominant clinical experience integrating Western and Chinese herbal systems into my practice, this, third one, on Ayurvedic Medicine, is written with my esteemed colleague, K.P. Khalsa, a well respected practitioner of Ayurvedic medicine.

Besides our close association as professional colleagues and friends in the

American Herbalists Guild (AHG), our background also shares similarities. Independently, we both first learned Ayurvedic medicine from our respective spiritual mentors- myself, with Baba Hari Dass, and for K.P., with Yogi Bhajan. In fact, these two Indian teachers were probably the first to introduce traditional Ayurvedic medicine to North America. It was a fortuitous time finding a reception during those soul searching decades of roughly the 1960's and 70's – a time when the world was living under the 'cold war' between Russia and the West and the eminent threat of nuclear annihilation, racial upheaval and the Vietnam war. It was a time when many of the values and institutions of the mainstream were being questioned, including Western medicine.

Many of us, in the midst of searching for more natural lifestyle alternatives, including older systems of natural healing with homebirth, herbs and acupuncture, also discovered the ancient treasures of healing wisdom from diverse ethnic groups. The reward of those "years of questioning and searching" resulted in learning Traditional Native American Medicine, Chinese Medicine and Indian Ayurvedic medicine.

For me, this was reflected not only in the many books which I wrote on herbal medicine, including my East West Herb Course, but also in the line of *Planetary Herbal Formulas*, which integrate under a single brand name effective herbal remedies from around the world. In fact, Planetary Herbal Formulas was the first to introduce to the North American herbal market such keystone Ayurvedic preparations and herbs as Triphala, Hingashtak, Guggul, Trikatu and Ashwaganda, to name a few. With the growing popularity of Ayurvedic medicine, Planetary Herbal Formulas is now launching an expanded sub line of Ayurvedic herbs and preparations.

Since 1978, in my clinical practice in Santa Cruz, California, I regularly recommend the therapeutic Ayurvedic diet of mung beans and rice, with certain herbs, together called *kichari*, prescribe and administer Ayurvedic preparations and therapies including shirodara (head oiling used for psychological disorders), incorporating all in a practice of integrated Western, Chinese and Ayurvedic medicines and acupuncture.

As with the two previous "*Way*" books, this one offers a good basis for the serious student as well as many simple and practical applications of common Ayurvedic herbs, such as turmeric, ginger, black pepper and many others that are commonly available for the lay person to safely assist in self and family treatment.

With the rise of globalization in the 21st century, it is inevitable that these ancient systems of natural healing should rise to the fore. It is also appropriate at this time that *The Way of Ayurveda* should be written and serve to not only advance the understanding and practice of the earth's oldest healing system, but by so doing promote its integration into other modalities with the evolution of Planetary Herbology.

Michael Tierra, OMD, L.Ac.,
Founder of the American Herbalists Guild, 2006

INTRODUCTION

Understanding Ayurvedic herbalism can keep you well. With the knowledge you are about to share, you can achieve balanced health. And balanced health can be a priceless gift.

Imagine a time in the near future when you're free from sickness, when you haven't been bothered by even a sniffle or a rash for a long, long time. Ayurveda helps that future become a reality.

Both authors are living proof of the power of natural medicine. We've seen thousands of patients regain vibrant health, and we're not alone. An entire new generation of natural medicine therapists is transforming the health care system in America. They are using ancient techniques, from around the world, right alongside modern ones.

These are hopeful signs at a time when future health conditions are reported to be harsh. Amid a rising wave of oddball bugs and scary epidemics, resistant to the best of conventional medicine, dread is running high.

We are sure you, like other Americans, want to know what you can do to protect yourself- not only against an unknown future of infectious disease, but the degeneration, aging and daily irritations that undermine the quality of our lives.

You are likely hungry for answers that offer promise. If the conventional treatments on which you have relied are failing you, there is no better investment you can make in your future than to learn and incorporate practical Ayurveda. In this book, we will make the rich, historically potent herbal traditions of India useful and constructive in an everyday way for everyday people.

Michael Tierra, L.Ac., O.M.D., A.H.G., is one of the founders of the North American natural health movement, and was one of the first acupuncturists to be licensed in the United States. He began his herbal and natural healing studies in 1968, while living in a community in the Klamath National Forest in northern California. There he learned the wild forest plants and healing ways of the Karok and Yurok Indians.

Starting in 1970, Michael studied and apprenticed with Norma Meiers and Dr. John Christopher in Vancouver, British Columbia, Canada, and began his Chinese medicine and acupuncture studies with Efrem Korngold, Foon Lee Wong and Mariam Lee in San Francisco. Soon his studies channeled into practicing and teaching in San Francisco. Additionally, he began studying Ayurvedic medicine and yoga with Baba Hari Dass, which later precipitated his move to Santa Cruz, California. In 1976, Michael started the first holistic health school in Santa Cruz, The Garden of Sanjivani, where he was the director and teacher in residence.

Michael Tierra's work spread and he began writing for numerous publications and teaching at many schools, including Norma Meiers' Herb School in Vancouver, British Columbia, The California School of Herbology, Heartwood College, Esalen Institute, American Herbal Academy, Santa Barbara Center for

Holistic Studies, Antioch University and Ojai Institute. Later he authored the nationally acclaimed herbal books, *The Way of Herbs*, *Planetary Herbology*, and *The Natural Remedy Bible* (co-authored with John Lust). His *East West Correspondence Courses in Herbology* has educated a generation of herbalists.

During those times, Michael received his C.A. and N.D. credentials, studied Ayurvedic medicine in India for three months and Chinese medicine and herbology in China for one and a half months. At the internationally recognized Herbal Symposium, in 1979, he received a distinguished achievement award as a Master Herbalist from Dr. Christopher.

In 1989, Michael Tierra founded the American Herbalists Guild, an organization whose goal is to establish standards for the professional practice of clinical herbal medicine in the United States. He received the degree of Oriental Medical Doctor (O.M.D.) from the San Francisco College of Acupuncture in 1987. Subsequently, he was part of the first group from the United States to study herbal medicine in China. He is co-founder of the American School of Botanical Medicine, and The East West College of Herbalism, which is recognized as an accredited professional herbal college in the United Kingdom. Each year, in the spring, Michael and his wife, Lesley, travel abroad to teach at the East West College. Michael still lectures throughout the world.

Karta Purkh Singh Khalsa is an herbalist, nutritionist, yoga teacher and educator. He has been making natural healing approaches palatable to the modern mind for over thirty years. His students find extraordinary benefits and reprieve from a vast range of health concerns by making these principles part of their lives. For the first thirty-two years of his career, he was the herbal apprentice of an Ayurvedic master, Yogi Bhajan. It has been his good fortune to have been involved in the American renaissance of modern herbalism, and particularly the introduction of Eastern ideas, from its beginning in the 1960s.

His interest in natural healing techniques developed because, as a child growing up in Oregon, he had a rare, serious disorder, and several serious illnesses. As a young adult, he studied a wide spectrum of physical and mental health care therapies from all over the world, and was successfully healed. He focused especially on Ayurvedic medicine and on the therapeutic value of yoga, meditation, and other studies of consciousness.

Khalsa is the author, editor or contributor to over 30 books on natural healing topics. He co-authored *Herbal Defense* (Warner Books), an exciting book for the popular market, on the use of herbs for staying healthy in modern times, and *Body Balance* (Kensington Publications), a guide to healthy body chemistry. With over 1,000 articles in publication, he is a frequent contributor to mainstream and professional publications in the natural healing field, and is a contributing editor for *Let's Live, The Herb Quarterly*, *Better Nutrition*, *Herbs for Health* and *Great Life* magazines.

Khalsa was the founder of Seattle's first multidisciplinary holistic clinic. A prominent member of the American Herbalists Guild, he served two terms on its governing council. He founded the first state chapter of the American Herbalists Guild, in Washington, and went on to found a second in New Mexico.

Khalsa's ongoing research and his vast knowledge of herbs from around the globe make him especially valuable to many herb industry businesses that call on him as an authoritative consultant. He has created over 400 of his own formulations for commercial applications, and works closely with companies that supply high quality herbal products to health professionals across the country.

He is on the faculty in the botanical medicine department of Bastyr University, a top naturopathic medical school. He is nationally certified in Therapeutic Massage and Bodywork and is a trainer for national certification in Ayurvedic massage.

For over three decades, he has spent his days involved with natural healing, and has observed how well it works with sick people in the real world. He has seen what works to confer long term, vibrant health. He has also seen what does not work. His specialty is making these natural healing concepts palatable to Americans.

Karta Purkh Singh and his wife, Jagdish Kaur Khalsa, are long time close students of Yogi Bhajan. Their unique experiences with Yogi Bhajan created a base of knowledge and an approach to life for which they will be forever grateful. It was by the grace of this master that they put their feet on the path of yoga and Ayurveda, and continued on that sacred path for a lifetime.

The Khalsas live in Eugene, Oregon, where they share a home with their teenage daughter. They have raised 3 children in Ayurvedic style, and lived to tell about it.

Interestingly, Karta Purkh Singh and Michael were both proficient musicians before taking up herbal medicine.

Yogi Bhajan was a dynamic teacher who taught in a traditional way, slowly developing the concepts of yoga and Ayurveda over decades. He was the first to teach Kundalini yoga, a previously secret science, openly in the West. Yogi Bhajan's teachings inspired thousands. Upon his death, the United States House of Representatives and Senate passed resolutions honoring his life and accomplishments, putting him in the rare company of such luminaries as Mahatma Ghandi and Martin Luther King, Jr.

Yogi Bhajan was active in promoting yoga and Ayurveda to the public. His most famous comment was, "I have not come here to create followers. I have come here to create teachers." He was the inspiration behind several now very successful natural food and medicine companies, including Yogi Tea, Ancient Healing Formulas, Herb Technology, Herbal Gems, Golden Temple Natural Foods and Peace Cereal. Karta Purkh Singh spent thousands of hours over more than thirty years working with Yogi Bhajan to collect his Ayurvedic knowledge. His contributions, begun long before Ayurveda became popular, contributed greatly to the birth of Eastern healing in America.

Baba Hari Dass is regarded as a living master and scholar of Ashtanga Yoga, also known as Raja Yoga. This is described as a scientific method of enlightenment first propounded by the ancient sage Patanjali in his *Yoga Sutras*. It is the Yoga that Baba Hari Dass has practiced since childhood. Since his arrival from India in 1971, Baba Hari Dass has been active in training students and teachers of Yoga in the United States and Canada. Through his compassionate example, young and old alike are learning the gentle art of peace. Baba Hari Dass is a mauni yogi, meaning he has observed for decades the austerity of non-speaking. He teaches through example, writing and discoursing with a small blackboard. As you will read, his aphorisms are potent, pithy and pointed.

Baba Hari Dass was one of the first to share the teachings of Ayurveda to Western students. While he always viewed enlightenment, as union with God, as the primary life goal, he also wisely recognized that at least in the early stages of seeking the physical body must be in a state of reasonable repair so as not to represent a distraction in our journey. His teachings embody the union of physical and the spiritual describing the body as a boat to carry one across the river of illusion and before undertaking the journey one needs to attend to repairing the leaks in the boat. This is also reflected in his statement, "The body is the temple of the soul, and the soul is the temple of God."

Michael Tierra says, "I was first directed to Baba Hari Dass based on the description that he was a great Himalayan healer. Later I came to appreciate and benefit from his spiritual teachings. Throughout my many years as his student, I carefully recorded numerous healing recipes with herbs and foods that he shared with me personally or with the group of us. Only later did I or anyone realize that Baba Hari Dass was deeply steeped in Ayurvedic medicine, then unknown in North America. To promote the teachings of Ayurveda in the west, Baba Hari Dass spent many long hours translating its ancient texts on healing into English. Eventually the Mount Madonna Center was founded, in Watsonville, California, dedicated to his teachings, which, since its inception in 1978, included the teaching and practice of Ayurveda. In January of 2006, the Mount Madonna Center has announced the founding of a state accredited Ayurvedic school as part of its offerings. The history of Ayurveda in North America will always owe a debt to the selfless contributions of Baba Hari Dass. Baba Hari Dass' teachings in this book were imparted in person to Michael Tierra while sitting in person or small groups.

Most of the ideas we present here are just common sense. If you had grown up in a culture, such as India, which still has an intact natural healing tradition, you would have been introduced to these ideas on your grandparent's knee. Growing up with these concepts and seeing the results all around you lets it sink in, so these ideas are not foreign, but beloved rules to live by. Ayurveda is not another intellectual theory, but a set of practical, well developed concepts with their roots in ancient traditions and their flowers in today's scientific discoveries.

Natural Medicine- Future Health Care

Natural medicine and self-care are leading us out of the flawed position that our present thinking and our systems of health care have created.

Ayurveda is the ultimate self-care system. Natural healing is all about prevention. The techniques of Ayurvedic self-care are geared toward never allowing you to have a symptom, and if you do, to bringing you back into balance quickly and effectively, so that you don't have another.

Ayurveda has a different vision of the healthy human- not just the gradually failing, getting through the day human, but a vibrant being with energy to excel. Prepare to explore how we can have that type of radiant good health.

In this practical guide to understanding and using this ancient healing system, we will also take a look at why Americans get sick and stay sick, and how Ayurveda can bring balance and keep them well for life. You may even be shocked at the breadth of knowledge and the extent of simple solutions.

How does your body work; how does it heal? What are the proper foods and herbs? Why use them? Why can herbs, foods, and spices heal? How does it all fit together? Understanding Ayurveda will put it all in perspective.

Why Ayurveda?

We're sure you've noticed that there are myriad natural healing theories and methods. And that they all seem to conflict with each other. How could they all be right?

They can and they are. But no one regime works for everyone. Individualization is the key. We are born into different bodies, each with a different heritage, and we have all lived different lives.

You may have heard of several systems. You may have practiced some. If you got well, you became a convert. If you didn't get well, you went on to the next theory. What we really need is a coherent, systematic way of understanding our individual needs and applying remedies to bring back health and happiness, in a body that works right year after year.

Traditional natural healing systems have already worked out this individualized approach. If we dig deep enough, we find them all dipping from the same stream. Ayurveda has worked out the idea that people are different and need to be treated differently. And it has worked out techniques to do just that- successfully.

Our research in the area of Ayurvedic medicine convinced us that this was an area that deserved serious attention. It is a coherent, cohesive theory that explains the success of the spectrum of effective health programs. Ayurveda gives us a measuring tool that people can master and apply. It explains the reason some people get better on one diet and others tolerate different foods. The overarching concept of energy balance is the glue that holds all the various theories, systems and techniques together.

According to the *Journal of the American Medical Association*, nearly half the people in the United States suffer from at least one chronic illness, and that, taken as a whole, these diseases account for three-fourths of all medical expenses in our country.[1] Crisis medicine reflects a crisis-based society. Unhealthy people make unhealthy choices, and create unhealthy environments, which create unhealthy people. Ayurveda helps us find, and stay in, balance.[2]

Alternative medicine has begun to achieve some degree of recognition in recent years, yet people are still confused about its basic concepts. Frequently, we speak with interested readers who have read half a dozen books on Ayurveda, and are confused, but still intrigued. Often, after we introduce them to Ayurveda, the light bulb goes off. "This isn't so obscure and metaphysical after all. I can do this," they say.

To quote author Khalsa's mentor, Yogi Bhajan, "Where's there's mystery, there's no mastery. Where's there's mastery, there's no mystery." How well this applies to natural healing. Tierra and Khalsa have spent their entire careers devoting themselves to demystifying these concepts. Ayurveda is systematic, organized, and straightforward to learn. We will put it in perspective.

A hundred doctors and healers can tell you that natural medicine is the way of the future and tell you what to do. We have done it (and thousands of our patients have as well). You can do it too- and it works. The wealth of information in this book makes sense. We hope it inspires you to action.

As we explore together, Ayurveda will get you out of the dark about the issues, bust some myths about diet and herbs in general and present science in everyday language that you can understand. We want to help you pursue optimal health so that it becomes a source of pleasure and energy instead of a problem. You will be able to make balanced foods and medicinal, healing, nourishing herbs a part of your entire life- as an everyday, lifetime tonic for better health, energy, stamina, and strength.

You will begin to take steps to live the life you can live- not only nourishing your body with the customized, individualized diet based on Ayurvedic principles, but also building on that foundation by using herbs, foods and teas to heal illness, soothe injury, and tip the odds against disease and degeneration in your favor.

The Ayurvedic perspective can be seamlessly integrated into your life. If you are of the people such as the mothers who believe that "all babies just get ear infections"; sinus sufferers who assume antibiotics and surgery are their only options; the arthritic, the allergic, the addicted who have been told there is no hope for their conditions, you are in for a great surprise.

Ever wonder if your skin rash, hemorrhoids, diarrhea, balding head and weak eyesight are connected? Ayurveda will give you the tools to reverse all of these and more with a new perspective on your life. Armed with the knowledge of how you are put together as an individual, you will be able to select your diet, know which herbs to take and what style of massage to have- even what temperature to keep your office.

Ayurveda is systematic and user friendly. You will find the methods in this book easy to understand and logical to apply. As we proceed, Ayurveda will come through as systematic, consistent and eminently useful.

There's much to learn- and it can be easy, fun and most importantly, effective beyond even what you might imagine. You will become more deeply committed to your health – and will have powerful new tools with which to do something about it. *The Way of Ayurvedic Herbs* will help Americans change the way they see health, disease, medicine and healing- and tangibly impact what they can do about it day to day.

Energetics

People of ancient cultures experienced the natural world in which they lived, and sought to develop a way to systematically understand their relationship to it. They reasoned that they were made of the same stuff as the rest of the natural world, and were subject to the effects of circumstances in their living environment. In culture after culture, often widely separated by distance and time, people came to remarkably similar conclusions about how their bodies responded to changes in the climate, diet, season of the year, and so forth.

Practitioners in these cultures put together systematic metaphors for how herbs, food and exercise interact with the body and mind, based on centuries of patient observations of their patients. Gradually a consensus emerged.

Fundamentally, these experts concluded that "like increases like." In other words, an external factor, when introduced to the body, will create a similar reaction in the body of the person experiencing the change. For example, going out into the cold weather will make the body cold. Eating heavy food will make the body heavy. This seems obvious on the surface, and it is ultimately pretty easy to grasp intuitively, but putting together all the intricacies of every possible effect of every possible herbal medicine on every possible person is a daunting task.

If we think of each of these possible effects, such as temperature or moisture, as an energy, we can put together a conceptual scheme that will explain the complexity of what it is to be a human being, while being consistent and systematic enough for people to learn and apply in daily life. The cumulative effect of these internal and external factors forms a complex metaphor that we call "energetics". This metaphor creates a conceptual model that is intricate enough to represent an entire human being, yet simple enough to be useful.

Energetic evaluation of the body is based on experiencing the body with the human senses. Since everyone experiences the world in subtly different ways, it takes centuries for a consensus to develop among practitioners about any given therapeutic procedure or remedy. It creates a structure in which remedies can easily be identified and understood. According to energetic systems, the sum total of the effect of a diet or supplement is what counts. For example, we may know from modern science that an herb contains antibacterial activity. We want to give that herb to treat an acute bacterial infection. But we also know that the herb tends to increase body temperature- it is "hypermetabolic, or "hot." If the patient has a fever, or is a person who is particularly prone to develop inflammation (heat) that is difficult to control, we would think twice about using that specific herb. It might kill the bacterium very nicely, and treat the infection, but the whole person would be worse off as a net total than before we started. Instead, we would seek out an herb that would kill the infection, but which had a "cooling" energy. This difference in approach can make a world of difference in clinical practice, and gives us an invaluable tool in managing a case for the best in the long term, and in treating the person as a whole human being. We don't want to make people worse while we think they are getting better.

Using an energetic model, the properties of foods and herbs are collated systematically according to their taste, temperature, effect before and after digestion, and similar factors.

While the modern method of nutrient analysis is to isolate and identify key active ingredients, which is incredibly complicated, and is far from complete, considering how recent the effort is, the art and science of energetics creates an impression from the whole, allowing us to grasp the overall nature of the remedy, and predict with great accuracy the expected consequences of its use.

Using a system of energetics allows the practitioner to match the actions and nature of the medicine to the individual patient. This categorization of the individual by energies is often referred to as "differential diagnosis." This term means something different than in conventional medicine. Rather than applying this process to diseases, to differentiate one from another, facilitating proper diagnosis, energetic systems understand this concept to mean the differentiation between individuals, all of whom might have the same diagnosis in the conventional sense. Line up ten patients with multiple sclerosis or chronic fatigue syndrome or pneumonia. Each of the patients in any group will have characteristics in common, but each case will be as unique as the person manifesting the disease. An herbalist using an energetic paradigm will choose the herbal prescription based on the uniqueness of the case, rather than the commonality of the medical diagnosis.

Various energetic systems carve up the spectrum of energies in the human body and mind in somewhat different ways. Basically, though, they are all looking at about the same things. The concepts that are common to just about all systems of herbal energetics are:

- Temperature. This implies body temperature, but also is generally construed to mean metabolic rate. The spectrum is from hot to cold.
- Weight. This is an observation of body weight, and also general density of the tissues.
- Moisture. This is an observation of the lubricious nature of the body fluids, and the degree of fluid retention.
- Taste. Taste is essentially a measure of biochemical composition. Generally speaking, we can divide tastes into energetic categories. Acid substances taste hot. Alkaline substances taste cold. Acid tastes are sour, pungent and salty. Alkaline tastes are bitter and astringent. Sweet taste is caused from carbohydrates, proteins and fats, which all produce acid reactions in the body.

A Note on Spelling

Sanskrit, the language of classical Ayurveda, is written in a script, called Devanagri, which is completely different from the Roman script in which English is written. It is difficult to match the Roman alphabet to the Devanagri alphabet. Furthermore, Sanskrit has some sounds not contained in English. It is difficult to adapt the Roman alphabet to the range of Sanskrit sounds. For example, Sanskrit, and other modern offshoots, uses aspirated consonants, which are separate letters from their unaspirated counterparts. A puff of air is released while pronouncing the consonant. The "p" in the English "put" is actually an aspirated consonant, but English does not represent it with a separate letter. These sounds are often transliterated into English with an additional "h," so "ph" in Sanskrit is not pronounced like "ph" in the English "philosophy."

Sanskrit words yield a dizzying array of Roman-alphabet spellings because of the many different schemes for transliterating Sanskrit. Although there are standardized transliteration methods developed for scholarly use, these systems have not been applied in a uniform fashion by past scholars in transliterating terms.

So transliteration is generally pretty unhelpful in conveying proper pronunciation.

British authorities introduced spellings that reflected what they thought a term sounded like.

Then there are the modern languages and dialects spoken in contemporary India. Any given herb might today be called by dozens of different, often somewhat similar names, with variant pronunciations. We have chosen consistent spellings throughout the book. The reader may come across many different names and spellings in the course of herbal study of other sources.

· ONE ·

THE PEOPLE'S MEDICINE

In a paper that confirmed the secret suspicions of many mainstream physicians, David Eisenberg revealed in 1993 that 54% of American adults had used at least one unconventional therapy in the previous year.[3] The researchers estimated that Americans made more visits to alternative health care practitioners in 1990, the year of the study, than to conventional primary physicians in the same period.

Then, a 1994 survey showed that over 69% of physicians recommended alternative therapies to their patients at least once in the previous year.[4] Twenty-three percent of these physicians had incorporated alternatives into their own practices. Forty-seven percent had used alternative therapies themselves.

It's estimated that 75% of all medical sessions are for symptoms of stress related disorders. Herbal medicine is ideally suited to these vague, non-lethal problems and patients like the results. Effective herbal medicine for these issues is relatively easy to learn and apply, albeit requiring a bit more time to administer and to educate, and has a bit of a learning curve for the health provider.

Humankind has been using herbal medicine since the dawn of the species to stay healthy and to treat disease. In every culture throughout the ages, herbal medicine was self-care. Most herbal use, even today, is by people in their own homes, successfully applying folk medicine principles to treat a large variety of diseases, and to stay healthy.

In our culture, nothing can beat modern medicine for crisis care- trauma, broken bones, auto accidents and heart attacks, although we would suggest that traditional Ayurveda has a lot to offer in those areas, as well.

For chronic, limited and pre-pathological stages of disease, herbal medicine works- without a doubt. In many situations, natural therapies not only work well, but are less expensive in the long run- and often in the short run, too.

What Are Medicinal Herbs?

Herbs are edible plants- in other words, concentrated foods. They are usually very safe, often nutrient-rich, and are useful for their content of compounds that can nourish tissues and support the body's own healing responses. They are often quite powerful, yet seldom habit-forming or addictive. Traditionally, herbal medicine has relied on these plants in their whole form- used in preparations that require minimal processing, including teas, powders and food ingredients.

There is no specific definition for what constitutes a medicinal herb. We find herbs somewhere in the middle of the continuum between food and drugs. Many herbs actually are nutritive, as food is, and essentially are used as food, consumed for nutrient content. Other herbs have high concentrations of compounds that are not nutritive in the usual sense, but which nevertheless have specific actions that can influence body processes to move them in the direction of healing. These herbs are used essentially for their targeted biochemical effect.

The Science of Life

Ayurveda is the holistic healing system of India. Translated from Sanskrit as "the science of life" (ayus = life, veda = knowledge, science), it is a huge collection of interrelated practices that oversee literally every aspect of a person's health and lifestyle. Ayurveda places particular emphasis on the science of longevity, of course focusing on promoting good health throughout that lengthened life.

Ancient Ayurvedic adherents observed and experimented with how people could best live to be as happy and healthy as possible. Over many generations of patient, careful observation and systematic exploration, they recorded in encyclopedic writings what they found worked and did not work about every aspect of living. Their culture at the time afforded the opportunity to closely observe the same people over very long periods of time- in extended families over generations, for example. There are documents in India filled with thousands of years' worth of written records- all in Sanskrit, of course.

Ayurveda is likely the oldest continuing healing system on the planet. It is said to be of divine origin, from Lord Brahma, and dates back to origin of human race According to these scholars of Ayurveda, this system is the origin of most healing systems on the planet today; all Asian medical systems evolved from the core of Ayurveda. Even acupuncture, largely thought to be a Chinese modality, may have originated from Ayurveda; archaeological digs in Northern India have unearthed accurate acupuncture maps.

Ancient Ayurvedic scholars were wanderers and traveled widely, sharing their knowledge of health and medicine. After Ayurvedic medicine was well developed in India, these scholars and practitioners traveled to gain and share knowledge- up over the Himalayas to Mongolia, China and Tibet, then down through Japan and Southeast Asia. They, or their ideas, eventually got to Southern Europe.

Although historians debate the dates surrounding Ayurveda, some authorities maintain that there is evidence for written records going back 5,000 years for Ayurveda and an oral tradition going back for thousands of years previous. Ayurveda offers the layperson a framework for understanding the body and how to best support its quest for balance.

Most of us have heard of the Vedas, the pillars of Indian philosophy and religion. We know of four Vedas: Rig, Sama, Yajur and Atharva. The Rig Veda is the oldest extant book in any Indo-European language, dating from about 3,000 B.C. It is an anthology of verses on the nature of existence (3000 B.C.), and describes the cosmology known as "Samkhya," which is the philosophical base of both Ayurveda and Yoga. This Veda includes verses on the nature of health and disease, pathogenesis and principles of treatment. This Veda includes discussion of the three doshas, and the practice of using botanicals herbs to heal the diseases of the mind and body and to cultivate longevity.

Another of the original four Vedas, the Atharva Veda, lists the eight divisions of Ayurveda, which are Internal Medicine, Surgery of Head and Neck, Ophthalmology and Otorhinolaryngology, Surgery, Toxicology, Psychiatry, Pediatrics, the Science of Rejuvenation (Gerontology), and the Science of Sexual Functioning.

In Vedic times, Vaidyas (Ayurvedic physicians) were sages and physicians, deeply devoted holy people, who saw health as an integral part of spiritual life.

In due course, Ayurveda grew into a respected and widely used system of healing in India. Around 1500 B.C., two main disciplines of Ayurveda had been established. The school of physicians bore the name of the presumed founder Atreya, and the school of surgeons was known by its founder's name, Dhanvantari. Dhanvantari is widely regarded as a divine figure.

Physicians and scholars from surrounding countries came to Ayurvedic schools in India to learn this medicine. Sages from China, Tibet, Greece, Afghanistan and Persia arrived to learn the wisdom and to return with it to their own countries. Ayurvedic texts were translated in Arabic, and physicians, such as Avicenna, who quoted Indian Ayurvedic texts, established Islamic medicine, which, through the passage of time, became popular in Europe, and helped to form the groundwork of the European medical tradition.

Paracelsus, a legendary figure in the history of modern medicine, who practiced in 16th Century Europe, developed and disseminated a system of medicine that borrowed heavily from Ayurveda.

During a period about 1200 years ago, Ayurveda underwent a systemic reorganization. (Some sources, including the Department of Ayurveda, Yoga and Naturopathy, Unani, Siddha and Homeopathy (AYUSH), of the Ministry of Health and Family Welfare, of the Government of India, say this occurred as early as 1000 B.C.)[5] The major figures of that movement, Charaka and Sushruta, wrote texts bearing their names, the *Charaka Samhita* and the *Sushruta Samhita*, which were master treatises on medicine and surgery, respectively. (Samhita means compilation.) These two compilations are dated to about 600-500 B.C. Along with the *Ashtanga Samhita*, a compendium of still earlier works, these books are still used today, and are the master source texts for the system.

The *Charaka Samhita* contains several extensive chapters dealing with internal medicine. About 600 drugs of plant, animal and mineral origin are described. It also covers other branches of Ayurveda, including anatomy, physiology, etiology, prognosis, pathology, treatment and medicine.

The *Sushruta Samhita* includes more than 100 kinds of surgical instruments, including scalpels, scissors, forceps and specula are described, along with their use. Dissection and surgeries are explained, making use of vegetables and dead animals. Incision, excision, extraction and bandaging are detailed. It also mentions such other topics as anatomy, embryology, toxicology and therapeutics, plus about 650 natural medicines. A rhinoplasty (nose job) procedure is described, that is used by surgeons today.

India was ruled from 1100 A.D. to 1800 A.D. by successive waves of Muslim invaders from the West- essentially Persians. Court life and government was controlled by Muslim colonial powers to various extents. The lingua franca in India was Persian, or similar variations, for about 600 years, so a good share of documentation from that time was in neither Sanskrit nor English.

The Muslim migration to India brought with it the system of medicine used in the Middle East, which was an amalgamation of Greek ideas and native pharmacopoeia. Cultures from south Asia to Europe, stretching from India to Greece, had been having some contact for centuries, and medical ideas certainly cross pollinated thought and practice in this entire swath of geography. Greek medicine, as practiced at the height of ancient Greek culture, substantially resembled Ayurveda. The Muslim introduction of these ideas was a return to India of Ayurveda by a circuitous route. In India, this Muslim medicine is called *Unani-Tibb*. "Unani" is a form of "Ionian," or "Greek."

Unani is essentially Ayurveda, with the texts in a different language, and some additional material medica imported from further West. In practical terms, Ayurveda and Unani are so blended, and so universally used, that there is no day to day difference. Texts from both systems are available in English translation.

In the 1600s, the British East India Company took control over India. By 1833, it took the initiative to ban all Ayurvedic colleges. The first Western style medical university was established. Ayurveda continued on only in rural areas, where local practitioners treated those who did not choose to use European medicine.

The awakening of nationalism and movement for self rule gathered steam in the early twentieth century.[6] The Indian cultural values and way of life, including interest in Ayurveda as a traditional health care system, surfaced again. In 1916, the Members of Imperial Legislative Councils pressed the British colonial government to accept Ayurveda, and develop it on scientific basis. In 1920, the Indian National Congress demanded Government patronage for Ayurveda, and provincial governments began to grant funding. Several states started training colleges for Ayurvedic practitioners. Mahatma Gandhi inaugurated The Ayurvedic and Unani Tibbia College in Delhi in 1921.

Ayurveda could not be taken from the people, since it was so much a part of the way they lived and cared for themselves. So it continued on as a grassroots, people-based folk healing legacy. After independence in 1947, the revival movement gained even more momentum. The first Health Ministers' Conference determined that Ayurveda should be developed for providing health care to the people. In due course of time, Ayurveda got official recognition and became a part of the National Health system. Gradually, the schools bounced back.

The English language arrived with the British. Whatever the benefits or problems of colonial rule, one benefit was a new lingua franca. Since India includes many scores of overlapping languages and dialects, most medical publication for the last 300 years has been in English, so it is readily accessible to global readers.

In Ayurveda, mind, body and spirit are inextricably entwined. Ayurveda and yoga are sister practices, two sides of the same coin. Ayurveda is the physical/health/medical side of the philosophies and guiding principles by which Ayurvedists live and teach while yoga is the science of spiritual development. Ayurveda looks to create a balance between body, mind, emotion, spirit and environment, and places emphasis on the ability of the human body to heal itself, with the assistance and support of a variety of non-toxic therapies, including medicinal foods, dietary programs and herbal medicines.

Today, many of the health and medical "discoveries" being heralded as breakthroughs by scientists every day were long ago observed and documented by the Ayurvedists. Modern science is now "discovering" the efficacy of healing foods, nutrients and herbs by the day—most of which were already "proven" in the eyes of the Ayurvedists to be useful and effective.

Today, well over 100 Ayurvedic colleges in India grant medical degrees. More than 300,000 Ayurvedic physicians are members of the All-India Ayurveda Congress, the largest medical organization in the world.

Certainly different cultures emphasized different aspects of the system of Ayurveda and interpreted it in their own ways, individualizing some aspects considerably. They employ different sets of herbs (usually those native to their own lands). We have something to learn from each culture and the way they use natural medicines for healing and prevention.

Ayurveda in India Today

Ayurveda is practiced around the world. The country from which it comes, however, has had some difficulties over the last several decades. During British occupation, Ayurveda was in somewhat of a state of decline in India, as the government was more supportive of Western high technology medicine.

After the Europeans left in the middle of the twentieth century, Ayurveda had an uphill battle to reestablish the schools, infrastructure and manufacturing pharmacies needed to deliver health care to a population that now numbers over a billion souls. Over the last decades of the past century, this all pretty much got accomplished.

Today, Ayurveda is undergoing a renaissance, comparable to that of natural healing, that started in the 1960s, here in America. Schools and hospitals are opening, and the knowledge of healing is starting to get the respect that it deserves. Interest from within and without Ayurveda is becoming trendy, in the land of its birth!

Today, specialists practice in these official categories:

1. Ayurveda Siddhanta (Fundamental Principles)
2. Ayurveda Samhita (Texts and Literature)
3. Rachna Sharira (Anatomy)
4. Kriya Sharira (Physiology)
5. Dravya Guna Vigian (Materia Medica & Pharmacology)
6. Ras-shastra (Mineral Medicines)
7. Bhaishajya Kalpana (Pharmaceuticals)
8. Kaumar Bharitya (Pediatrics)
9. Prasuti Tantra (Obstetrics & Gynecology)
10. Swasth-Vritla (Social & Preventive Medicine)
11. Kayachikitsa (Internal Medicine)
12. Rog Nidan (Pathology)
13. Shalya Tantra (Surgery)
14. Shalkya Tantra (Eye & ENT)
15. Mano-Roga (Psychiatry)
16. Panchkarma (Detoxification)

The legal system in India differs from the American system, and conditions are favorable for the practice of Ayurveda.

Yogi Bhajan said, "So in India you will find it's not like America, where only an M.D. can practice and nobody else. There are three systems practiced with equal grace. They have hospitals, they have dispensaries, they have practices, they have their medical men, they have medical associations, and they don't bug each other. There are certain diseases for which neither in allopathy and nor in homoeopathy there is a treatment."[7]

· TWO ·

THE FIVE ELEMENTS AND THE BASIS OF AYURVEDA

Our life is an existence, including the body, together with mind and the spirit- the soul, the pure consciousness. Every individual is indivisible. Each person is a unique phenomenon. To understand your individuality is to know yourself, what you are. Knowing yourself is the foundation of life and the foundation of health and happiness. If you do not know what you are, your life becomes a meaningless game. The creation of the universe and creation of man are the same, says Ayurveda.[8] Yogi Bhajan is fond of saying, "As above, so below."[9] Each person is a reflection of the divine.

That divine consciousness, that divine awareness,
which exists in every human being,
is called purusha.
Yogi Bhajan puts it this way,
Ang Sang Waheguru
My every limb belongs to God

Ayurvedic Energetics

Ayurveda is a complete approach to health and lifestyle management. This system incorporates diet, exercise, life activity routines, psychotherapeutic practices, massage, and, of course, botanical medicine, which is the foundation of Ayurvedic therapeutics.

People of ancient cultures experienced the natural world in which they lived, and sought to develop a way to systematically understand their relationship to it. They reasoned that they were made of the same stuff as the rest of the natural world, and were subject to the effects of circumstances in their living environment. In culture after culture, often widely separated by distance and time, people came to remarkably similar conclusions about how their bodies responded to changes in the climate, diet, season of the year, and so forth.

Healers in these cultures put together systematic metaphors for how medicines interact with the body and mind, based on centuries of patient observations of their patients. Gradually a consensus emerged. To understand Ayurvedic treatment and health management, we need to understand the underlying physiological concepts that form the Ayurvedic worldview.

Fundamentally, the ancient sages concluded that "like increases like." In other words, an external factor, when introduced to the body, will create a similar reaction in the body of the person experiencing the change. For example, going out into the cold weather will make your body cold. Eating heavy food will make your body heavy. This seems obvious on the surface, and it is ultimately pretty easy to grasp intuitively, but putting together all the intricacies of every possible effect of every possible natural medicine on every possible person is a daunting task. This metaphor of *energetics* creates a system that is complex enough to represent the tremendous complexity of the human being, yet simple enough in concept to be useful.

Energetic evaluation of the body is based on experiencing the body with the human senses. Since everyone experiences the world in subtly different ways, it takes centuries, potentially, for a consensus to develop among practitioners about any given remedy. It creates a structure in which herbs can consistently be identified and understood. According to energetic systems, including Ayurveda, the sum total of a medicine, say an herb, is the important consideration.

For example, we may know from modern science that an herb contains antibacterial activity. We want to give that herb to treat an acute bacterial infection. But we also know that the herb tends to increase body temperature–it is "hypermetabolic," or "hot." If the patient has a fever, or is a person who is particularly prone to develop inflammation that is difficult to control, we would think twice about using that specific herb. It might kill the bacterium very nicely, and treat the infection, but the whole person would be worse off as a net total than before we started. Instead, we would seek out an herb that would kill the infection, but which had a "cooling" energy. This difference in approach can make a world of difference in clinical practice, and gives us an invaluable tool in managing a case for the best in the long term, and in treating the person as a whole human being. We don't want to make people worse.

Using an energetic model, the properties of herbs are collated systematically according to their taste, temperature, effect before and after digestion, and similar factors.

Ayurveda is based on the concept of five primal elements, or "states of existence," which make up all interactions of matter and energy in the human body and in the surroundings. These five elements ("*mahabhuta*" or "*tattva*") are the basic foundation of the theory of anatomy, physiopathology and pharmacology. Ayurveda assigns all matter/energy interactions in the world to this scheme of five primal elements (metaphorical concepts that describe physiological processes and environmental interactions): earth, water, fire, air and ether.

These five "states of existence" describe the ways that matter and energy can interact. Like increases like, so if your body contains an excess of earth element, and you eat food in which earth predominates, you will become more like earth–heavy, stable and solid.

In therapy, it's necessary to know only the state of proportionate balance of the elements in all parts of the body to shape an accurate diagnosis. In practice, Ayurveda does name diseases, but only for the convenience of discussion; all diagnosis is based on the energetics of each individual case. As the body is composed of the five elements, all other substances on the planet are likewise composed. Nutrition or botanical medicines interact with the tissues of the body according to innate characteristics of their five-element profile.

Ayurveda is based upon a universal notion, expressed in nature in bi-polar terms (Shiva-Shakti). Diseases, herbal medicines and therapies are similarly classified in a bi-polar scheme as "heating or cooling," "strong or weak" and so forth. We further subdivide natural energy into the concepts of "five elements" and "three humors," the latter of which assumes a central position in Ayurveda.[10]

FIVE ELEMENTS

	Ether (Space)	Air (Gas)	Fire (Power)	Water (Liquid)	Earth (Solid)
Name	Akasha	Vayu	Tejas	Jala, or Apas	Prithvi, or Bhumy
Nature	Vacuum (distance without physical existence)	Mobile, dynamic (existence without form)	Trans-forming (Form without substance)	Flux (substance without stability)	Fixed, rigid (stable substance)
Qualities	Soft, light, subtle, smooth, sound promoting	Light, dry, cold, rough, clear, subtle, soft, oily, touch promoting	Hot, intense, subtle, light, dry, clear, sharp, oily, vision promoting	Liquid, oily, cold, slow, soft, smooth, dull, slimy, strong taste	Heavy, rough, hard, slow, stable, gross, tough, dry, dense, smelly
Pharmac-ological effects	Softness, porosity, lightness	Roughness, dryness, lightness, aversion	Heat, oxidation, metabolism, luster, radiance, color	Stickiness, oiliness, compactness, softness, moisturizing, contentment	Plumpness, heaviness, compactness, stability
Sense & Organ	Hearing Ear	Touch Skin	Seeing Eye	Taste Tongue	Smell Nose
Action & Organ	Speech Mouth	Holding Hand	Walking Feet	Procreation Genitals	Excretion Anus
Positive Effect	Illumination of silent mind	Vigor	Clarity	Juicy	Stability
Negative Effect	Ache of Hollowness	Exhaustion	Manipulation	Sticky	Petrify

Figure 1 The Five Elements

· THREE ·

THE THREE DOSHAS

For ease of conceptualizing the actions of these five element energies, and for therapeutic application in diagnosis and treatment, the five elements, as they manifest in the body, are further condensed into three primal metabolic forces, called *doshas.* These forces underlie all of the theoretical foundation of Ayurvedic diagnosis and therapeutics.

These "master forces" of well-being are responsible for promoting and sustaining balance in the daily and life-long health of the individual. Ayurveda defines disease as an imbalance in the doshas.

The term "dosha" is often translated as "fault." The doshas represent the ways that a particular type of energy tends to go out of balance. The term has also been translated as power, essence, influence, humor, and transporter.[11] They are "master tendencies" that can go out of whack in the body at any given time, if allowed to do so. Each dosha tries to overwhelm the other two and dominate. The other two resist and try to restore equilibrium.[12]

The ultimate task of a human is to attain the goal of pure undifferentiated consciousness (nirvana). The human body exists as a physical entity because of the mixing of the five elements with the soul, the mind, the cycle of rebirth and the senses. The doshas "bind the Five Great Elements down into living flesh." [13] Seen this way, the doshas are rightly understood as the three faults.

Kapha dosha maintains structure, solidity and lubrication in the body, forming connective and musculoskeletal tissues. It is wet/oily, cold, heavy, slow and stable, and, in the body, manifests those qualities. It is *anabolic* (tissue building) in function.

Pitta dosha maintains digestive and glandular secretions, body heat and metabolism, including digestive enzymes and bile. It is wet/oily, hot, light and intense. It is *metabolic* (tissue fueling) in function. Pitta predominates in the small intestine, the most intense region in the body, with the highest metabolic rate. Really, it is describing intensity. It is a metaphor for destruction, especially the destruction of the digestive process. Ayurveda says that bile is the most concentrated essence of pitta. Of course, the bile is the most alkaline fluid in the body. The stomach acid, the most acid fluid in the body is also a site of pitta.

Vata dosha maintains movement in the body, such as respiration and joint mobility. It is dry, cold, light and irregular. It is *catabolic* (eliminative) in function. Vata predominates in the large intestine. The fecal contents are supposed to be slightly acidic, but generally we can consider the effect of cooling vata throughout the body to be slightly alkaline.

From the Ayurvedic point of view, all functions occurring in your body at any moment are a result of the doshas. Every single action affects their balance. The three doshas are ebbing or flowing in the body at any given time.

The fundamental concerns, then, when looking at health from an Ayurvedic approach are:

- *Vikruti*. The relative balance of the doshas at a given moment (the short-term issue- symptoms and disease), and;
- *Prakruti*. The *constitution*, defined by our primary dosha, and what it will tend to do over the rest of our lives (the long-term issue).

According to Dr. Lad, "Health is a state of perfect, state of awareness, and Ayurveda defines health as:

Samadoshaha samaagnischa, samadhatumalakriyaha,
prasannaatmindriyamanaha

"Swastha" means health. 'Swa' means cell, 'stha' means situated- located, grounded or anchored. When you are totally anchored within your true self, it is called "swastha," the happy state, the healthy state.

DOSHAS- GENERAL CHARACTERISTICS

	Vata	Pitta	Kapha
Elements	Air + Ether	Water + Fire	Earth + Water
Function	Movement, nerve regulation, respiration, circulation, excretion	Digestion, metabolism, assimilation, body heat, glandular secretion	Solidity, stability, lubrication, tissue building
Moisture	Dry	Oily (wet)	Oily (wet)
Temperature	Cold	Hot	Cold
Density	Light	Light	Heavy
Viscosity	Mobile Rarified	Fluid	Viscous Dense
Action Tendency	Irregular	Intense	Stable
Texture	Rough	Liquid Malodorous	Smooth
Energy State	Kinetic	Balancing	Potential

Regulates (Physical)	Movement Breathing Natural urges Tissue transformation Motor & Sensory Functions	Body heat Temperature Digestion Hunger Thirst	Stability Energy Lubrication Slipperiness
Effect on Tissues	Destructive to all Dhatus	Enhances Blood Tissue	Enhances all Dhatus
Produces (Emotional)	Spaced-out Fear	Perception Understanding	Forgiveness Greed Attachment Possessiveness
Initiates Disease Process	80% of cases	15% of cases	5% of cases

Figure 2 Dosha Characteristics

Subdoshas

Each of the doshas is further reduced into 5 subdoshas, based on the locations and actions of the energies. These sugcategories help further define energy imbalances.

DOSHAS- ENERGIES, LOCATIONS AND SUBDOSHAS

Dosha	Vata	Pitta	Kapha
Function	Movement	Digestion, metabolism	Solidity, stability, lubrication
Elements	Air/ ether	Fire/ water	Water/ earth
Organ systems & Concentration	Respiratory, Head (strength, determination), Peristalsis, Excretion (feces, urine, fetus flatulence, semen, menses,) Circulation (nerve, lymph, blood), Colon, Thigh, Bones, Ears, Skin	Small intestine (bile, chyle), Skin, Eye, Liver, Spleen, Mind (digestion of sensory input), Blood, Sweat	Joints (synovial fluid), Tongue (saliva), Stomach (mucus), Brain (cerebrospinal fluid), Chest (lubricate lungs, heart), Fat
Treatment	Oil	Ghee	Honey
Subdoshas	Prana (vital) Heart, mouth cavity, brain, face, thorax, ear, nose, tongue Nervous system, mind, senses	Alochaka (seeing) Eye Vision	Tarpaka (pleasing) Head- cools Eye, ear, nose

Udana (upward) Thorax, throat Sound, speech	Sadhaka (fulfilling) Heart Intellect, memory	Bodhaka (feeling) Root of tongue Appetite, moistens food
Samana (even) Intestines Movement of body fluids	Ranjaka (coloring) Liver, spleen Blood	Avalambaka (supporter) Thorax Cools system
Vyana (diffused) Throughout body Distributes nutrients	Pachaka (dig. juice) Duodenum Digestive fire	Kledaka (moistener) Stomach Moistens stomach
Apana (downward) Colon, urinary, reproductive Elimination	Prajaka (shining) Skin Healthy glow	Sheshaka (phlegm) Joints Lubricates

Figure 3 Subdoshas

Tridosha and the Mind

The Ayurvedic worldview is closely associated with Samkhya philosophy, one of the classical schools of philosophy in Indian thought. It posits that Purusha (formless, male) and Prakruti (form, female) are cosmic forces that create the world and everything in it. And within the creative force, prakruti, are three gunas, or qualities.

Sattva (essence) is creative potential. It represents contentment, joy, peace and harmony. Rajas is active vital force. It represents energy, change, emotion and turbulence. Tamas is potential destructive force, often described as inertia. It represents rest, dullness, inertia, depression, spoilage and resistance.

Each guna is necessary to be a successful human living on Earth. The challenge is to be flexible enough to use the correct guna for the activity of the moment. For when asking your boss for a job, you want to use rajas. You need to be a little aggressive! On the whole, the goal of yoga and Ayurveda is to move toward being in a sattvic state of mind, and to lead a sattvic life, as much as possible. The objective is harmony. We can keep a pinch of rajas and tamas to accommodate movement and rest.

Prakruti creates cosmic intellect (mahad). From mahad comes ego (ahamkar). Ahamkar divides into the three primal gunas of the universe- sattva, rajas and tamas. From the three gunas comes all the manifestations of the organic and inorganic universe, including the five elements, the five motor organs and the mind.

In the West, the mind is thought of as a single entity, essentially divorced from the body, but somehow somewhat associated with it. The body and mind may influence each other. An increasingly popular alternative view is that the mind is simply a set of chemical reactions in the brain, and therefore the mind is only physical.

Ayurveda categorizes the mind into various aspects:

- Chitta, mindstuff
- Manas, the emotional, formless aspect of chitta, connected to the senses
- Buddhi, formed structures in the chitta (the intellect
- Vritti, bubbles in chitta (thought)
- Samskaras, subtle residues of a thoughts, actions or events
- Vasana, an accumulation of samskaras that modifies thoughts and behaviors
- Manas srotas, the subtle channels of chitta in the entire organism

According to Yogi Bhajan, the mind produces one thousand thoughts per blink of the eye. Few ever bubble up to the level of conscious awareness.

Yogi Bhajan describes the mind as being three separate entities:

- Negative Mind- acts first to calculate danger in any situation, takes immediate action to avoid danger, assesses the possible negative outcomes of any action, brings the character trait of obedience.
- Positive Mind- acts second to calculate benefit in any situation, takes action to derive benefit, assesses the possible positive outcomes of any action, brings the character trait of optimism.
- Neutral Mind- takes the information from the negative mind and the positive mind and calculates the net consequences, brings the character trait of service (Attaining the neutral mind is the goal of yoga).
  Aspects of the mind are often categorized in terms of the three gunas.

Medhya is a concept that implies intellect, or wisdom. It is mental development, or mental therapy. Medhya means something that is mighty, vigorous and pure, as well.

There are many ways to bring medhya into play in the mind. Anything that promotes the sattva guna can be applied. The yamas and niyamas of yoga are aimed at this. Ayurvedic herbal medicines play a role, and bhasma preparations containing emeralds, gold and diamonds are important.

Medhya herbs and therapies are typically thought of as those that promote the capabilities of the Western world calls the mind. Medhya herbs engender and summon intelligence, memory and mental perception. They make the mind worthy of sacrifice to the Divine.

· FOUR ·

THE WAY OF HEALTH AND DISEASE IN AYURVEDA

Ayurveda is a complete approach to physical, mental and spiritual health. The goal is to preserve what we have been given, and work consistently to create the perfected human. Ideally, we would like to start with someone who was conceived by, and born to, a healthy mother, and started life with the gift of robust health. Then we could concentrate on building reserves for later life. If we are constantly treating disease, we are practicing an inferior form of Ayurveda.

To understand Ayurvedic treatment and health management, we need to understand the underlying physiological concepts that form the Ayurvedic worldview. The Ayurvedic system of energy is based on human sensory experience and the intuition and insight of experts. It is an eminently usable and practical way of understanding and predicting how a person's health will benefit from things we can offer.

Ayurvedic Anatomy

In modern practice, Ayurveda understands and acknowledges contemporary ideas of anatomy and physiology. But Ayurvedic physiology is much more ancient. These ideas came from a time before microscopes and modern chemistry. They came from centuries of patient observation and endless experimentation. They are based in practical clinical knowledge.

The concepts of Ayurvedic anatomy are energetic, and they give an accurate impression of what happens in the real world with real patients.

Ayurveda conceptualizes a scheme in which food is consumed and broken down in successive steps, until the energy is processed and dispersed to all the body's tissues.

The individual soul is signified by fire in Vedic thought. This spiritual fire is called Agni, which means inner guide. The ultimate goal of all Yoga and Ayurveda practices is to develop the inner agni into its full glory. The fire of agni, the very spark of life, manifests in many forms in the human body.

Fire in the stomach (jatharagni) begins the breakdown of food. Fire in the liver (bhutagni) extracts the energy of the elements from the food.

At each stage, the appropriate agni (metabolic tissue process) acts to form a tissue, and then to pass on the metabolic products to the next tissue. The process starts with rasa, and gets progressively more refined as the metabolic actions persist. Ultimately, the most refined essence of prana in the body is involved in forming the reproductive secretions."

The Seven Tissue Types (Dhatus)

A unique feature of Ayurvedic physiology is a concept of tissue formation in which each human tissue is formed from the previous tissue in ascending order of complexity. The word "dhatu" means "support, that which bears."

When food is digested until, it becomes chime, *ahara rasa*, or food essence. Ahara rasa is converted into Rasa dhatu (blood plasma), the simplest tissue. Rakta converts into mamsa (muscle tissue), and so on.

Each dhatu consists of countless infinitesimal subunits of cells and channels, which are units of structure and function. The status of each dhatu as well as its relative energy level is evaluated.

Another classified group, the *upadhatus*, includes hair, nails and ligaments. They are structurally important, but usually are not incriminated in disease conditions. The dhatus and upadhatus as a whole comprise the physical bulk of the body.

THE SEVEN TISSUE TYPES (DHATUS)

Tissue	English	Function
Rasa	Plasma	Menstruation and lactation
Rakta	Blood	Tendons and blood vessels
Mamsa	Muscle	Muscle and skin
Meda	Adipose	Fat and sweat
Asthi	Bone	Teeth, nails and hair
Majja	Bone Marrow and Nerves	Tears
Shukra	Reproductive tissue and semen	Sexual organs

Ama

This idea is a key concept. When you take substances into your body, mainly through food, and they don't get processed correctly, the incompletely processed particles don't get metabolized or eliminated properly. This accumulated waste is *ama*. This very general concept of *ama* covers just about any substance or energy that originates from improperly digested or metabolized particles. It's very similar to the Western natural healing idea of "toxicity."

These improperly digested toxic byproducts clog the channels (srotas) in your body. Commonly observed obstructions of the srotas or nadis are in the liver (reducing the passage of bile), urinary tract, fallopian tubes, blood vessels and respiratory tract.

Ama toxicity tends to accumulate wherever there is a weakness in the body, which will result in disease. This idea is exemplified in osteoarthritis, which is called *amavata,* signifying that it results from the accumulation of vata and ama in the joints. The term "sama" means "with ama."

Low digestive agni (Agnimandya) will create ama, as food cannot be completely digested. Low tissue agni (Dhatu-agnimandya) will retard formation of that particular tissue, and ama is produced. Also, during the catabolic process, the disintegration of tissues, minute, or subtle, waste products (kleda) are formed. They are called subtle waste products or kleda. This is normal, and the excess is excreted from the body. When this excretion becomes insufficient, due to excessive production of kleda or its faulty excretion, it gets accumulated in the body, and becomes transformed into the toxic substance, ama. Ama often obstructs vata, so movement and nerve impulses to that part of the body are obstructed.

Characteristics of ama:

- Always incompletely digested substance, so non-homogenous
- Very bad or foul odor (experienced only when ama combined with excretions- sweat, urine, and feces- or in sputum or vomit
- Very sticky

Symptoms of ama accumulation include:

- Coating on the tongue, especially upon awakening
- Frequent fatigue, lethargy
- Obstruction (Srotorodha) - stagnation and disturbance in transport in any size srota, even at the cellular level
- Fuzzy thinking
- Aches and pains
- Bloating and gas
- Skin blemishes
- Stickiness of bodily fluids
- Bad breath

A great deal of the therapeutic focus is on procedures to cleanse the body of ama. Of course, it's best to prevent it from forming in the first place. When ama becomes mixed with unbalanced doshas, disease is not far behind.

Optimum Digestive Health

As polite topics of conversation go, constipation, gas, diarrhea and irritable bowel syndrome probably don't even make your list. You're probably too busy thinking about your face or waistline to reflect on your colon. But Ayurveda says you had better think about your digestion- it's the most important system in your body, and the starting place for good health or a lifetime of health problems.

Fortunately, you can perfect your digestion ("panchan") and elimination by following a few basic lifestyle rules. And if you do have a few troubles along the way, some straightforward and effective natural Ayurvedic remedies can put you back in balance.

Ayurvedic herbalists are as interested in what comes out of the human body as what goes in. If food doesn't get properly digested, or the waste products of digestion can't get out, it hardly matters what you put in your mouth.

The stomach is where the first real action is. This first stopover in the digestive journey mixes powerful chemicals with the food mass. If these digestive juices, including hydrochloric acid and bile, are in short supply, the whole process gets off to a poor start.

Traditional herbalists around the world agree that herbs with bitter taste promote digestive secretions and speed up digestion. Ayurvedic cuisine often includes a small serving of an intensely bitter condiment to be consumed before the first bite of a meal, to stimulate digestive secretions and keep food passing through at a good clip. Bitter melon or fenugreek chutney might be used. Bitter herbs reduce gas, bloating, symptoms of food allergies and indigestion. Gentian root is a popular "digestive bitter" in Ayurvedic and Western herbalism. Other bitter digestants include barberry root, dandelion and chiretta.

Agni is the fire energy of metabolism and digestion. Every organ, and for that matter, every cell, has an agni. In normal discussion, the term is used to describe the collected energies of the digestive tract, which are responsible for breaking down and absorbing food during the process of digestion. The agni in the stomach is jatharagni, the gross digestive fire. This agni is works on the nutrients in the stomach and small intestine to assure that food is thoroughly digested and assimilated.

All energy from the outside of the organism must be transformed to be usable on the inside. That is the job of agni, in all its forms and subdivisions. Just about every quality of health is a function of agni, the heat of life, and the metabolic force that creates the vital energy at every level. Agni is said to regulate, in addition to digestion, vision, body temperature, complexion, bravery and anger. Since all bodily functions depend on metabolism, agni is paramount in health and homeostasis. Fundamentally, all pathology is due to impairment of agni in some manner.[14]

There are four variations of digestive agni, which are classified by their origins and qualities.

Mandagni (low, weak digestive fire) produces ama due to an excess kapha condition. It produces slow metabolism, overweight, allergies and mucus diseases. Tikshnagni (too intensive digestive fire) produces ama due to an excess pitta condition. It may cause hyperacidity, heartburn, hypoglycemia and inflammatory diseases. Vishamagni (imbalanced digestive fore) produces ama due to an excess vata condition. The gastric fire becomes suppressed, causing irregular appetite, indigestion and gas. Due to the nature of vata, this results in anxiety, insecurity, fear, and neurological problems. Samagni is the result of balanced doshas. Having this type of agni allows a person to eat almost any type of food without problems. Digestion, absorption and elimination function properly.

THE 13 AGNIS

Agni	Location	Function
Jatharagni, or Pachakagni	Stomach	Initial Breakdown of Food
Akasha (ether) mahabhutagni	Liver	Fine molecular metabolism & assimilation
Vayu (air) mahabhutagni	Liver	Fine molecular metabolism & assimilation
Agni (fire) mahabhutagni	Liver	Fine molecular metabolism & assimilation
Jala (water) mahabhutagni	Liver	Fine molecular metabolism & assimilation
Prithvi (earth) mahabhutagni	Liver	Fine molecular metabolism & assimilation
Rasa (Plasma) Dhatvagni	Plasma	Provide tissue energy
Rakta (Blood) Dhatvagni	Blood	Provide tissue energy
Mamsa (Muscular tissue) Dhatvagni	Muscles	Provide tissue energy
Meda (Adipose tissue) Dhatvagni	Fat	Provide tissue energy
Asthi (Bone) Dhatvagni	Bone	Provide tissue energy
Majja (Bone marrow) Dhatvagni	Marrow	Provide tissue energy
Shukra (Semen) Dhatvagni	Reproductive tissues	Provide tissue energy

Figure 4 The 13 Agnis

The stomach is the seat of kapha in the body, so this organ is a prime place to manifest kapha symptoms.

For the cold kapha stomach, carminative herbs warm up the digestive tract, speed up and increase the thoroughness of digestion and reduce gas. Fennel, cardamom, dill, cumin and caraway seeds are carminative. Ginger reduces spasm, absorbs and neutralizes toxins in the gastrointestinal tract and increases the secretion of digestive juices, including bile and saliva.[15] Ginger contains ingredients that soothe the gut and aid digestion by increasing peristalsis. Warming cinnamon bark is another mild but useful remedy for sluggish digestion.

When the food mass reaches the small intestine, nutrients will enter the bloodstream with the help of the liver. In the very hot and active liver, metabolism is governed by the bhuta agnis. Food is made up of the five elements. Bhuta agni assures the processing of adequate amounts of the elements to nourish the tissues. There are five bhuta agnis, each associated with an element. Baba Hari Dass says that sweet craving is a sign of liver weakness.

It's time to talk about the ideal bowel movement. The proper stool is like a peeled, fully ripe banana, in size, shape and color. And it floats. If your stool is sinking, you're sinking!

Regular, bulky, soft and comfortable bowel movements are vital to good health. But something must be seriously wrong, since four and a half million Americans say they are constipated *most* or *all* of the time. Constipation is medically defined as passing stools less than 3 times a week, or in low quantity.

Proper bowel timing includes the key concepts of transit time and regularity. The time it takes for a meal to go in the mouth and come out from other end is referred to as "transit time." For a person who eats a healthy diet, free of refined, processed foods, 30 hours is an average transit time. Ayurveda says the ideal transit time is 18 to 24 hours. In our constipation-prone society, 48 hours, or considerably more, is commonplace.

The hitch with lengthy transit time is that the longer the end products of digestion stay in our system, the more chance they have of decomposing into unhealthy compounds. And, if bowel transit time is slow, increasing the time that fecal matter spends within the colon leads to greater absorption of water from the feces. More water is absorbed, resulting in harder, smaller stools that have more difficulty moving forward. Increasingly, evidence implicates slow transit constipation in the development of gallstones.[16]

Measure your transit time by swallowing something that colors the stool. Mark the time that you see the color in the feces. Charcoal powder, beets and chlorophyll all work well.

Regularity is the interval between bowel movements. A bowel movement every day is essential. A bowel movement for each meal is even better. A proper bowel movement depends mainly on three factors: peristalsis, fiber and moisture.

Fiber absorbs moisture, increasing stool size, giving the muscles in the intestinal walls something to grab onto, making the stool softer. Natural bulk laxatives provide soluble fiber to slow intestinal motility. Psyllium seed, a bulk fiber laxative form Ayurveda, balances bowel function and relieves pain in irritable bowels.[17]

Proper moisture content is critical for good elimination. Mucilages are herbs that create a healing slime that coats and soothes the gut wall and keeps the stool moist and slippery enough to exit smoothly.

Ayurvedic examples are shatavari root and bala root. Marshmallow root, a similar herb better known in Europe, closely related to the Asian bala, is used for inflammation of the stomach membranes.[18] To use bala, marshmallow or a similar lubricating herb, take 1 Tablespoon of powdered bulk herb per meal (stir into a bite of food, like applesauce, to swallow).

When the food nutrients enter the dhatus, the second stage of metabolism, vipak begins in the tissue systems. Each dhatu processes the nutrients necessary for its own functions. Each dhatu has a respective agni, for a total of seven dhatu agnis. Nutrients feed each dhatu in sequential fashion. First, rasa dhatu takes what it needs. Then, rakta dhatu extracts its required nutrients and passes it along to mamsa dhatu. This process continues through the seven dhatus, ending with the production of ojas.

Malas

Through digestion, we generate different kinds of waste materials, *malas*, which must be eliminated. Malas are of two types. *Ahara malas* are wastes from food, while *dhatu malas* are wastes from the tissue metabolism.

The main malas come from food. The ahara malas are feces (*purisha*), urine (*mutra*), and sweat (*sveda*). The dhatu malas are the numerous secretions of the nose, eyes, ears, plus lactic acid, carbon dioxide, and other metabolites, plus exfoliated hair, skin, and nails. If the malas become abnormal in some way, they disturb the doshas and become involved in creating disease.

THE THREE MALAS

Mala	Elements	Vriddhi (increase)	Ksaya (decrease)
Feces (purisha)	earth	Heaviness Flatulence Abdominal pain	Bloating Abdominal pain Low back pain Weakness Asthma Osteoarthritis
Urine (mutra)	water and fire	Urinary frequency Bladder disorders Urinary tract infections	Reduced urine Chronic thirst Kidney stones Lower abdominal pain
Sweat (sveda)	water	Copious perspiration Skin fungus and itching Constipation Body odor	reduced perspiration Hot, dry skin Burning sensations

Figure 5 The Three Malas

Natural Urges

In order to facilitate the elimination of wastes, the body is equipped with urges that appear naturally. There are two types of natural urges- suppressible and nonsuppressible.

There are thirteen natural urges in the body that should not be suppressed. These are the natural calls that appear in order to maintain the balance. We must not be embarrassed to answer these calls when they come. Suppressing any of these urges can cause dosha imbalances and problems with the organs involved. In our culture, holding a bowel movement is extremely common, and often leads to constipation in later years.

The thirteen non-suppressible natural urges are:

- Urination
- Bowel movement
- Releasing semen
- Passing gas
- Vomiting
- Sneezing
- Burping
- Yawning
- Hunger
- Thirst
- Shedding tears
- Sleeping
- Breathing heavily after exertion

· FIVE ·

THE WAY OF AYURVEDIC DIAGNOSIS

Health is that state in which the structure and function is operating optimally and in a state of physical, mental, and spiritual equilibrium. Specifically, there are some signposts:

- The three doshas are in equilibrium with respect to the constitution
- All dhatus are in the proper state of strength and balance
- All agnis are balanced, giving rise to proper appetite, digestion, and assimilation
- All malas are being produced (and eliminated) properly
- The sense organs are functioning normally
- The mind is in equipoise
- The person is living in contentment

Ayurveda purports the principle of *svabhavoparamavada*, that everyone has an inherent tendency to move in the direction of balance, with respect to the constitution, and that the body has the inborn wisdom to heal itself. If we can live a natural, clean life, the momentum will be in the direction of health.

Disease arises from disturbance in the balance of the doshas. Ayurvedic medicine stresses the necessity for an extensive and precise evaluation of the disease process. Ayurveda has developed a unique approach to diagnosis (*rogi-roga pariksha*), that involves ascertaining the energy of the patient (rogi) and the disease (roga). We are concerned about a person who happens to have a disease, rather than a disease that happens to be in a person. In any person, aspects of health always remain alongside the disease state, and the reservoir of prana is the foundation for her eventual recovery.

When properly supported, the tendency of the body is to eliminate the root of a disease and to heal itself. Without balance, we can go from yogi (spiritual aspirant) to rogi (patient).

Ayurveda gives equal weight to diagnosis of the patient and diagnosis of the disease.

The Healer in Ayurveda

The healer is a facilitator of balance. Ideally, she preserves the stability that is already there. Usually, though, she assists the return to balance of the doshas. Creating a plan, executing the plan, and sticking to the plan- that's what it takes. Ayurveda is a no nonsense system. The object is to get back to balance by the quickest feasible means. If a patient is out of balance, laws of the universe were broken somehow, by somebody. To restore health, we do what it takes to get back to balance as fast as possible, short of creating any more damage. Personal preferences, and wishing it weren't so, and wanting to do otherwise, are issues we all deal with. But none of us can change the laws by which we were created. It would be nice to be able to eat an entire chocolate cake every day with no consequence, but, alas, it cannot be. So, we have a little bitter digestive herb mixture, detoxify a bit, and go about our days.

Yogi Bhajan lays it out.

"From the very first conception of the man there has been a fight between the health and the disease. In our own body we have a healthy bacteria and anti-health bacteria. We have a system to preserve our body and recuperate our body."

"Along with the time, as the humanity progressed, there were very different systems ofhealth. One is called the Ayurvedic system. Then comes the naturopathy system, then comes the Greek system, then comes homeopathy and then comes allopathy, including surgery. So, somehow these five or six systems exist today in their complete form. Every system has advantages and disadvantages. The Ayurvedic system is very sharp and cute, but there is no system to take the diagnosis and call it authentic, in the sense that, in the allopathy, we can take the x-rays and other so many tests to come to a conclusion. Homeopathy has a problem, because the person who is concerned in the disease is not in a position to tell the symptoms correctly, and the symptom investigation sometimes causes a lot of problems."

"Then comes the system of healing. Healing. Everybody I know wants to become a healer, but actually, those who want to become a healer never end up becoming a healer. And it is a first step to be a failure as a healer. 'Healers' are those fakes between a spiritual demagogue and an egomaniac. If you put the wording of spirituality over it as a cover, that's all it is about."

"To become a real healer is a long road, and a very heavy development of the self is required. Healing is a process, not a gimmick. I have seen people who are natural healers. They study almost every system, and they have a very sensitive consciousness. There is a lot of divine power in them."

"Actually, a healer has not only to have knowledge, he has to have his own psyche to substitute the psyche, the faltering of the psyche, on the correct path of the person who is going through the problem. So to be a healer you have to not only become spiritually very powerful, you have to become very giving and you have to become a very authentic human being, deeply sensitive."

"The depth of your sensitivity can unite you with a person in pain, and you will be in a position to understand the pain of the person, and you will be in a position to share, through your life energy, to bring comfort or health to that person. Actually, a spiritual healer is not a miracle, it is just a divine person who gives his part of life to give comfort to somebody."[19]

Diagnosis of the Patient

This process, *rogipareeksha*, is the true majesty of Ayurvedic diagnosis. It includes holistic findings regarding the patient- his personality, moods, habits, digestion, intelligence, heredity, finances, family, community, desire to heal, and constitution. We use a ten part system to gather the details of these factors.

1. Constitution (Prakruti) - physical and mental characteristics established by the time of birth
2. Current dosha balance (Vikruti) - the extent of deviation from original proportions of the doshas (Prakruti)
3. Tissue State (Sara) - quality of the seven dhatus and the mind
4. Body Compactness (Samhanana) - solidity and physique
5. Stature and Proportionality (Pramana) - presence of well proportioned frame
6. Physical Strength (Vyayama Shakti) - physical exertion and exercise endurance
7. Adaptability (Satmya) - capacity for maintaining homeostasis
8. Emotional Balance (Sattva) - capacity to remain even-minded and calm
9. Digestive Capacity (Ahara Shakti) - appetite and capacity to ingest, digest, and assimilate food
10. Rate of Aging (Vaya) - comparison of chronological age with apparent age

Constitution

This system of understanding your body and mind is incredibly valuable because it is an excellent predictor of how your body will grow and change over the course of your lifetime. When you can predict with great accuracy the types of diseases to which you are most susceptible, you can act well in advance to prevent them. It lets you develop preventive living. Your constitution establishes the long-term likelihood for your body to slip into ill health in very particular ways. By understanding those ways, you can live in ways that prevent problems, and draw the most on your inherent gifts.

Determining your body type

The constitution (*prakruti*) is already determined by the time birth occurs. Characteristics of a particular constitution are already evident in infancy.

There are endless possible body types, because not all bodies manifest the tendencies of one primary dosha. There are dual-dosha types and even a tri-dosha type in which all three- vata, pitta and kapha- are about equally strong. For example, your baseline biochemistry might be anywhere on the pH spectrum, from extremely alkaline, through neutral, to extremely acidic.

For convenience, Ayurveda commonly divides body types into seven categories.

It is possible to be:

1. Vata
2. Pitta
3. Kapha
4. Vata-pitta
5. Pitta-kapha
6. Vata-kapha
7. Tri-dosha (or, balanced- *Sannipatha*, or *Sama Prakruti*)

Fortunately, here is no "best" body type to be. Each has its advantages and disadvantages- its own strengths and weaknesses. Single-dosha constitutions tend to have fewer, but deeper, serious health problems. Dual-dosha types and the tri-dosha type will tend to have a wider variety of less severe problems.

The constitution verifies not only characteristics of the body.[20] The mind, of course, is also a part of the whole person. The constitution predicts personality characteristics.

The earth, kapha, type is destined to be down-to-earth: conservative, loyal, slow, calm and steady. The fire type, pitta, tends to be fiery. They are likely to be a leader, passionate, colorful, argumentative, competitive, decisive and convincing. The air type, vata, is the creative, nervous type. They are restless, disorganized (in other words, "spacey"). The very descriptions- earth, air and fire- evoke perceptions that influence our perceptions of people to a large extent.

On the planet as a whole, there is thought to be roughly an equal number of the constitutional categories present in the population.

Questionnaires

Using a questionnaire to determine your constitution is inherently problematic. It's reductionist, and, if not taken in the context of all the other diagnostic information, can end up being frustrating.

The usual prakruti questionnaires are, by necessity, oversimplifications, and often lead to errors. Success with Ayurveda requires that the entire patient be understood, in health and in disease. Questionnaires are valuable to help you get a basic understanding of the dosha balance you were born with. Understand that the quiz is just the beginning. As you soak up the feel of Ayurveda, your self understanding will become deeper, and will continue to become more profound and subtle as the years progress.

Physical features, such as bone size and eye color, are pretty good tools for prakruti assessment. Disease tendency is trickier. People tend to develop certain categories of diseases, and the *tendency* is part of prakruti. Actually *developing the disease* is part of vikruti. Kapha prakruti people have a tendency to develop mucus diseases. Anyone may develop pneumonia, however. Just because you had pneumonia doe not mean you have a kapha constitution.

Any given person can have any combination of constitutional factors in the body, mind and senses. More important than the total average score on a quiz is the understanding of which part of the person is infused with which dosha, and how it can be kept in balance.

CONSTITUTIONAL OVERVIEW

	Vata	Pitta	Kapha
(Primary Location-main problem area)	Large intestine	Small intestine	Chest & stomach
General Nature	Variable, weak, frail	Intense, aggressive, athletic, leader	Solid, smooth, slow, lethargic, slimy
Temperature	Cold	Hot	Cold
Moisture	Dry	Oily (wet)	Oily (wet)
Frame	Slender, tall or short, disproportionate, visible veins, tendons	Medium, pronounced muscle definition	Thick, large, no definition
Weight	Low	Moderate	Heavy, obese
Skin	Rough, dry cool, dark	Red, yellow moles, freckles, rashes warm, soft, perspire	Thick, oily, cool, pale
Hair	Dry, kinky	Scanty, bald grey, red	Thick, dark
Appetite	Variable generally low needs frequent meals (hypoglycemia)	Sharp, large	Regular, steady slow to hunger (hyperglycemia)
Digestion	Irregular, gas	Rapid, hot, acid	Smooth, efficient
Feces	Constipation Dry, hard	Diarrhea Oily, burning	Mucus, thick, heavy regular, slow
Mental	Fluctuating, moody euphoria relentless, curious	High intelligence sharp, irritable	Well considered conclusions placid, calm, receptive
Memory	Generally poor, short good, long poor	Good	Prolonged

Emotional Strengths	Creative, artistic	Productive, intelligent, determined	Loyal, calm, stable
Emotional Weakness	Anxiety, fear, insecurity	Jealousy, aggression, judgmental	Depression, greed, attachment
Sleep	Insomnia, erratic	Sound	Prolonged, deep
Dreams	Flying, jumping, running, tall things	Fiery, passionate	Water, romance
Habits	Hasty, erratic, moving, traveling	Volatile, foolish, hunting	Regular, considered, water
Profession	Plays, drama, dance	Sports, politics	Business, cosmetics
Activity	Restless	Athletic	Slow
Menstruation	Irregular, missed, scanty, dark blood, cramps	Regular, profuse bleeding, bright red blood, PMS, moderate cramps	Easy, regular, light blood, edema
Sexual	Variable, low libido, deviant, fantasy, desire strong, energy low, low fertility	Moderate libido, passionate, domination, moderate fertility	Strong, sensual, low but constant libido, devoted, high fertility
Disease Tendency	**Pain (all types)** Headache, osteoarthritis	**Inflammation** Hypertension, fever, liver, acid, skin, hemorrhoids, irritable bowel, rheumatoid arthritis	**Mucus** Strong immune system, sinus/respiratory, kidney/edema, tumor, abnormal growth or secretion

Figure 6 Constitutional Overview

Personal Constitution Test

Take the following test to assess your constitution. When you have a pretty good idea of where you stand in terms of the dominant dosha in your makeup, you can begin to recognize and even predict some of your health issues. Many people are amazed at how neatly this explains their health history, and how consistently their most nagging problems are predicted by their body types. Then you can begin to apply specific natural healing techniques with more discretion, choosing certain remedies over others for their precise usefulness with your particular type of body.

Occasionally, some people will find that their answers clearly fall into line within one dosha column. There are 20 questions, and if more than two-thirds, or 14, of your answers fall in one column, that's a good indication of a single-dosha constitution. For example, if someone takes the test and scores 14 out of 20 answers in the pitta column, with five kapha and 1 vata answer, she clearly has a pitta constitution.

If your answers are almost evenly divided among the three columns, you are most likely the tri-dosha type. If you have 9, 9 and 2 (or something similar to that), then you are a dual dosha constitution, with the two dominant ones representing your constitution. For instance, 11 vata answers and 9 pitta answers would probably make you vata-pitta.

Answering truthfully

If you have difficulty deciding on answers for some of the questions, either about your body or your personality, it may be because time and the standard American way of living have distorted your experience of your true constitution. Our modern lifestyle and habits can alter you in a way that conceals the real you, so to speak. Our constitution represents tendencies that include gifts and potential, but a poor lifestyle that abuses your health may mean that potential is never realized and the gifts get buried. Tendencies are just that—natural inclinations. They are not fixed. They can be masked by other developments as time progresses.

A classic example of this is the pitta type, normally a naturally muscular and medium body type, which may have a great deal of fat piled on top of its underlying medium-sized frame, and whose muscles may be poorly developed despite their natural tendency to be very developed. We would call such a person a pitta-type constitution *with* kapha *(earth)* temporarily in excess. A high-fat, poor quality diet and sedentary lifestyle make this pitta constitution drift in the direction of larger, slower kapha, screening the fundamental constitution.

Most Americans require some work just to get back to exhibiting the normal tendencies of the primary dosha. Usually, at first, you have to deal with things as you find them, scraping away layer by layer till you hit bedrock—the bottom line dosha that determines the constitution. Once you reach that point, you can work on yourself constitutionally for the rest of your life—as fortunate people in some other cultures do from the very beginning.

A good rule of thumb for many people, if an essential aspect of your constitution is not clear, is to think back to what you were like as a young child. Ask your parents or friends if you cannot remember. These masking symptoms often start early, so you might have to go back quite a way. Often, by three years of age, lifestyle practices and diet have begun to overshadow the true expression of the constitution.

How did you compare to other kids? If you were strong and muscular until your 20s, then spent the next 30 years in a sitting job and eating burgers for lunch every day, you may look and feel and act like a kapha, but you probably are actually a pitta, like the example above. If you were quick, light and creative as a child, but now find yourself working 16-hour days with three kids at home, you may not look or feel like the vata you are. Your child self—as you or a parent will remember you—can often provide clues to the true constitution underneath the current signs and symptoms.

Constitutional Questionnaire

This is a very quick summary test of constitution. It is not designed to be thorough. It is designed to bring your dominant constitutional dosha to the forefront- to increase your self-awareness. It will give you a beginning for exploring the complex concept of Ayurvedic constitution. See the appendix for a longer test with more detail.

Instructions:

- For each category, put a check in the box that most represents you. You may have characteristics of all three choices. Make a choice, and decide on the box that is the closest to the way you have been the most consistently throughout your life, especially your earlier years
- Remember back to your earliest childhood years, and compare yourself to other children at that age. For example, were you in the chubbiest third, the skinniest third, or the middle third, of, say, 3 year olds? Ask your parents.
- Ask the advice of a friend or spouse, especially for negative characteristics, which can be difficult to self-assess.
- Make only 1 check for each category Do not split answers. Put a check in each category.
- Do not overrate yourself as pitta. Since pitta is in the middle column, many people check the pitta column as a compromise.

Add the checks in each column. The total of all three columns should equal 20.

CONSTITUTIONAL QUESTIONNAIRE (SHORT FORM)

Body Characteristics	Vata	√	Pitta	√	Kapha	√
Frame	Thin, poorly developed, tall or short		Medium frame, moderately developed, muscles visible		Large frame, stout, thick, muscles not visible	
Body weight	Low, prominent bones		Moderate		Heavy, obese	
Disease Tendency	Pain, nerve diseases		Inflammation, infection, heat, fever		Mucus, congestion, water	
Skin	Dry, rough, cool, thin, cracked, veins visible		Moist, soft, oily, warm, moles, freckles, acne, pink		Thick, oily, cool	

Complexion	Brown, black, dull	Fair, red (ruddy, flushed), yellow	Pale, white
Hair	Brown, black, dry, kinky, wavy, scanty, coarse	Soft, oily, fine, yellow, red, early graying, balding	Thick, oily, wavy, dark or light
Joints	Thin, crackling, unstable	Medium, soft, loose	Thick, moves smoothly
Teeth	Protruded, cracked, spaces, thin and receding gums	Moderate size, soft, pink bleeding gums	Large, white, full
Eyes	Active, dry, brown, black, small, thin, unsteady	Medium size, penetrating gaze, green, gray, red or yellow sclera	Big, wide, prominent, blue, thick, oily, white sclera
Elimination	Constipation, hard, dry, Pain	Loose, soft, oily	Oily, thick, slow, heavy
	Body Total	Body Total	Body Total

Behavior Characteristics	Vata √	Pitta √	Kapha √
Activity	Active, talkative, nervous, short bursts	Moderate, mid-length, purposeful, goal setting	Lethargic, stately
Appetite	Variable, erratic, low	Excessive, strong	Slow, steady
Thirst	Variable	Excessive	Slight
Sleep	Insomnia, light	Short and sound	Heavy, deep, long, excessive, difficulty waking
Mind	Restless, curious, short attention	Aggressive, perceptive	Calm, slow, steady
Personality Strength	Creativity	Leadership	Loyalty, calm, contentment
Personality Weakness	Anxiety, insecurity, fear	Jealousy, irritability, aggression	Greed, attachment, self-centered
Memory	Generally poor, short term good, long term poor	Moderate, clear	Slow to memorize, good retention
Dreams	Active, flying, fear, involved, nightmares	Angry, passion, color, fire, conflict	Water, romance, few dreams
Speech	Chaotic, continuous, quick, talkative	Cutting, incisive, argumentative, convincing	Slow, melodious, definite, reticent
	Behavior Total	Behavior Total	Behavior Total
	Grand Total	Grand Total	Grand Total

Figure 7 Constitution (Short Form)

Making the best of your constitution

Use foods, teas, herbs and nutrient substances to enhance your gifts, those aspects of your constitution that are advantages. It's also important to offset your constitution's potential shortcomings. At any given time, you might be eating, supplementing or following some other lifestyle practice to address a specific, current issue of balance (vikruti). Concurrently, you would also be doing things that enhance the benefits of your long-term constitution, and to ease and soothe the natural tendencies of the body you inherited in order to stave off health problems of the future.

When you have one dosha that is clearly dominant, your entire health maintenance scheme spotlights the suppression of that one dosha. If you are vata constitution, than vata is what wants to get inflated in comparison to the other two, and bring you out of balance; your vata tendencies will cause certain fundamental vulnerabilities to flare up or show themselves as symptoms. The way you eat, exercise, supplement and live should be slanted toward keeping vata under control.

In a tri-dosha person, all three doshas are continually trying to conquer the other two. Balancing this body type can be challenging; it's for sure a tightrope balancing act.

Mental Constitution

The body and mind are inextricably interlinked. We have a mental constitution (manas prakruti), just as we have a physical constitution. While the mental tendencies are as permanent as the physical, it may be a bit trickier to ascertain the patterns, as the mind can shift more easily than, say, the bone structure.

Dr. Lad has said "Manas means the mind should be balanced. So, when we have balanced mind, balanced bodily three humors - vata, pitta, kapha, balanced state of three doshas - balanced state of three malas - urine, feces, sweat, there is no constipation, no diarrhea, no bloating. Then last state that you are in the pure state of witnessing awareness, then in that state your true nature of happiness, bliss, joy, peace, love, manifest, then you are healthy."[21]

We use somewhat different terms to describe mental attributes. Sattvas means pure, true and balanced. Rajas means active. Tamas means inertia, implying spoiled.

MENTAL CONSTITUTION (MANAS PRAKRUTI)

Characteristic	Sattva	√	Rajas	√	Tamas	√
General Behaviors	Calm, gentle		Intense, aggressive		Destructive, stuck	
Communication Style	Clear		Controlling		Resistant	
Commitment	Complete		Partial		Never	
Concentration	Good		Fluctuating		Fuzzy, distracted	

Will Power	Strong	Fluctuating	Limited
Knowledge	Good, consistent	Variable	No interest
Memory	Good, sustained	Variable	Limited, lack of retention
Forgiveness	Easy	Difficult, conditional	Holds a grudge
Cleanliness	Good	Moderate	Poor
Sexual Activity	Moderate, spiritual	Variable, controlling	Physical, urges
Charity	Anonymous, selfless	Attachment, recognition for contribution	For personal gain
Depression	Never or infrequent	moderate	Frequent, prolonged
Emotional Expression	Honest, sincere	Denial	Repressed
Attachment	Rarely	Moderate	Very attached
Fear	Infrequent	Medium	Frequent, prolonged
Anger	Uncommon	Intense	Frequent, prolonged
Greed	Rarely	Moderate	Frequent, pronounced
Confusion	Infrequent	Moderate	Frequently dull, confused
Pride	Uncommon	Moderate	Self-involved
Hate	None	Moderate, but intense	Deep, holding
Grief	Rarely	Moderate	Often, prolonged
Love	Unconditional, universal	Selfish, personal	Obsessive
Sensory Perception	Clear	Agitated	Blocked, suppressed
Speech	Calm, peaceful, clear	Restless, agitated, rapid	Slow, monotonous, dull
Sleep	Light, sound, peaceful	Interrupted, disturbed, angry	Deep, dull, difficulty waking
Waking	Fresh, alert	Disturbed, aggressive	Drowsy, heavy, dull
Physical Activities	Alert, aware	Hyperactive, aggressive	Slow, sluggish, dull
Exercise	Daily, gentle, yoga, walking, swimming	Aggressive, intermittent	Heavy, difficult, resistant
Facial Expression	Happy, contented	Mixed	Dull, dreary
Eyes	Clear	Restless	Dull
Diet	Vegetarian, all 6 tastes in moderation, 1 - 2 meals/day	Occasional meat, hot, spicy, 2 - 3 meals/day	Heavy meat, sweets, cheese, 4 - 5 meals/day
Digestion	Normal	Variable	Sluggish

ELIMINATION	Consistent	Irregular	Slow
DRUG, ALCOHOL USE	None	Social, moderate	Frequent
MENTAL CLARITY	Easily achieved	Moderately ease to achieve	Difficult to achieve
MENTAL PEACE	Consistently at ease	Moderate, sometimes	Infrequently
LIFE SATISFACTION	Typically satisfied	Sometimes, partly satisfied	Rarely satisfied
SPIRITUAL PRACTICE	Consistent	Sometimes	Never, rarely
SPIRITUAL POWER	Humanitarian	Selfish, personal	Destructive
TOTAL (39 TOTAL)			

Figure 8 Mental Constitution Test

Diagnosis of the Disease

Diagnosis of the disease, rogapareeksha, is aimed toward assessing the nature of the disease and is divided into three main activities. Interrogation (Prasna) involves taking a very complete history, including symptoms, history and lifestyle. Palpation (Sparsanam, or Panchendriya pariksha) is a complete physical examination involving the practitioner's five senses. Inspection (Darsanam, or Ashtavidha pariksha) involves an intricate process of experiencing the patient's urine, feces, tongue, body and voice sounds, eyes, tastes and odors. This three fold process is sometimes referred to as Darsan- Sparsan- Prasan.

Everything in the body and behavior is significant when we are seeking to determine where the imbalances lie in the doshas. Ayurveda uses many methods of observation and assessment to gather knowledge about the patient. The practitioner will assess everything that goes in or comes out of the patient. Ayurveda pays particular attention to feces, urine and sweat (the 3 malas).[22]

Ashtasthana Pareeksha (eightfold examination)

Principles to observe:

1. Pulse- the principle diagnostic technique
2. Urine- color, density
3. Feces- consistency, smell
4. Tongue- color, size, shape, and taste ability
5. Sound- breath, voice, body sounds
6. Touch- temperature, moisture, texture
7. Sight- eyes and vision
8. Form- shape and size of various body parts

Lifestyle details and overall impressions are added.

Dasavidha Pareeksha (tenfold examination)

1. Structural and functional abnormalities
2. Home location- neighborhood conditions
3. Physical strength and stamina
4. Season and Climatic Conditions
5. Digestive capacity
6. Constitution
7. Age
8. Mental status
9. Personal habits and lifestyle routines
10. Dietary habits

DIAGNOSIS

Principle	Vata	Pitta	Kapha
Urine	Scanty Painful or difficult urination Gray	Colored Burning Blood	Large quantity Cold Pale
Feces	Hard Dry Impacted Dark Gas	Loose Yellow Green Black Red	Well formed Mucus Light color Large Wet
Tongue	(Back area) Black Dirty	(Middle area) Yellow or Green Ulcers	(Front area) White Thick
Sound	Crackling Raspy breath High	Moderate Hot voice Intense	Deep Full Rich
Eyes	Dark Purple	Bright Green or Hazel	Light brown Blue
Taste/ Odor	Putrefied	Fermented	Overripe or Sweet

Figure 9 Diagnosis

Symptoms

Symptoms can tell us a lot about what's going on in the body, and how the doshas are behaving. Certain symptoms are associated with excess energy in certain doshas. Pain means vata excess. Heat means too much pitta. Mucus and edema signifies excess kapha. Use this table for an overview.

	VATA	PITTA	KAPHA
PRIMARY	Pain (generally)	Inflammation	Mucus
PAIN	Cutting, pricking	Burning	Dull
OTHER	Cracking Crackling Dryness Stiffness Tension Immobility Hoarseness Gas, constipation Worry Fatigue Emaciation Insomnia	Redness Blisters Green color Yellow color Angry Argumentative Heartburn Diarrhea Bad breath Sour taste Night sweat Bloodshot eyes	Phlegm Mucus Itching Heaviness Cold Greasiness Pallor Sweet taste Drowsiness Indigestion (slow/ full) Edema Obesity

Let's take an example. Cancer is not, in any medical system, a discrete disease entity. Rather, it is a group of related conditions. From the Ayurvedic perspective, the principal characteristic feature of cancer is the cells' mutiny against the body's own self-identity ("ahamkara" in Sanskrit), typically when *ahamkara* has been weakened by repeated damage to the immune system.

Cancer is an allopathic, reductionist concept. While Ayurveda recognizes conditions essentially like what we call cancer, treatment is based on balancing the *dosha*s in the individual.

Cancer cells have lost touch with the body's basic intelligence. Svoboda says of cancer that it might as well be called 'giving up,' since your 'I-ness' gives up its responsibilities and allows a new center of self-awareness to arise within you.

Cancer of any type may, and usually does, involve all three *dosha*s. Such a serious degenerative disease only manifests after the balance of the *dosha*s has been seriously disrupted for an extended time. Typically the process starts with the predominance of one of the *dosha*s. The digestive fire (*agni*) is low, as are the other metabolic processes, allowing toxins to accumulate in the tissues.

Ayurveda views cancer of any type as a psychological disease, at least partly stemming from negative life energy, including poor self-image. Often suppressed or stagnant emotions are a major factor. This basic problem usually comes from excess of *apana*, or downward moving vata, the energy which balances *prana*, or energizing, upward moving vata. Ayurveda treats cancer with emotional therapies and meditation to balance the psychological side.

In addition, cancer can be promoted by environmental toxins, devitalized food, sedentary lifestyle, and lack of spiritual purpose in life.

Vata cancer includes emotional symptoms of fear, anxiety, depression, and insomnia. The skin is gray or brown, with the growths being dry, hard, and variable in size, shape, and consistency.

Pitta cancer includes emotional symptoms of anger, irritability, and resentment. The growths are inflamed, infected, burning, and bleeding, and the skin is hot, oily, and spotted. Most skin cancer is pitta type.

Kapha cancer includes emotional symptoms of depression, lethargy, and fatigue. The skin is cold, pale, and oily. The growths are often benign at first, becoming malignant over time.

After a thorough analysis, a treatment plan will be established. In general terms, Ayurvedic treatment progresses through three stages: elimination of accumulated toxins in the body ("*ama*") (providing the patient has sufficient vital energy to tolerate detoxification - otherwise, small incremental steps of alternating rebuilding and detoxification is used), balancing the *doshas* proportionately, and finally tonification. As cancer is fundamentally a disease characterized by material that should not be there, detoxification is paramount.

Cause of Disease

The cause of disease (nidana) is examined very holistically.

In contemporary Ayurvedic thought, in the West, much emphasis has been placed on the doshas. True, the root cause of disease is always an imbalance in the doshas. But what brings about that imbalance? Often that concern is in fact more critical in the long run.

The microcosm (the human being) and macrocosm (the universe) are in a constant and infinite interaction with each other. In this situation, like increases like. When there is deviation between the individual and Nature, harmony is lost and a disease can arise. The intellect, the material world and natural rhythms must be in synch with the universal flow of energy.

According to Charaka, improper use of the intellect (wrong understanding), or a volitional transgression against what one knows to be correct and true leads to wrong conclusions, and hazardous actions. If an otherwise intelligent person participates in an unhealthy habit or abuse, it is the result of improper use of the intellect. These actions may be verbal, mental or physical. Smoking cigarettes despite health warnings on the packet is a good example. Too much thinking, talking, reading, mental work or physical activity, gossip, lying, inciting violence and irrelevant, illogical or harsh speech, or suppressing natural urges all count too.[23]

Unwholesome sense perceptions disturb the mind and can be the root causes of disease. Staring for a long time at the television or computer, listening to very loud music and eating when not hungry are examples.

Being out of harmony with the rhythms and cycles of Nature can also initiate imbalance and bring sickness.

· SIX ·

FOOD AND DIET IN AYURVEDA

Diet is the first, and most basic, building block of good health, and can be an effective treatment for disease, even when used alone. It is the safest therapy, and can be used by anyone as self care. Of course, the results can materialize more slowly than more directed methods, such as herbal medicine.

Improper diet is the main underlying physical factor that induces disease. So, when we modify the diet, we also get at one of the underlying problems. Ayurveda primarily evaluates the diet based on the energetic qualities of the food, and its effect on the doshas, not necessarily on the chemical nutrient content.

Digestion begins when you first begin to think of food. When your grub is well selected, properly prepared and presented beautifully, your senses will aid digestion. All of you- your body and your mind- are receptive. Flavors, aromas, colors, and textures make the experience of eating an agreeable and creative time.

Keep the dining table dedicated to eating. Only your food should be in front of you. Use appetizers and appetizing aromas 30 minutes before your meal to get the digestive juices flowing. Eat in a serene atmosphere so your body can give its full attention to making you healthy.

We should eat when feces and urine have been eliminated, the emotions are calm, the doshas are balanced, belching has no foul smell or taste, we are truly hungry, gas is moving downward, digestive firs is high, the sense organs are clear and the body feels light. After a proper size meal, the stomach should be half filled with food, one quarter filled with liquid and one quarter empty.[24]

Eat heavy, oily and sweet food, if it is served, at the beginning of the meal. Consume sour and salty tastes in the middle of the meal, and dry, light and bitter foods at the end of the meal.

Eight important rules (*Asta Ahara Vidhi Visesayatana*) are involved in proper diet. They must be considered in order that the diet can be nurturing and nutritive.[25]

EIGHT FACTORS OF DIET AND DIETETICS

Factor	English	Detail
Prakruti (or Svabhava)	Nature of the food	Basic energetics, ex., heavy
Karana (or Samskara)	Processing method	Modifications, ex., decoction, roasting, churning
Samyoga	Food combining	Avoiding improper combinations
Rasi (or Matra)	Food quantity	Appropriate amounts for health
Desa	Habitat, climate	Appropriate for season and location
Kala	Current state of patient or disease (lit., "time")	Effect of food on that stage of disease
Upayoga samstha	Rules for eating	Personal tolerances
Upayokta	Wholesomeness of patient	Readiness to eat

Figure 10 Dietetic Factors

Personalizing the Diet with Ayurveda

Each of us is unique. As different as our body type is, so, too, are our nutritional requirements. Ayurveda recognizes this, and emphasizes the correct diet for each individual.

To achieve balance, the diet for treating each dosha will have the characteristics that are opposite that of the dosha that is dominating and causing the problem.

Dosha	Qualities	Diet Should Be
Vata	Cold, Dry Light	Warm, Moist, Heavier
Pitta	Hot, Wet, Light	Cool, Dry, Heavier
Kapha	Cold, Wet, Heavy	Warm, Dry, Light

Taste represents a sensory way of determining the chemistry of food. The significance of taste is further discussed in the herbal therapeutics section.

In daily food, the tastes must be consumed in appropriate proportion. Each taste has a measure of potency, or intensity of metabolic effect. Sweet is the least potent taste. Everyone will eat the vast majority of the diet as sweet (neutral, bland) tastes, as those are the macronutrients- necessary for nutrition, but minimally impactful in metabolic action. Sour is the next most potent taste, although it should be consumed in much lower amounts than sweet. Sour is a great taste for vata, as it promotes digestion. Salty is next in power of action. In general, we will eat only small amounts of salty. Pungent, then bitter, and, finally, astringent are the three most potent tastes.

Vatas should strive to concentrate on sweet, sour and salty tastes- the anabolic, building tastes. Salty is best for vata because it promotes moisture retention in the tissues.

Pittas should use mainly sweet, bitter, and astringent- the cooling tastes. Bitter is best for pitta because it is the most cooling.

Kaphas will primarily consume pungent, bitter and astringent- the catabolic, detoxifying tastes. Pungent is the best for kapha because it is warming and drying.

The table below lists the tastes in order of potency. The proportion of the diet, in general, that should be made up of each taste is indicated.

TASTES PROPORTION IN DIETARY THERAPY

			Least Potent	Most Potent		
	Sweet	Sour	Salty	Pungent	Bitter	Astringent
Vata	(3rd best)	(2nd best)	(best)			
Pitta	(2nd best)				(best)	(3rd best)
Kapha				(best)	(2nd best)	(3rd best)

Often, the diet that is best for you will be the same as the diet for your prakruti, but remember, any dosha could be out of balance at any given time - treat what you are like now.

For example, if you are a thin framed, always cold person with dry skin, you have a Vata constitution, and should eat a Vata-balancing diet as your lifetime program. However, if this week you are retaining water, feel sluggish, and have a chest full of mucus, you are experiencing a Kapha imbalance, and should use a Kapha balancing diet until your body is again balanced and healthy.

According to Tillotson, here is the proper proportion for a meal:[26]

Vegetarian meal
4 parts grain
1 part beans
1 part milk products
1 part vegetable or fruit
1 part liquid drink

Meat meal
3 parts grains
1 part fruit or vegetable
1 part meat, eggs or milk product
1 part liquid drink

Vata folks who eat meat might increase the meat portion to two parts. Ideally, a meal, or at least the day's diet, will contain all six tastes, in proper proportions. Altering the taste proportions can be used to shift the doshas back into balance.[27]

Food Qualities for the Doshas

The food you eat will act in your body based on its energy properties, such as temperature, weight and moisture. The inherent taste will be important, as will caloric content, preparation method, serving size, moisture and density.

We can evaluate these qualities for any food, and for any food program. On the whole, we can average the net effects of a food, and get an idea about whether any given individual should avoid or emphasize that food in her diet. The following table gives an overview of idealized dietary choices. Choose the diet that lowers the dosha that is currently in excess.

FOODS FOR BALANCING VATA

Energy	Warm, Moist, Heavier (Avoid Cold, Dry, Light)
Tastes	Sweet, Sour, Salty
Strategy	Nourishing, easy to digest, warm, filling, heavy, moistening, strengthening, small frequent regular meals, mild warming spices, calm and concentrate while eating
Emphasize	Sweet fruits Cooked vegetables Cooked grains (oatmeal) Nuts Natural sweeteners Mild warming spices (basil) Milk products in moderation, especially warm
Avoid	Dry fruits Dry grains (rice cakes) Raw vegetables Cabbage family (broccoli) Beans in general Any food which causes gas

FOODS FOR BALANCING PITTA

Energy	Cool, Dry, Heavier (Avoid Hot, Wet, Light)
Tastes	Sweet, Bitter, Astringent
Strategy	Mild, bland food, served cool, raw, no hot spices, low oil, eat when calm, three regular meals

EMPHASIZE	Sweet fruits Sweet and bitter vegetables (greens) Beans in general Natural sweeteners (maple syrup) Mild cheeses (cottage cheese) Sweet and cooling drinks (apple juice)
AVOID	Sour fruits Pungent vegetables (onion) Nuts Hot spices (chilies) Fermented milk products (yogurt) Oils

FOODS FOR BALANCING KAPHA

ENERGY	Warm, Dry, Light (Avoid cold, oily, heavy)
TASTES	Pungent, Bitter, Astringent
STRATEGY	Eat less total food, low fat, low calorie, hot spices, occasional fasting, less frequency, largest meal midday
EMPHASIZE	Dry and astringent fruits (apple, raisin) Vegetables, especially raw Dry grains (rice cakes) Hot spices (black pepper, chilies) Cooked beans with warming spices Spicy herbal teas (ginger)
AVOID	Sweet fruits Nuts Milk products Oil

Figure 11 Foods for the Doshas

Fasting and Detoxification

Terry Picard, a client of Khalsa's, had been noticing sores on his knees and elbows for about a year. But when the sores turned to crusty scabs, and more sores began to pop up behind his ears, he knew it was time for a change in his routine. His skin problems were a perfect opportunity to do some fast detoxification, and he was up for it. At 39, he was still pretty healthy, and pretty adventurous. So we used a gentle program of herbs and juices that got quick results.

We worked out a program that included the cleansing herbs violet leaf and amla berry. He used magnesium and the herb haritaki to keep the bowels open, and ate a diet rich in root vegetables and cooling juices.

After 6 weeks, Terry wrote to report. "Here's an update - the knees are completely cleared, the elbows are 95% cleared, and the ear is about 30% better - it's still scabbing up but not as badly." All in all, a good start.

Of course, prevention and clean living is the first resort, but what if the damage is already done, and the body is stuffed with noxious gunk? There is still something you can do. You can detoxify.

Alas, the Ayurvedic concept of detoxification is a bit hard to define in medical terms. The traditional concept is metaphorical, not a well defined process of physiology. The signs of a need to detoxify are well known, the practical process of "detoxification" is well understood, we know when it has been accomplished, because the signs go away, people feel a lot better after being "detoxified," and, on the whole, clinical and laboratory signs of disease improve with the process.

Fluids can congregate where they don't belong. Edema, eye bags and fluid filled cysts are inappropriate collections of fluid that often contain high concentrations of damaging waste molecules. Blood can collect in stagnant areas, where it impedes the smooth movement of normal body fluids. Bruises, blood clots and blood congested in the endometrium are good examples of congested blood. Minerals, even normal ones, can accumulate, and if in excess, cause problems. A bone spur is an example of an unhealthy mineral deposit. Toxic minerals such as lead and cadmium are damaging when they accumulate. Microbial by-products can be negative. Yeast, a normal inhabitant of the colon in appropriate numbers, produces alcohol as a normal byproduct of its own metabolism. We all absorb small amounts of alcohol from our own intestinal yeast as a matter of course. But when the yeast reaches excess proportion, the alcohol can impact our normal metabolism.

Normal body chemicals in excess can be a problem. Glucose, our normal blood sugar, causes diabetes when it's too high. Even normal body wastes can become problematic if they accumulate in excess. If urine concentrates in the bladder, it can irritate and weaken the bladder tissue. Even constipation can be considered a type of toxicity.

Detoxifying the body is frequently the first phase of natural therapeutic work. It is often seen as central in the treatment of chronic, degenerative diseases. A detoxification program can involve the use of homeopathic medicines, targeted dietary changes, nutritional supplements and lymph stimulation therapies that focus on the elimination of toxins and waste products from the body at the cellular level.

Tillotson says, "In my experience, untreated dysbiosis can be a causative factor in a multiplicity of difficult disease conditions, including thyroid problems, eye inflammation (uveitis), chronic fatigue and others. I almost never start treating the thyroid or the eye or the muscles or the emotions or any other part of the body until existing gut inflammation is cleared. Not that it's a big deal - it is a basic Ayurvedic concept. I learned decades ago to fix the stomach first."[28]

Signs of the need for detoxification

So, how do you know that you need to be detoxified? Well, it's a safe bet, that if you live in an industrialized society, you do. Since ama is at the root of nearly all chronic conditions, the symptoms are so common as to seem vague. Nonetheless, when you engage in some of these therapies, and see the results, you will see for your self that these lifelong signs, so normal for most of us, really can disappear. Consider yourself "toxic" (full of ama) if you have fatigue, swelling (eye bag, prostatitis, etc.), masses (cyst, fibrosis, stones, clots), edema, skin disorders, especially inflammation (eczema, acne), headache, joint pain (and much other chronic pain), foul odor in general (stool, breath, perspiration), constipation (regularity or transit time), tissue discolorations (yellow skin, purple lips, brown mucus, etc.), tongue coating, sclera color (yellow or brown in the "white" of the eye), excess mucus (lung/sinus congestion or in the stool), concentrated urine, or conditions caused by natural chemical accumulations (gout, etc.).

Getting it Out

One way or another, we can get all the eliminative channels cleaned out. Aerobic exercise increases circulation, increases metabolic rate, and stimulates the exit of body byproducts. We can also eject these materials more directly by using the body's own expulsion mechanisms - purging, diuresis, diaphoresis, expectoration, vomiting- all of which propel wastes out with immediacy. These direct methods tend to be less popular with Western people.

Generally, the body goes through cycles of food processing (usually during the day, and detoxification (usually during the night). When the body does not get food for a while, it goes into detoxifying mode. That's the theory behind fasting. Temporarily reducing calorie intake, to whatever degree, will speed up detoxification. Upping water intake promotes fluid exchange and urination, so many experts recommend substantial water consumption while detoxifying. Heat will increase circulation and urination, so crank up the sauna!

Fasting is widely promoted for detoxification. And there are many kinds of fasting, from water only regimes to limited intake strategies, such as juice diets. On the whole, Ayurveda does not advocate water fasting. The drastic lack of food makes the body think it is starving, and the body attempts to preserve its resources, which actually impedes detoxification. Yogi Bhajan said, "I do not doubt people who can go forty days on pure water fast, or those seven days, or fifteen days. I cannot match with them, but we believe fasting and normal eating is a very unique situation."

Folks with less robust health, and those with excess vata, especially, will not do well on this rigorous regime. More robust, kapha types may do fine with occasional extended water fasting. While it's generally effective, in order to work properly, the eliminative mechanisms have to be working properly to empty the wastes that are released from the tissues.

Most Americans are not in that boat. If the typical modern person attempts even a single day water fast, the discomfort by evening time will make her question if she ever wants to try that again. And the blood sugar mood swings will make everyone else around question it, too!

Perhaps it's better to detoxify a little less drastically by following a monodiet. In a monodiet, the diet is limited to specifically therapeutic foods for a short period of time to reduce the stress on the digestive system while keeping fuel coming in for the health and comfort of the person. Monodiets should be individualized to the person and/or condition, and are best undertaken with the advice and supervision of a trusted and experienced natural health practitioner. Yogi Bhajan was a great advocate of monodiets, and frequently recommended them. He said, "Whatever we want to do with the body, and with our system, it does depend on something, and that is called the cleansing week. In twelve months we require a feast and fast together. And if you really want to live healthy and long, then you have to go through what we call a forty day fast."

"But what we suggest that a person should start with watermelon so he can get rid of his kidney deposits, gallbladder this and that- we call it clogged up system, the digestive system. We want him to go three days on pure watermelon, provided he is a normal, healthy person. If we want the colon and the heart and the arteries and blood proprietary portions to come through, then we expect him to go on melon for three days."

"Then we want, if there is any poison and toxin in the body, to clean that out. We expect him to go three days on papaya. I am explaining to you the fast. Whether you have it or not, I am not worried about that. There are lots of things that we don't have in America that we have it in India, but nothing will substitute."

"And then after that we want him to go lemon, water and honey for three days. Then we want him to go on lemon and water only for three days, and then we want him to go three days only on water. After one does this one should come back the same way; three days water, it means six days continuous water in between- that's all. But three days you are on water, three days you come on water and then you have lemon and water, then you have honey and lemon and water and that way, count how many days it is total."[29]

Cantaloupe is warming and laxative. Watermelon is cooling, and cleanses the kidneys and large intestine. Papaya assists the body in removing excess protein substances. Baba Hari Dass expressed it by saying that papaya is good for the liver.[30]

Yogi Bhajan gave several versions of this famous melon diet. Some included other melons, and varied in the length and directions. Essentially the idea is to work into the fast with melon, then reduce to water, and come back out. Break this fast, over a period of 3-4 days. Add other fruits, then add yogurt, and finally vegetables, to allow a transition to a more typical diet. Avoid excessive oil for a few days.[31]

This is an example of a very extreme fast. Depending on the version you use, the entire process takes about 40 days. As Yogi Bhajan says, only healthy people should try it. This should not be the first fast one tries. Work up to this very long and deeply cleansing fast over a period of time with shorter, less rigorous, progressively longer fasts.

Yogi Bhajan giving an example of a grain based monodiet, says, "A person will go on mung bean and rice. The first three days- pure mung bean and rice, and then mung bean and rice, and include vegetables in it. People who have done it have found it very fascinating, very cleansing and very healthy."[32]

Most people do better to gradually work into fasting by starting with a single day of slightly more digestible food- say, steamed vegetables- only for the day. Next week, try it again. Over time, one can slowly increase the interval of he fast, and increase the intensity of the restriction, going through vegetable and fruits to juice, tea and water.

Many people with chronic diseases are very full of waste materials. They are often cold, sluggish and usually constipated. Traditional healing systems do not advocate fasting for these people, at least not until they have developed some robust stamina, and succeeded in clearing out the eliminative organs.

The root vegetables are unparalleled for liver support and detox. Beets, carrots and radishes are the best for this job—raw, cooked or juiced. Their properties in this regard have not been studied, but they have a long history of traditional use in other cultures for this purpose.

Beet juice is the king of liver detoxifiers; in fact, it's so powerful that it must be used carefully. It detoxifies the liver so quickly it must be mixed with other juices so that all the toxins don't get blasted out into your bloodstream at once.

Beet root is the time honored Ayurvedic treatment for hemorrhoids. It stimulates the liver to produce more bile, promoting circulation through the liver and reducing pressure on the portal vein at the site. Just eat a very large quantity of beet root or beet greens until the pain and itching lessen. Continue until you get complete relief. Carrot is milder, but will also work. Try carrot juice mixed with fresh gobo juice- delicious.

I (Khalsa) remember a time I happened to bump into someone who wasn't aware of this. In the checkout line in a health food store, a young woman was chatting with the checkout clerk. She was wielding an empty container and proudly announcing, "I just drank 16 ounces of beet juice!" I turned to the clerk and asked, "Do you have a bed or couch somewhere in this store?" The clerk responded, bewildered, "Sure, why?" I explained, indicating the woman, "Because she's going to faint." Right then, the woman slumped to the floor, caught just in time by the clerk. She slept for an hour in a back room of the grocery. The problem was that such a large quantity of pure beet juice emptied all of her liver ama into bloodstream at once, and it couldn't all be eliminated at once.

Green vegetables are widely regarded in natural medicine as the most cooling, anti-inflammatory treatments. They also happen to be detoxifying, so they work for healing *and* to treat symptoms. Wheat grass is especially good, but broccoli, cucumber and dark leafy greens will do the trick. Juice is the best way to get enough green vegetables in you—after all, how many cucumbers or celery stalks can you eat? If you can drink a quart of vegetable juice a day, you will rapidly detoxify. Baba Hari Dass mentioned that cooling cucumber cures drug intoxication.[33] As they say, what goes in has to come out. Detoxification might not be they most fascinating cocktail party conversation, but it's a fact of life. Maybe Grandma, with her "spring cleaning," had it right, after all.

Yogi Bhajan Melon Fast
Eat only one indicated food per day. Consume as much as desired.
3 days cantaloupe
3 days watermelon
3 days papaya
3 days water with lemon and honey
3 days water with lemon
6 days water
3 days with lemon
3 days water with lemon and honey
3 days papaya
3 days watermelon
3 days cantaloupe
Figure 12 Melon Fast

Foods that produce or assist detoxification

Onion/Garlic/Ginger (sulfur-containing, circulation-enhancing)
Watermelon (antioxidant compounds)
Chiles (increase circulation)
Pineapple (proteases reduce excess protein accumulation and toxic by-products of protein breakdown)
Yogurt (good bacteria keep toxin-producing "bad" bacteria at bay)
Papaya (proteases reduce excess protein accumulation and toxic by-products of protein breakdown)
Crucifer family (cabbage, kale and broccoli, among others contain sulfur compounds; also antioxidant compounds)
Turmeric (antioxidant compounds)
Green vegetables (especially raw, are the most overall detoxifying vegetables available)
Citrus (antioxidant compounds, including vitamins, minerals and phytonutrients)
Figure 13 Detoxifying Foods

Milk Products

In the vegetarian diet of yoga, milk products are a significant source of protein, so milk forms an important part of the diet.

Cow's milk is cold, heavy, sweet and slimy, so it tends to promote kapha excess if taken cold. When cow's milk is heated and taken warm, it breaks down the long chain proteins that are difficult to pass through the liver. Thus it seems to not cause the adverse congesting effects of cold, unprocessed liquid milk. Milk is never taken cold except as yogurt (where presumably it is somewhat predigested).

Bringing milk to the scalding point makes it more digestible, presumably by breaking down the long chain proteins. In general, Ayurveda maintains that warm food is more easily digested, as it is less likely to suppress digestive agni. We recommend using this scalded milk as a source of digestible protein.

Milk does not combine well with tastes other than sweet. Do not consume it at a typical meal, which has all six tastes. Use milk products alone as a meal, or combine milk products with sweet ingredients, such as cereal or toast.

It is likely that some nutrients are lost in this procedure, but the increased digestibility makes it worth the effort.

So where does this put us on the issue of pasteurized milk? On the surface, it would seem like the heat of pasteurization would be a plus, from the Ayurvedic point of view. Ironically, however, we prefer to recommend raw milk because the cows are treated better, are given little or no growth hormones, antibiotics, and, perhaps of equal or greater importance, are likely to have less stress hormones in their milk. We know from our experience that an upset mother can adversely affect her milk and cause an infant to have colic. Thus the 'sacred cow' idea is not so strange, considered in this light. "Don't upset Bessie or she will poison her milk."

We have had numerous cases of infants and adults who have had cow's milk intolerances exhibit no problems when given scalded warm milk. Warming spices (cinnamon, clove, ginger) and honey add to the digestibility of milk, especially for those sensitive vata folks, but just scalding it is usually sufficient to offset milk sensitivities.

In a traditional country, such as India, where refrigeration has been a problem, milk is taken directly from a cow, kept warm and immediately sold to the consumer. Consider the safety issue before using raw milk.

For vegetarians, we recommend that tonic herbs, such as ashwaganda, shatavari or ginseng be taken with ginger and honey in scalded warm milk daily. It is a great way to promote a building or roborant program with severely depleted patients who are suffering diseases caused by deficiency. In emergency circumstances, Ayurveda will recommend meat broth soups for this purpose.

We don't think that a tonic, such as ashwaganda, Asian ginseng or American ginseng, when it is called for, is sufficient, if there are not tonic foods in the diet. The two together, herbs and protein foods, makes a superior tonic combination. Licorice powder with milk is a rasayana that promotes the intellect.[34]

Milk products are used in an astounding number of ways. And not just cow milk! Milk from literally any animal you can imagine has been investigated, and may be prescribed.

Yogi Bhajan says, "This is a Geet, this is folklore. It says if I eat yogurt and make it sweet with dates (khaaj, khajoor), I need not care for God because He can't give me sickness. Can you believe it? This is folklore, coming from heart to heart. Yogurt is a self-digestive perfect food. When added with the dates, provided they don't have sulfur on them, a man can recover his health under any circumstances and it is a beautiful, beautiful food which can cure you of anything. Of anything. Let us add to our diet from today onwards one meal of dates and yogurt. But don't be cheap, add as many dates as possible!"[35]

"The people, who are above forty, like me, old people, should boil the dates in milk and make a sweet out of that. Don't worry that boiled milk doesn't have vitamin D. So what we have to do is we have to age that milk by boiling it. Over a low fire, put lot of dates in a glass of milk and let it boil."

"You should boil the milk. There is nothing wrong in that. Boil the milk. Don't you see the boiled milk and the dates have taken away all the mucus from the body? Do you want more practical proof? That is true. Yogis, I say, 'Then please boil the milk.' What should I do? That is the way the system, as we know, we practice." [36]

Yogi Bhajan once gave a diet that was milk boiled with pistachios, dates and saffron. He was asked if it was a good general formula to give to people.

His response was, "Yes. That is an energy formula. It is a high potency situation. You can take milk, you can boil pistachio nuts, dates and saffron in it. It can make the dead speak! It is very powerful. Normally people who have problems in their later years of life, sexual problems, ejaculatory problems, and those kind of things, if they take this drink, and after sex they drink it and then go to bed, it is very regenerating, very very good."[37]

Milk does not combine well with fish, eggs, yogurt, or salty, sour, bitter, pungent or astringent tastes.[38] Milk does combine with sweet, including wheat, rice, honey, sugar and dates. Generally, it's better to drink milk separately from meals.

Ghee and Butter

Ghee is the best of all oily foodstuffs, and is used to cure disturbances in pitta and vata. Ghee is thought to have the healing benefits of butter, with the impurities (saturated fat, milk solids) removed. The *Susruta Samhita* claims ghee is good for all parts of the body, and it is the ultimate overall remedy for pitta (inflammatory) problems, and is the medium of choice (anupan) for mixing medicines for these conditions.

Specifically, ghee is said to promote memory, intelligence, quantity and quality of semen, and to enhance digestion. We do know from modern science that ghee is rich in phenolic antioxidants.[39]

Dietary fats regulate a wide variety of T cell functions. A 1996 study in mice showed that a diet containing ghee prevented T cell mediated contact hypersensitivity in the skin.[40]

Ghee's benefits increase with its age. Aged ghee (up to a hundred years) reduces all three doshas and dispels blockages in the srotas.[41] It treats alcoholism, fever, and vaginal pain. Since it has a special ability to clear the manovaha srota (mental channel), it used issued for mental diseases, namely epilepsy and psychosis.

Ghee is lauded for sexual vitality and for building nerve and brain tissue. Long a favorite of yoga practitioners, it lubricates the connective tissues and promotes flexibility.

I (Khalsa) remember a client of mine, an extreme pitta ("fire") type, who, at age fifty, the prime of high pitta midlife, was a walking ball of inflammation from accumulated past athletic injuries. Every joint, every muscle was sore. He undertook to use ghee to treat his condition. After working up to one cup (!) of ghee per day, his inflammation was completely under control. Much to my surprise, he gained not one pound, and his cholesterol went down, not up. Same for triglycerides.

Medicated ghee, clarified butter in which herbs have been extracted (*ghrita* in Sanskrit), is a famous preparation method for treating pitta conditions. For example, the well-known *Brahmi Ghrita* contains the popular herb gotu kola, and is used for a broad variety of brain conditions in a dose of 1 Tbs. per day.

Shatavari ghrita is made by decocting 1 part shatavari root in 4 parts ghee and 8 parts water and 8 parts milk (or just 16 parts water), over a low heat, until all the water is evaporated and only the medicated ghee remains. After it cools, vitamin E can be added to preserve it, if desired.

Ghee is also used externally. Ayurvedic beauty consultant Pratima Raichur suggests it as a massage base to benefit sensitive (pitta) skin. Ayurveda is known for recommending ghee, sometimes mixed with honey, as an application for wounds, inflammation, and blisters. A special preparation, *hundred-times-washed-ghee*, is applied topically for wound healing, and to calm pitta.

Ayurveda suggests that natural milk products are superior to margarine. A 1991 study by the Medical Research Council showed that eating butter created half the heart disease risk, compared to polyunsaturated margarine, which contains risky *trans* fats.[42] Ghee in actual diets also produced less heart disease than *trans* fat containing diets.[43] When all is said and done, though, ghee is fat, and only a certain amount of total fat is necessary in the diet. If you would like to switch to ghee, make sure you reduce your total fat intake proportionately.

To make ghee, place 1-2 pounds of butter in a saucepan on the stove top. Melt at low heat until white curds separate and sink to the bottom. When a drop of water flicked into the pan boils immediately, the ghee is done. Decant the butter oil from the pan, discarding the curds at the bottom. Store in a clean jar in the cupboard. If kept clean and water free, ghee needs no refrigeration.

Ghee and butter have essentially the same healing properties, but ghee is more digestible. Where ghee is warm and light, butter is said to be cold and heavy. Butter is tonic and building. It treats anorexia, enlargement of the spleen, hemorrhoids and facial paralysis. It increases vision, memory, gastric fire and semen. It is good for muscles, mental disorders, swelling and lethargy. Butter increases kapha, and reduces vata and pitta.

Honey

Honey, *madhu*, is sweet, astringent, heavy, dry and cold. Due to its dry and astringent nature, it is the treatment par excellence for kapha disorders, for which it thins mucus and other kapha accumulations. The older the honey is, the better, for kapha. It is the main anupan for kapha. Its coolness subdues pitta. As it is sweet, it can be good for vata, but the cold, dry and astringent properties make it problematic. Honey is yogavahi, a substance that is capable of penetrating the deepest tissue. Ayurveda distinguishes types of honey based on the type of collector bee, and classifies them somewhat differently.

Honey is sedating. Use it for bedwetting, thirst, diarrhea and nausea. For weak eyesight, use it with carrot juice. For lung disorders with mucus, mix honey with equal amounts of ginger juice. Asthma benefits from equal parts of black pepper, ginger juice and honey.

Honey is also a mild laxative, when taken in a glass of warm water.

Apply astringent, antimicrobial honey to wounds to seal the tissue, promote healing, stimulate granulation and prevent infection. It makes the skin soft. A combination of honey, turmeric, and garbanzo flour is very good face pack. Apply it and leave for 20 minutes. Wash off with water.

Ayurveda recommends using unequal amounts of honey and ghee if they are mixed (such as 2 parts ghee, one part honey).[44] Although this is contemporary teaching, there are many formulas in various sources in the literature and recent references that include equal parts.

According to historical Ayurveda teaching, honey should not be cooked. Stirring a little into tea that has cooled is OK. For sweet cooked dishes, use a variety of unrefined raw sugar, in reasonable quantities, or another whole, natural sweetener. The seriousness and reasons behind these prohibitions are somewhat vague, and are followed because they are mentioned by the ancients.

We discussed this with Dr. Tillotson. According to him, quoting his mentor, Dr. Mana, "The idea is that, in ancient times, honey pollen was sometimes collected by bees from poisonous plants, and if heated or mixed with ghee, the poisons would get activated and come out. This was probably due to experience, not logic. Anyway, in modern times, since honey is made by bees collecting from safe plants, we don't have to worry about it."[45]

Lemon

This zesty citrus fruit is a very common in Ayurvedic home medicine. Fresh lemon juice, in moderation, is healing for all doshas. (Like all acids, it will aggravate pitta, in excess.) Lemon is antibacterial, so reduces disease causing bacteria in the digestive tract. It is an an acidic digestion enhancer that eases bloating. Lemon ups agni, so is just right for a lethargic appetite. It's high in antioxidant flavonoids, and therefore fights disease-causing free radicals. It keeps your skin clear and your eyes luminous.

Mix the juice of a freshly squeezed half lemon to a large glass of warm water, and drink it first thing each morning as an aid to internal cleansing.

Add lemon juice to your herbal tea, and to your beans and lentils, and, of course, to your salad.

Salt

Ayurveda does not have the aversion to salt that is common in American health food circles. Rather, each person should do what her body requires. People with excess kapha will retain water and get too slimy with excess salt. Those with excess vata will benefit from the moisturizing and blood volume increasing properties of salt. The chlorine in salt will contribute to the stomach hydrochloric acid, and increase digestive fire.

Ayurveda mentions many types of mineral salt, each of which has different composition, and different properties. Rock salt is preferred.

Indian Black Salt (also called Nirav Black Salt, Sanchal, or Kala Namak), is a volcanic, rock salt, or saindhav, mined from the earth. It is pink, from the presence of trace minerals and iron. This salt has a strong sulfur taste. It is used in Indian cuisine as a condiment, especially in raita (yogurt with cucumbers and tomato). Black salt is recommended for people with high blood pressure, because it is lower in sodium. It is also know for reducing intestinal gas, indigestion, and heartburn.

According to Baba Hari Dass, for swollen tonsils, mix chimney soot with black salt directly press with the thumb on the tonsils.[46]

You can drink water according to your thirst and eat salt according to your taste. If you do not crave, or have an aversion to, salt, you are probably salt deficient. The same is true for water. Test this by starting to eat a little more salt than you do now. Increase the daily amount a little at a time, without using so much that it ruins the taste of your food. If you keep increasing your salt intake, you will eventually develop a desire for salt.[47]

If salt makes you retain water, you may be eating too many carbohydrates- or not enough protein.

In a recent challenge to medical dogma, a Canadian researcher from Toronto's Mt. Sinai Hospital, Dr. Alexander Logan, reviewed 56 studies and decided that, surprisingly, sodium intake has no noteworthy effect on blood pressure. Instead, he found a number of negative effects from restricting salt intake, including disturbances in cholesterol and calcium metabolism.[48]

Protein

While Ayurveda comes from a culture that is now primarily vegetarian, Ayurveda is not in and of itself a vegetarian system. Ayurveda does not prohibit meat. The *Charaka Samhita* includes guidelines for eating vegetable and animal products. It does not affirm or recommend routine or excess meat eating. It opines that meat is nutritious for the relief of certain diseases, and when the patient dehydrated, emaciated, weak or convalescing. Dr. Marc Halpern, of the

California College of Ayurveda, says, "Some people benefit from meat while others thrive as vegetarians."[49]

Yoga, on the other hand, promotes vegetarianism for spiritual and health reasons. Ayurveda always recommends doing what works for you. Well cooked meat broth, for example, is suggested for those with high vata or those who are severely depleted.

One of the authors, Khalsa, is a long time vegetarian, who follows a yoga (lactovegetarian) diet. The other, Tierra, is a meat eater. The point is to honestly assess how your body is coping with your lifestyle, health history, and dosha balance today. Then make adjustments. It is essential to consume and digest enough protein. Both authors have seen patients who eat and digest too little protein, and are depleted from their diet. Both have also seen people who consume excess protein and do not digest it, resulting in a buildup of ama and the need for detoxification.

Swami Sadashiva Tirtha says, "Ayurveda suggests using meat only as a medicine since meat does not actually rebuild and regenerate the cells and tissues. In the case of extreme weakness, such as advanced cases of anemia, red meat (or its substitutes like liver pills) and bone soups are useful to take until the anemia is treated."[50] *If meat is to be consumed, it is best taken during the day, when agni is high, and prepared by being well cooked to promote digestion.*

Dr. Virender Sodhi, an Ayurvedic physician in Washington state, says that, "It was essential for certain treatments. The animal was sacrificed for the patient, and it involved a ritual of gratitude for the animal."[51]

Moral issues aside, the main practical objection to meat is that it is dense and heavy, so hard to digest. It is essential to cook it properly and to assure that agni is up to the job. Yogi Bhajan said that, from the point of view of physical health, you could eat anything you want, if it would come out within 24 hours. His opinion was that meat usually would not.[52]

Interestingly, the pitta type person is the most likely to be able to digest meat, but may be the type that benefits least from it, as it is usually hot, and tends to increase aggression.

According to Dr. Gaby, the American diet tends to contain too much protein. He claims that studies have indicated that excessive protein in the diet may encourage bone loss.

Beans, peas and other legumes, including lentils, are an excellent source of protein. If you include these in your diet, and also eat whole grains such as whole wheat, oats, corn, barley, millet, buckwheat and, rice, these two food groups together will provide the entire assortment of essential amino acids you need for protein. Legumes are high in the alkaline minerals calcium, magnesium, potassium, iron, copper, zinc and vitamin B-complex, all nutrients that benefit strong bones. As an added benefit, legumes are high in soluble fiber, the kind that lowers cholesterol.

Having said this, remember- it's still necessary to consume enough protein.

Decreased density of the femur is associated with the amount of protein in the diet. The bone is composed of a very important protein matrix, in which minerals are deposited. Unless there is sufficient dietary protein, the body cannot preserve its protein matrix. So, as with most things, balance is the key- we need neither too much nor too little protein.

Recall that Ayurveda says that meat is not to be consumed with milk, yogurt or eggs.

Meat builds blood. Other blood building options include black sesame seeds, pomegranate, black grape juice and molasses. Chyavanprash, turmeric and ghee help. Iron supplements should be taken with ginger or cinnamon to aid assimilation.[53]

The text in the *Charaka Samhita* states that meat is 'unwholesome' if it comes from an animal that has been raised in surroundings that is not its natural or native environment. Meat is toxic if the animal has consumed food not its natural diet or environment. In present day industrialized countries, meat is produced in unhealthy ways, and contaminated with many drugs and hormones. Probably, wild game, or meat from organically raised animals, would be preferable.

MEAT ENERGETICS

Meat	Tastes	Temperature	Vipak	Dosha Effects	Properties
Beef	Sweet	Heating	Sweet	PK+V-	Heavy, Thick
Buffalo	Sweet	Cooling	Sweet	VP-K+	Heavy, Dull
Chicken, Light	Sweet Astringent	Heating	Pungent	VPK=	Light, Oily, Strengthening
Chicken, Dark	Sweet	Heating	Sweet	V-PK+	Heavy
Duck	Sweet Pungent	Heating	Sweet	V-PK+	Heavy
Eggs	Sweet	Heating	Sweet	V-P+K=	Heavy, Oily
Egg Yolk	Sweet	Heating	Sweet	V-PK+	Oily
Fish	Sweet	Heating	Sweet	PK+V-	Heavy, Oily, Smooth Promotes Heat
Lamb	Sweet Astringent	Heating	Sweet	VPK+	Heavy, Strengthening.
Pork	Sweet Astringent	Heating	Sweet	VPK+	Heavy, Oily, Smooth Appetizing Diuretic
Rabbit	Sweet Astringent	Heating	Pungent	V+PK-	Light, Dry, Rough

MEAT BY DOSHA

Vata		Pitta		Kapha	
No	Yes	No	Yes	No	Yes
Turkey Rabbit Pork Lamb	White Meat Chicken Broth	Meat Chicken Ducks Eggs Pork Salmon Sardines	Moderate Fowl, Fish	Beef Buffalo Chicken Duck	Fresh Water Fish Shrimp Rabbit Venison White Meat (small amount)

Figure 14 Meat Properties

Beans

In Ayurvedic cooking, legumes (beans, peas and lentils, collectively called *dal*) constitute an important source of nutrition. Beans are rich in protein, complex carbohydrates, including soluble fiber, and vitamins. Beans are particularly good sources of significant minerals- folic acid, calcium, zinc, iron, and selenium. They are versatile and delicious, and are used to make salads, appetizers, soups, main dishes, condiments and desserts. They combine well with many ingredients, such as grains and vegetables, and are good main ingredients for dishes spiced with herbs.

Adding warming carminative spices, such as cumin, black pepper and ginger to beans helps the process of digestion.

Mung Beans and Kicharee

Mung beans are small, cylindrical beans with a dark green skin. They are used whole or split and hulled. They are tridoshic and very easy to digest, especially as compared to larger beans. They have astringent and sweet qualities, and a cooling energy. Easier to digest than most other beans, mung beans are a good source of vegetarian protein. They detoxify the blood and neutralize toxins, especially pitta. By neutralizing toxins throughout the body, they are able to calm the mind, relieve hypertension, clear the accumulation of excess cholesterol and other lipids from the veins and arteries of the body, and promote the healing of all diseases. This bean is a real star of Ayurveda. Baba Hari Dass opines that the combination of dates, mung beans, rice and ginger powder is cooling.[54]

Mung beans go well with many grains and flours, vegetables and greens, plus tart fruit, other sprouts, spices, and soy or nut milks. When cooked, mung dal has the consistency of porridge. It can be used to create suppers, salads, soups, spreads, snacks, smoothies and sweets.

Rinse and clean the beans well before cooking. Dried mung dal does not usually require soaking.

Kicharee is the most famous nutritive food of Ayurveda. It is gruel, cooked to butter-soft consistency, made from a grain (almost always rice) and a small, easily digested legume. Lentils are often used, but it could also contain split peas, urid dal or mung beans. Even without a pressure cooker, kicharee will cook on the stovetop burner in about half an hour.

The stew is pre-digested, and is usually very mildly spiced. It will contain, perhaps, a little pepper, and a little cumin. There are many simple recipes for kicharee.

This one pot meal is the main convalescent food of Ayurveda. When folks are hospitalized, it would be common to eat nothing but kicharee for the duration of the hospital stay. Frequently this hospital kicharee is nothing but lentils, rice and a little salt and pepper. Usually it is a thinner gruel consistency, using perhaps 10 parts water to 1 part grains. Sometimes disease is treated with nothing more than a kicharee diet for up to several weeks. Kicharee fills the bill for amino acid balance with beans and grains.

Tierra and Khalsa both regularly recommend this dish for a deep cleansing and rejuvenation diet. Kicharee makes a good base for medicines. Cook in or stir in the desired herbal foods for a convenient way to ingest large quantities of nutritional medicine.

Kanji

Kanji is very thin gruel. It is given in cases of very low agni, when a lighter diet is needed, such as during a cold. Kanji water may be made from split mung beans, cracked barley or rice. The usual dose is one or two quarts per day. Kanji is usually made by cooking one part grain in 14 parts water until the soup is very thin. Ginger, cumin and salt may be added for taste. Strain the gruel if desired.

Kanji can be a digestible, low fat dish for the third trimester of pregnancy.[55] It can be a vehicle for medicine, or a base to disguise medicinal tastes to improve compliance. The water can be substituted with herb decoction.

Kanji is sometimes fermented, which is less suitable for pitta.

Chinese medicine uses essentially the same gruel, where it is called "congee."

Karela

Karela (*Momordica charantia*), also known as balsam pear or bitter melon, a vegetable widely cultivated for food in Asia, Africa and South America, is widely known as a bitter folk remedy.

This melon is green and covered with gourd-like bumps. It is very bitter, and somewhat pungent. It is light, dry, and warming. This melon reduces kapha and pitta. It is a good source of bitter taste, and a convenient way to get this taste into the diet. Bitter is not ideal for vata, so use caution in high vata, although the digestive benefit might be of help in vataja conditions, if use is not excessive. In high pitta conditions, it can be used with a bit of ghee.

Bitter melon can be steamed or sautéed and eaten as a food. The fresh juice, dried herb, and water decoction (tea) are all active. Clinical reports show good results with 2 ounces of juice per day. This vegetable is widely available in Asian food stores. The juice is difficult to make palatable, so plug your nose, and take a two ounce shot - down the hatch!

Many studies have demonstrated the hypoglycemic effect of this herb. Karela seems to have some action on the pancreas, as well as on other tissues involved in diabetes, including a constituent with insulin-like action, making Momordica a possible insulin substitute.[56] Researchers have coined the term *plant insulin* to describe karela. The insulin-like molecule in karela is almost identical to bovine insulin, widely used by diabetics.

Bitter melon contains potent detoxifiers that protect the pancreas from free radical damage, which is widely thought to be a cause of type I diabetes. Karela is used for amenorrhea, worms and obesity. It increases appetite and stimulates digestive agni.

Karela is as easy to grow as cucumber. If you are a gardener, this would be a great addition to your backyard patch. The young leaves can be used as green vegetable.

Eggplant

Eggplant, known as "elabatu," is called "God's ovaries" by Yogi Bhajan. It is sweet, astringent and pungent. Khalsa learned about eggplant for women from Yogi Bhajan. It's a warming circulation enhancer, excellent for physiologically "cold" women. It is an emmenagogue, diuretic food that increases pitta and pacifies vata. In our experience, this is one of the greatest foods for women's healing. Eggplant has not been studied much, as far as we know, so the mechanism is unclear, but eggplant may contain phytohormones, like those being discovered in many other foods. Eggplant can be helpful in chronic PMS treatment.

Khalsa's colleague, Robyn Landis, used eggplant to naturally stimulate the onset of menses that had ceased for over two years.[57] For amenorrhea, it needs to be eaten regularly- half of an eggplant daily- to produce results. Based on these properties, it is contraindicated in pregnancy.

Eggplant increases appetite, and it may increase gas in some. It increases semen and muscular strength, while treating gallstones. It also finds use in asthma, cough and chronic pain.

Eggplant is a nightshade. Sensitivity is rare, but some folks who have trouble with nightshades may have to avoid it. Many people with nightshade sensitivity are vata types. Generally, eggplant is not compatible with yogurt, milk, melon and cucumber.

Onion

The onion (palandu) is a pungent edible of the lily family, and one of the oldest cultivated vegetables. Its properties are very similar to garlic, albeit a bit less concentrated. This bulb affects virtually every tissue and forms the basis of every strong herbal program (except for celibate yoga practitioners). Onions are tonic for the hormone-producing endocrine glands, which increase stamina, vigor, alertness and sexual performance. They also reduce blood pressure and cholesterol and increase circulatory health. They enhance digestion, strengthen the joints and support the immune system. The characteristic smell of onion comes from the active sulfur compounds.

Onions are excellent anti-allergy and respiratory food, especially for asthma. They thin phlegm and promote expectoration. Equal amounts of onion juice and honey should be mixed and three to four teaspoons of this mixture should be taken daily for cough.

Onions increase sexual energy, libido, and sexual secretions. They are good aphrodisiacs, but, since they promote sexual desire, they may lead to excessive sexual activity, which may offset the gains of the rejuvenation.

Onions are significantly hypoglycemic. The active properties are thought to be the sulfur containing compounds (disulphides), such as allicin. Evidence suggests that these compounds lower glucose levels by competing with insulin (also a disulphide) in the liver. The well known cardiovascular benefits of these herbs alone (regulating blood pressure, cholesterol, and platelet aggregation) justify their use in diabetes. Ayurveda considers onion to be a multipurpose heart medicine. However, even at moderate dietary levels, this food has potent effects. Diabetics should use them liberally.

A study performed at Cornell University found that several spices, including garlic and onion, kill every bacterium tested, even anthrax.[58]

Onions are valuable in bleeding hemorrhoids. About one ounce of onion should be mashed in water and 2 ounces of sugar added, and taken twice daily. It will bring relief within a few days.

Onions are one of the richest sources of flavonoids.[59] Onions contain the bioflavonoid quercetin, They also inhibit an enzyme, lipoxygenase, which generates an inflammatory chemical.[60] They possess a high level of antioxidant activity. Pungency and flavor of onions are influenced by the bitter, astringent flavor of flavonoids. Scientists investigated the total phenols content, flavonoids content, antioxidative activity and anticancer activity of shallots and 10 onion varieties differing in color, pungency and bitterness. For all varieties, the total phenols content and flavonoids content were strongly correlated with total antioxidative activity.[61]

Yogi Bhajan mentioned the value of the onion, garlic and ginger combination, which he called trinity roots, countless times. "I said, in this universe, in Ayurveda, the basic method of healing, there are only three things. Ginger, garlic, onion. These are called Triyajhad, three roots. And we have 3R (the three root combination).

"We know 3R works with spinal column and it keeps the tattvas together. I was feeling miserable about many situations. Now everybody asks me, 'How do you drink this milk?' I take a glass of goat milk, in which, at night, we boil garlic, ginger, onion in the raw state and put a lot of water in it, on slow fire. By the morning it is done. And people ask me, 'Doesn't garlic bother you? Don't you smell onion?' No, I don't smell anything. Doesn't bother me, I can work the whole day as a young man and each day is better than yesterday."[62]

"Chop raw onion. You know one raw onion a day can keep you as long you want to live? Are you aware of that fact? One raw onion a day can take care of man's every problem. One raw onion a day is equal to ten apples plus lot of zucchini. I am not kidding, I am just telling you what exactly it is."[63]

"So take a big bucket of chopped onions and- you know this server spoon?- nine server spoons of crushed chilies, red. Then apple cider vinegar- five cups will do. You can add little salt if you are crazy about salt. Normally we don't add it. And concentrated tamarind- two bottles. In case you don't get tamarind, you can take half a bucket of lemon with skin."

"I'll tell you one thing. If you have cancer in your intestinal system, cancer in your stomach, just take the orange peels and put olive oil in it and put water on it, and boil it and live on it- you will be cured. So chop it up, and then put olive oil, and then put water in it. I made like a vegetable and I ate it. You cannot imagine what it does to you. And if you sleep at night, the bathroom door should be open."

"You will get up by nature's call, so you don't worry, it will be very early hours. That is the beauty, my dear, of olive oil and orange peels, very finely chopped up."

"So, what they do is chop them up, and take onion, and put in rice- put those chopped peels in the rice- and then we put some green vegetables and we put in that oil- sesame oil- in that rice. A beautiful dish is prepared and it is perfect. You can use it anytime you like it."[64]

· SEVEN ·

THE WAY OF AYURVEDIC TREATMENTS

Ayurveda takes a very holistic approach to treatment. Every aspect of the patient, the disease, environment and lifestyle are considered as ways to bring balance back to the body, mind and spirit. Similar to modern medicine, the ancient classics divided Ayurveda into 8 branches of treatment (*Ashtanga Ayurveda*).[65 66]

These divisions are not mutually exclusive, and are all based on the same underlying concepts. The 8 branches are quite recognizable, even to modern readers.[67] They are Internal Medicine (*Kaya Chikitsa*), Pediatrics (*Kaumar Bhritya*), Psychiatry (*Bhoot Vidya*), Otorhinolaryngology and Ophthalmology (*Shalakya*), Surgery (*Shalya*), Toxicology (*Agad Tantra*), Geriatrics (*Rasayana*), Sexual Life and Aphrodisiacs (*Vajikarana*).

AYURVEDA BRANCHES

Branch	Name	Comments
Internal Medicine	Kaya Chikitsa	General medicine for adults
Pediatrics	Kaumar Bhritya, or Bala Chikitsa	Prenatal, postnatal baby care Care of woman before and during pregnancy Diseases of children
Psychiatry	Bhoot Vidya, or Graha Chikitsa	Mental diseases and treatments Improve mental function Methods include medicines, diet, yoga, mantra Includes spiritual alignment and right practices

Otorhinolaryngology and Ophthalmology (ENT)	Shalakya Chikitsa	Diseases of head and treatments Ear, nose, throat
Surgery	Shalya Tantra, or Shalya Chikitsa	Surgery per Sushrutha "Shalya" is a foreign object that gets lodged in the body, in a penetrating wound. Shalya Tantra evolved from removing penetrations. Also includes removal of tumors, etc. Now, modern day surgery
Toxicology	Agad Tantra, or Visha Chikitsa	Toxins from vegetables, minerals, animals Includes bites of snakes, inscets, food poisoning Epidemiology
Geriatrics, Antiaging	Rasayana	Disease prevention Promotion of long and healthy life Increase health, intellect, beauty
Sexual Life and Aphrodisiacs	Vajikarana	Increasing sexuality vitality

Figure 15 Ayurveda Branches

Of course, Ayurveda uses diet and medicinal food as the basis of health. Added to that, herbs are the foremost method for impactful treatment. Ayurvedic treatment tends to use highly refined products and processes, based on low technology methods, such as decoction, juice extraction and roasting.

Ayurveda considers the possibility of many approaches to the goals of treatment. Ayurveda has classified these approaches, enumerating several ways to reestablish health and relieve suffering.

These are:

- *Shodhana* therapy (Purification)
- *Shamana* therapy (Palliative)
- *Pathya Vyavastha* (Prescription of diet and activity)
- *Nidan Parivarjan* (Avoiding disease causing and aggravating factors)
- *Satvavajaya* (Psychotherapy)
- *Rasayana* therapy (Rejuvenation)

Ayurveda Treatment Categories

There are many ways to approach a case. In the case of disease, the best general method, to get to long term balance, if purification, either mild methods with diet and herbs, or more aggressive clinical methods. Since the basis of most disease can be traced to ama, this makes sense.

If the patient is not robust enough to tolerate detoxification, we could also begin with palliating the symptom, allowing the person some measure of temporary comfort. Usually this involves acute care herbs and some moderate lifestyle or diet changes.

We might also recommend long term diet changes, or adjustments to daily activity routines. We could clean up the person's life, to prevent problems. Psychotherapy and antiaging regimes might also come into play.

AYURVEDA TREATMENT CATEGORIES

Therapy	English	Details	Used Mainly
Shodhana	Purification	Internal and external detoxification Purvakarma Panchakarma Metabolic purification	Neurological Musculoskeletal Vascular Respiratory Metabolic (Diabetes, similar)
Shamana	Palliative	Superficial rebalancing of doshas Food, lifestyle Acute care herbs	Alleviate symptoms Weaker patients
Pathya Vyavastha	Prescription of diet and activity	Indications and contraindications in diet, activity, habits, emotions	Enhance therapeutic measures Impede pathogenetic processes Optimize digestion Build tissue strength
Nidan Parivarjan	Avoiding disease causing and aggravating factors	Refrain from disease precipitating factors	Prevention
Satvavajaya	Psychotherapy	Restrain mind from desires for unwholesome objects Cultivation of courage, memory, concentration	Mental illness
Rasayana	Rejuvenation	Promote strength, immunity, vitality, youthfulness	Antiaging

Figure 16 Ayurveda Treatment Categories

Massage Therapy in Ayurveda

Ayurveda has a long history of using unique sophisticated massage techniques as integrated parts of a total healing system. Massage is used for even the most serious conditions and can be a pillar in an effective holistic management program.[68 69]

All therapy revolves around the behavior of the doshas. Our goal is to find the offending dosha- the one that has become overactive, and balance it by offsetting the energetics. So, for example, if kapha is the culprit, the symptoms will involve cold, slow, wet, heavy conditions (obesity, chest congestion, diabetes, etc.). Our massage strategy will then be to offset the kapha energy with warming, active, rough, dry techniques and lubrication media.[70]

Ayurveda uses massage therapy as a foundation treatment for virtually all conditions, not just musculoskeletal disorders. Depending on the specifics of the treatment, such as the precise oil, often with infused medicinal herbs, the temperature of the treatment room, the depth and intensity of the treatment, the body region worked and the session length, Ayurvedic massage can treat just about any tissue or function.

Oil massage, *abhyanga*, is performed with much larger quantities of oil than Western styles. This oil is very important to the medicinal aspect of the therapy. The oil is food and medicine, and must nourish the tissues properly. The oil is chosen specifically as the medicine, and is usually an herb infused variety. The goal is to get as much medicated oil to penetrate the tissues as possible to pacify the dosha being treated.[71] Ideally, Ayurveda recommends a massage with oil before exercise, to increase lubrication in the tissues before the movement. After exercise, when you are cooling down and kapha is again accumulating, you could have another massage with a dry powdered lubricant, such as selected powdered herbs, to absorb the wastes on the skin and stimulate the tissues. Follow the massage with a shower to remove the herbal powder.

The doshas vary in their predominance depending on the time of the day. To best control kapha, have massage between 6:00 and 10:00 am or 6:00 and 10:00 pm. For pitta conditions, apply the massage therapy in the hottest part of the day, from 10:00 am to 2:00 pm. To aid in controlling excess vata with massage, schedule the therapy in the afternoon, from 2:00 to 6:00 pm.

Ayurveda gives special care to selecting oils and other massage media. Each oil is seen as having specific therapeutic properties, and is chosen according to the individual client and her relative dosha balance at the time.

MASSAGE MEDIA FOR DOSHAS

Vata	Pitta	Kapha
Base Oils	Base Oils	Base Oils
Almond	Almond	Almond
Avocado	Calendula	Corn
Castor	Coconut	Jojoba
Olive	Pumpkin seed	Mustard
Sesame	Rice bran	Olive
Wheat germ	Safflower	Safflower
	Sandalwood	Sesame
	Sunflower	Vitamin A
Infused Oils	Infused Oils	Infused Oils
Narayan	Eclipta	Narayan
Bala	Neem	Eucalyptus
Amla	Brahmi	Calamus root
Dashmula	Guduchi	Rosemary
Ashwaganda	Amla	Bhumy amalaki
Ashwaganda- Bala	Brahmi-Amla	
Guduchi	Bringraj	

MAJOR MASSAGE OILS

Oil	Energy/ Doshas	Uses
Castor	Hot, Sweet V↓P↑K↑	Best overall for vata Swellings, benign masses
Ghee	Hot P↓V↓K↓	Best overall for pitta (Tridoshic) Inflammation, skin rash
Mustard	Hot V↓K↓P↑	Best overall for kapha ÐBody temp, wounds, stiffness, bronchitis, blood purifier, arthritis, earache (in ear)
Olive	Hot V↓K↓ P↑	Arthritis, Gout
Sesame	Hot, Sweet, Heavy V↓P↓K↓	Superior Massage Oil- swelling, pain, stiffness, skin, hair, specific for breast, semen, hair color (especially black sesame)

AYURVEDA THERAPEUTIC SETTINGS

VATA	PITTA	KAPHA
Warm- blanket, hot water bottle	Cool, open, luxurious, elegant	Warm, stimulating, exciting, lively
Cozy, homey	Lightweight sheets	Red sheets, bright colors
Color- gold	Colors- light blue, silver	Light wool fabrics
Relaxing, slow	Green plants	Copper vessels, etc.
Silk fabric	Flowers- white rose, pink rose	Flowers- red, bright
Soft light, quiet sound/ music	Cool eye pillow	Aromas-
Flowers- deep, rich colors	Aromas-	Basil
Aromas-	Gardenia	Camphor
Geranium	Jasmine	Eucalyptus
Juniper	Lavender	Frankincense
Lavender	Lotus	Lemon
Myrrh	Rose	Peppermint
Patchouli	Sandalwood	Rosemary
Sage	Vertivert	Sage
Basil		

Figure 17 Therapeutic Settings

Panchakarma

After determining a dosha imbalance, an appropriate counterbalancing dietary, herbal medicine and therapeutic regime is undertaken. The most profound therapy is *panchkarma* (five internal cleansing methods). These consist of varying processes of vomiting, purging, enema, nasal medication and bleeding.[72]

It is customary to prepare for panchkarma therapy with a combination of oiling and sweating (*purvakarma*), to loosen ama and drive it toward the digestive tract for elimination.[73] A special diet of kicharee is often taken exclusively or primarily during the program, since this food is both nourishing and detoxifying.[74]

Unfortunately, some therapies are difficult to perform in America today, so are often neglected. Emesis (vomiting) is extremely important in the elimination of mucus. In India, bleeding is often done painlessly with the aid of leeches that selectively extract the toxic blood from a particular area. Presently, many American Ayurvedic centers may not administer these therapies because of certain legal restrictions and liabilities. Individuals may be directed to vomit at home, which can be quite problematic and scary to the uninitiated, or to donate a quantity of blood at the local blood bank. (This is a reasonable substitute, but does not have the specificity by which Ayurveda chooses where to withdraw the venous blood, which may be extracted in small quantities from a few different locations.)

Panchakarma, the Five Cleansing Therapies for Chronic Diseases

First, apply therapies (*purvakarma*) to prepare for pancha karma:

1. Panchana- Preparatory diet

- Medicinal foods to cause doshas to liquefy and come to digestive tract
- Ex: yogurt with salt
- Ex: Banana and milk with raw sugar

2. Snehana (Oil- internal and external)
   Abhiyanga- Oil Massage
3. Swedana (Steaming and Fomentation)
   - Steam box or tent
   - Use hose to direct herbal steam (can use pressure cooker with hose)
   - If robust enough, proceed to pancha karma. If fragile, medicines only

Then, apply panchakarma therapies.

Therapy	Process	Dosha Treated	Benefit
Vamana	Vomiting	Kapha	Respiratory diseases
Virechana	Purgation	Pitta	Inflammation
Basti	Enema	Vata	Gas and Nerve diseases
Nasya	Nasal Wash	Vata & Kapha	Sinus and sensory diseases
Raktamokshana	Bloodletting	Pitta	Blood disorders

TYPICAL DURATION

1st cycle	2nd cycle	3rd cycle
1st-7th days- oelation, fomentation and nasal therapies 8th day- emesis therapy 3 days off	1st-7th days- oelation, fomentation and nasal therapies 8th day- purgation therapy 3 days off	1st-7th days- oelation, fomentation and nasal therapies 8th day- enema therapy

Figure 18 Panchakarma

Then, apply post-treatment (Paschat Karma)

- Samsarjana Karma- restore digestion through specific diet
- Rasayanadi Karma- rejuvenation therapy
- Samana Prayoga- specific disease treatment as necessary
  Then, procede with after care
- Oleation therapy for the same number of days as the pancha karma
- Warm water for drinking and bathing
- Celibacy
- Avoid:
- Suppressing natural urges
- Speaking loudly.
- Anger and anxiety.
- Exposure to sunlight and cold breeze
- Walking or driving long distances
- Exposure to smoke and dust

Herbs for the Mind

Ayurveda is nothing if not holistic. It encompasses positive and negative sides of every aspect of living, including behavior and conduct. These principles are designed specifically to achieve and maintain internal and external balance. Given due importance are the body (*sharira*), the senses (*indriya*) and the mind (*manas*).

Herbs are very powerful tools to heal the mind and emotions. Yogis have classified certain herbs that have a particularly positive effect on the mind. They can open the heart, balance anger and enhance communication. According to Baba Hari Dass, "to fix the head, cure the stomach first."[75]

"Losing connection with our inner beauty is par for the course in our hectic, day-to-day world," says *Better Nutrition* magazine.[76] Beauty is in the things we invite into our minds, bodies and lives. True beauty isn't about doing the right things. It's a quality-of-life issue. "To be sexually appealing, to look good for a lingerie shoot, to win the modeling job, to be lean and mean for the corporate machine--they're all motivations that keep us at war with who we are."

Beauty director Mikki Taylor, of *Essence* magazine, says that an Ayurvedic health regime produced fascinating results. Her energy level is at an all-time high, she has no more postmeal bloating and her aggravating sinus headaches have disappeared.[77] She learned that the routine takes commitment. She says that Ayurveda gives us a deeper understanding of our essential selves. Turning within through this ancient practice helped me her reach higher ground. In her opinion, many of us are seeking to understand ourselves better and to truly reach total well-being. Ayurveda helps her make this connection.

According to De Jager, we should take it with a grain of salt when the classic texts talk about curing "insanity."[78] Nonetheless, many of these therapies are very effective, and can help substantially in managing mental illnesses. Perhaps a better way to interpret this translation would be an effort toward "brain balancing." Khalsa has found many of these remedies that refer vaguely to insanity to be applicable in the vata/kapha derangements of epilepsy and autism, when applied with proper differential diagnosis.

Bitter taste, for example, is composed of air and ether elements, the same elements that predominate in the mind. Herbs with bitter taste generally open the mind, increase the sensitivity of awareness and improve mental function. Bitter tasting herbs are cooling, calming and mind expanding, so they combat mental dullness. Bitter mind herbs are chamomile and gotu kola.

Sweet taste, composed of earth and water elements, is grounding and calming. Sweet herbs for the mind include ashwaganda and licorice.

Traditionally, Ayurveda uses many herbs to help us become more accepting of ourselves and others, and to open the heart, manage anger and enhance communication.

When seeking herbs to open and balance the mind, four herbs stand out- gotu kola, brahmi, shankpushpi and jatamansi. Most folks would profit from long term use of one or more of these at modest doses.

Mental difficulties can arise from any dosha, but commonly vata dosha is the culprit. The thrust of many mind therapies is to control vata, the dosha that regulates the nervous system. Dashmula is a prime vata pacifying remedy, taken as powder, tea or as an enema. Dashmula decoction, with ghee or meat soup, or with white mustard is useful for the ambiguously termed "insanity."

Baba Hari Dass talked about consuming pumpkin seeds for craziness.[79] Of course, now that we know that the brain is a tremendous user of essential fatty acids, we can see how right he was.

Brahmi and gotu kola are the foremost general herbal medicines for the mind. Old ghee, processed with brahmi juice, vacha, Kustha (*Saussurea lappa*) and shankpushpi, assuages "insanity," epilepsy and tough karma in life.[80] Let's say that brahmi eases the mental tendency to create problems in our lives.

Baba Hari Dass mentioned brahmi often. Again, for the rather vague "craziness," he used it with calamus and shankpushpi.[81]

Jatamansi is an outstanding sattvic rasayana herb that opens and cleanses the srotas and brings in prana. The five parts of the lotus- stem, seed, stalk, stamen, and leaves, especially when taken with gold and milk, promote strength and intelligence.[82]

Amla is a first rate general herb for the mind. Many authorities say that amla is the best for preserving youth and preventing senility.[83] Used with sesame, honey and ghee in morning, it is a rasayana that heightens the intellect. One of its names is Dhatri, the nurse, a nod to its broad healing effects. Another triphala herb, haritaki, brings long life and a happy mind. Use it with raw sugar, honey, dried ginger, pipali and salt.

Ashwaganda, used consistently over years, brings a calm and grounded quality to thinking and to life. Ashwaganda and shatavari, mixed with mandukaparni and shankpushpi, represents a classic combination to promote the intellect over the long term. [84] You can think of bala as a cooling version of ashwaganda.[85]

Guduchi is tridoshic, and therefore a widely useful herb. As it is a cleansing and building herb, it can be given in almost every case. It has a prabhava as 'nectar' to the body and mind. The juice of the whole guduchi, along with gotu kola, the paste of shankpushpi, and powdered licorice promotes the intellect.[86] Kustha is an herb better known in Chinese medicine. It is also generally indicated for a wide array of mental disorders.

A few other miscellaneous herbs are worth mentioning. Juniper berry with barley, cooked in milk and water, with added ghee, honey and oil is employed as an enema to enhance digestion, strength and intelligence.[87]

Saffron (*kesar*) is a tridoshic nervine that treats depression and melancholy. Yogi Bhajan prepared this as a tincture with camphor, and dispensed it by the drop.

Finally, an Ayurvedic tip. Use shirodara, a slow, relaxing stream of warm herb oil on the forehead. It is relaxing and helps to manage stress. Bring back that beautiful inner glow.

Nasal Rinsing- Spring Cleaning for your Nose

Call it spring cleaning for your nose. Neti (nasal rinsing, nasal douching or sinus irrigation) is a simple, ancient technique. A warm saltwater rinse of the nasal passages takes a few seconds a day and pays off big.

Yoga breathing practices require a clear nose, so yoga, and its sister medical science, Ayurveda, refined the procedure. Yoga cleansing practices have utilized the nasal rinse for thousands of years. The Ayurvedic version uses a neti pot. It is a small pot with a spout, designed for efficient and easy cleansing of your nasal passages- Aladdin's lamp for the sinuses. It will hold around 10 ounces of water to cleanse both nasal passages. Traditionally made from metals such as copper and silver, or clay, modern designs are usually made of stainless steel, ceramic or even plastic. The procedure is sometimes called "jal neti"- "jal" means water.

When we are exposed to irritants, such as allergens, pollution, debris, microbes and smoke, the mucus membranes of our sinuses swell, leading to increase in mucus production, thicker, stickier mucus, clogged mucus flow and decrease in nose hair function. Next step: congestion, infection and medication use. (Mucus that stagnates is an important cause of sinus infections.)

Neti washes out accumulated mucus and debris before they can cause trouble. This simple maneuver washes particles out, shrinks nasal membranes, increases the nose hair function, thins secretions and opens the tiny sinus openings. The salt reduces swelling. The gentle blast of warm water works like a hose rinsing old leaves off a sidewalk.

The result? Less money spent on drugs, reduced allergy misery, decreased congestion and a healthier sinus for the future. It may not be pretty, but neti opens up the head and often does what sinus surgery, antibiotics, decongestants and antihistamines don't. And neti is safe and natural.

The usual solution, so called "isotonic," is close to the salinity of human tissues. Use one cup of water to one teaspoon salt. You may use many types of natural medicines in the neti water, including decocted, strained herbal teas or ghee. To make a solution for use in the neti pot, brew an herbal tea from 1 teaspoon of herb in one cup of boiled water.

Ayurveda sometimes recommends using potassium alum and salt for brushing the teeth. One year, when a bad flu was making the rounds, Yogi Bhajan suggested using the combination (2 parts alum, 1 part salt) in the neti solution, replacing the plain salt. Now hear this- alum is extremely astringent! So folks had a big surprise when they squirted it up their nostrils. But, boy, did it dry out those soggy sinuses. You've been warned.

In the neti, a strained triphala decoction will shrink swollen membranes, eucalyptus will thin mucus and goldenseal will kill bacteria. Gotu kola, scullcap and calamus are traditional nasal application herbs for sinus conditions.

Warm milk or glycerin in the neti will be soothing.

Neti Tips:

- Boil the water (ideally purified, or distilled) first.
- Use body temperature water. It should feel neutral in the nose.
- Use unprocessed, non-iodized salt, if available. Optional: add baking soda.
- Use a heaping quarter teaspoon to one half teaspoon of salt per neti pot.
- Increasing the salt content creates a slight stinging feeling, but cuts mucus better.[88]
- Thoroughly wash the pot before and after each use.
- Neti use might not be advised for those with nosebleeds, after surgery, or with an impaired gag reflex.

Optional neti medicines:

- Warm milk- soothing
- Glycerin- soothing
- Ghee- anti-inflammatory
- Triphala decoction- astringent, anti-inflammatory
- Brain herb decoctions- gotu kola, scullcap, calamus

Figure 19 Herbal Neti

· EIGHT ·

AYURVEDIC MATERIA MEDICA

Herbs are the foremost medicines of Ayurveda. We make very little distinction between food and medicine. We put herbs in food for taste, and for medicinal effects. We mix food into herbs to make them palatable. Ultimately, herbs work their way into everyone's health program.

Herbs are taken for acute illness, to maintain balance and to prevent disease. Their use depends on sharp differential diagnosis procedures. By narrowing down herbal energetics, we can design herb regimes with power, potency and targeted effects.

Temperature

Ayurveda classifies herbal actions based on temperature, a concept that includes influence on metabolic rate and effect on actual body temperature.

A good way to understand the broad concept of temperature (*virya*) is a spectrum from hypometabolic (cold) to hypermetabolic (hot). As the metabolic rate increases, more calories per minute are burned. Temperature and all other biological processes increase. The opposite is true for the cold direction.

	Examples	Action	Promote	Dosha Effects
Heating Herbs	Mustard, clove	Increase circulation, increase appetite, raise body temperature	Digestion, dizziness, thirst, fatigue, sweating, burning sensations	P↑ KV↓
Cooling herbs	Dandelion, Sandalwood oil	Slow down the metabolism, reduce inflammation and treat fever	Refreshing feeling, tissue firmness, calm, clarity	P↓ KV↑

Taste

In Sanskrit, the word for taste, *rasa,* has many meanings. The interrelated nature of the definitions helps us conceptualize the importance of taste. *Rasa* means "essence," a window into the Ayurvedic idea that taste is perhaps the key factor in understanding the qualities of a plant. *Rasa* also means "sap," a metaphor for the taste of an herb reflecting the qualities of the sap that nourishes the medicine when it is growing. In addition, rasa can mean "appreciation," "artistic delight," or a "musical note"- same idea.

Taste directly affects our nervous system through the *prana,* the life force. Taste stimulates the nerves, the mind and the senses-it makes us lively. Through stimulating the gastric nerves, taste enhances digestion.

Physiological effect is caused by the intrinsic biochemical makeup of the food or medicine, which can be identified by taste, of which there are six- sweet, sour, salty, pungent, bitter and astringent.

Sweet, or bland, tasting plants' active compounds are often carbohydrates, fats or amino acids (proteins). These foods are macronutrient builders, promoting tissue mass and health, and they form the bulk of most diets around the globe. Most general long-term nourishing tonics are sweet; research is revealing that many immunostimulant tonics have in common a certain kind of long-chain carbohydrate called *polysaccharides*. Eating foods with sweet rasa may increase heaviness, coldness, yet increase physical stamina. Sweet foods are useful in easing bowel movements, have a diuretic effect and are calming for the brain. However, an excess can lead to lethargy, emotional withdrawal, obesity, feelings of fullness with loss of appetite, diabetes and edema and swelling in various tissues.

All grains and nuts are predominantly sweet. Shatavari, the root of an asparagus plant, is a sweet herb that is used for kidney and lung problems. Licorice is a classic sweet herb.

Carbohydrates, proteins and fats must be balanced by other, more potent tastes, those contained in the micronutrients.

Foods with a sour taste produce their action through organic acids and cleanse the body of toxins and promote digestion. Acidic foods tend to be high in vitamin content, such as vitamin C in lemons. Citrus peels are, in fact, used herbally to promote digestion and stimulate appetite. Rose hips are sour therapy, contain vitamin C and are used for the respiratory tract.

Salts are mineral compounds that help the body retain fluids, and improve digestion and bowel action. They add savor to food and activate the flow of saliva and gastric juices. Salty foods and herbs, like kelp, act to control gas, and are given for coughs. Most salty taste comes from sodium chloride (table salt). This chemical is necessary for nutrition, but contributes to the acid load. Other minerals, less abundant in our diet, also usually have a salty taste.

Salty taste can contribute to pitta symptoms. But, since it promotes water retention, it is very salubrious for vata. On the other hand, retaining that water is disagreeable for kapha, and excess salty energy can lead to obesity and other disorders of heaviness.

Pungent, comprised of the elements of fire and wind, increases digestive secretions. These foods usually contain volatile oils—ginger, for example. These pungent foods heat up the body. The fire tattva in pungent opposes the cold nature shared by kapha and vata, but only kapha truly benefits from pungent alone, due to the drying quality of this taste.

Pungent is detoxifying in the tissues. This taste makes body fluids like sweat, tears, saliva, mucus and blood flow freely. Black pepper is an excellent pungent medicine, and is used in Ayurvedic therapy as a digestive tonic and blood purifier. Asafoetida is another. The "herbs of life," as Yogi Bhajan terms them, include pungent marjoram, rosemary, oregano and thyme.

For vata, pungent needs to be modified in order to avoid aggravation from its dryness. For vata, use pungent with fat, which has a 'guru' or heavy property, or sweet, which is wet and heavy. A few pungent herbs are sattvic in nature, because they tend to not aggravate vata. Ginger, cardamom, and other mild aromatics are good compromises for vata when heating energy is needed. These sattvic pungent herbs can even be used in small amounts in the presence of pitta, as they are not hot enough to derange the hot dosha. Pitta problems tend to be set in motion by deranged vata, so often these mild sattvic pungents can balance the underlying vata imbalance that is propelling the pitta.

Bitter foods and herbal preparations often contain alkaloids and glycosides as constituents. Polyphenols, including those found in grapes and black tea, also often contribute to bitter taste. Leafy greens are mildly bitter. These medicines are cleansing and can remove toxins from the tissues. Many pharmaceutical drugs that have been created from plants come from this bitter category, such as digitalis from foxglove. From folk use, people in India know that, when the body becomes toxic, hot or itchy, bitter taste is the best corrective measure.

In many regions of Asia, a small serving of bitter condiment is consumed at the beginning of a meal since it activates and speeds up digestion. However, take care that excessive bitter taste is not included in the diet as it is catabolic can lead to appetite loss, weight loss, dry skin or headaches.

Bitter is a detoxifying taste, but, due to its drying nature, it creates difficulty getting the ama to actually exit the body by shutting down the circulation necessary to flush out the wastes. They combination of bitter taste, along with a heating energy, such as a pungent tasting herb, is a very valuable combination to remember for clinical purposes.

Astringency, the tightening, drawing, puckery sensation produced by the presence of tannins, a subcategory of polyphenols, is not really a taste in the biochemical sense. There is no taste bud on the tongue for astringent. It is characteristic of those herbs and foods that are used to promote tissue contraction and fluid absorption. Astringent rasa is cooling and constrictive, stopping metabolism and the flow of secretions, such as sweat and tears. Emotionally, it reduces anxiety and excitement. Too much astringent tasting food in the diet (not likely!) may lead to constipation and dryness of the mouth.

Astringent herbs are used in the treatment of diarrhea, hemorrhage or excessive urination. The astringent leaves of strawberry, raspberry and blackberry are used as toning herbs for the mucous membrane of the digestive tract, the uterus and the kidneys. Plant gum resins, such as frankincense, myrrh and guggul, treat by drying areas as skin and sites of inflammation.

Since most Americans need to detoxify, we encourage almost all of them to concentrate on increasing bitter and astringent tastes.

THE SIX TASTES AND THEIR PROPERTIES

	Sweet (Madhura)	Sour (Amla)	Salty (Lavana)	Pungent (Katu)	Bitter (Takta)	Astringent (Kashaaya)
Elements	Earth + Water	Earth + Fire	Water + Fire	Fire + Air	Air + Ether	Air + Earth
Composition	Carbohydrates, proteins, fats	Organic acids	Minerals	Capsaicin & similar	Alkaloids & other principles	Polyphenols (tannins)
Characteristics	Pleasing, brain tonic	Digestive, sialagogue	Moistening, expectorant	Detoxifying, cardiac	Appetizer, drying	Stiffness, absorbent
Temperature	Least Cold	Medium Hot	Least Hot	Hottest	Coldest	Medium Cold
Post-digestive Effect (Vipak)	Sweet	Sweet	Sour	Pungent	Pungent	Pungent
Moisture	Wettest	Least Wet	Medium Wet	Driest	Medium Dry	Least Dry
Weight	Heaviest	Lightest	Medium Heavy	Medium Light	Lightest	Least Heavy
Food Examples	Wheat, rice, milk, sugar, dates, licorice, peppermint	Yogurt, cheese, green grapes, lemon, hibiscus, rose hips, tamarind	Salt, kelp	Onion, chilies, ginger, garlic, radish	Turmeric, rhubarb, fenugreek, dandelion root and leaves	Unripe banana, pomegranate, goldenseal root, alum
Actions	Increases: rasa (juiciness), water, ojas, strength relieves thirst, creates burning sensation, nourishes & soothes, cools	Stimulates appetite, sharpens mind, strengthens sense organs, cause secretions & salivation, light, hot, unctuous	Promotes digestion & salivation, anti-spasmodic, laxative, nullifies other tastes, retains water, heavy, unctuous, hot	Cleans mouth, Promotes digestion & absorption of food, purifies blood, cures skin disease, reduces blood clots, light, hot, unctuous	Promotes other tastes, antitoxic and germicidal, antidote for fainting, treats itching and burning sensations	Sedative, onstipating, Vaso-constricting, Coagulation of blood, dry, rough, cold
Dosha Effects	↓V, ↓P, ↑K	↓V, ↑P, ↑K	↓V, ↑P, ↑K	↓K, ↑V, ↑P	↓P, ↓K, ↑V	↓P, ↓K, ↑V

Disorders Produced by This Taste	Obesity, excess sleep, heaviness, lethargy, loss of appetite, cough, diabetes, abnormal growth of tissue & muscles	Increased thirst, teeth sensitivity, eye closure, liquefaction of kapha, blood toxicity, edema, ulceration, heartburn, acidity	Blood disorders, heat disorders, fainting, skin diseases, inflam-mation, digestive ulcer, rash, pimples, hyper-tension	Heat, sweating, fainting, burning sensation in throat, stomach, heart, digestive ulcer, dizziness, uncon-sciousness	Roughness, emaciation, dryness, reduced bone morrow & semen, dizziness, uncon-sciousness	Dry mouth, distension, onstipation, speech obstruction, heart disorders
Tissue Effect	Anabolic	Anabolic	Anabolic	Catabolic	Catabolic	Catabolic
Emotion	Satisfaction	Envy	Enthusiasm	Extro-version, anger	Dissatis-faction	Introversion

Figure 20 The Six Tastes and Their Properties

The aim of Ayurveda is to restore proper harmony to the doshas. By understanding the energetics contained in the food or medicine, we can offset the accumulation of energy characteristic of the offending dosha, thus restoring the condition to its original proper functioning.

Gurvadi Gunas

There is a total of ten pairs of energy characteristics on which any given remedy can be classified. These attributes are the gurvadi gunas. The main energetics, temperature, moisture and weight, are the primary gunas- the upakarmas. The remainder are further subtle distinctions that help us to narrow down herb use in clinical application. For example, an herb with a slimy guna would help heal a fracture.

GURVADI GUNAS

English	Sanskrit	Properties	Dosha Effect	English	Sanskrit	Properties	Dosha Effect
Main gunas (upak-armas)							
Heavy	Guru	Heav-iness, induces fatigue, impairs digestive functions, increases waste	K+PV-	Light	Laghu	Purifi-cation of channels, increase agni vigor, joy	K-V+

Cold	Shita	Decrease heat, increase strength, stamina	VK+P-	Hot	Ushna	Increase heat, metabolize Rasa, rakta promote sweating	VK-P+
Oily (Wet)	Snigdha (or, "sneha"-love)	Develop soft & smooth, generate strength, com-plexion, aphr-odisiac	KP+V-	Dry	Ruksha	Dry, hard, rough, reduce secretions, an aphr-odisiac	KP-V+
Other gunas							
Smooth	Slakshna	Pleasant touch (Smooth due to lack of water- like polished metal)	KP+V-	Rough	Khara	Un-pleasant touch, scraping emaciation	V+KP-
Slow, dull	Manda	Dullness, de-pression, slow, pacifi-cation, sup-pression, weak action	K+PV-	Fast, sharp	Tikshna	Pene-trating, purifying, evac-uating, burning, secretion, scraping	PV+K-
Solid (Dense)	Sandra	Repl-enishing, increase dhatus	K+VP-	Liquid	Drava	Micro-scopic, flowing, through entire body, increase rasa	KP+V-
Soft	Mrudu	Promote laxity, reduce secretions	K+PV-	Hard	Kathina	Make body firm and hard, dry, stiff excretions (mala)	V+KP-
Static (Stable, Im-mobility)	Sthiram	Stability, hold, obst-ruction	PV-K+	Mobile	Chala	Promote defe-cation, flatus Release waste products (mala)	VP+K-

Subtle, Minute	Sukshma	Dis-coloration, absor-ption micro-scopic Mala, easy digestion	V+PK-	Gross (obvious)	Sthula	Large size, obst-ruction, sleep, dull thought, good digestion, strong joints	K=VP-
Friction (Clear, clean-liness)	Visada	Remove stickiness, heals ulcer	K-PV+	Slimy (Smooth due to water)	Picchala	Joining, Jeevan (life), Bala (strength), Sandhan (to join), Uplepa, Shaitya (coldness), Tantul (fibrous) and Gurupaka (difficult to be digested)	KP+V-

Figure 21 Gurvadi Gunas

Special Potency

Some herbs manifest special characteristics that are not predictable by their energetics. They are used therapeutically for these special properties, and since these actions fall outside the scheme of energetics, they must be learned as exceptions. This uniqueness is the special potency, or prabhava.

Sometimes, an herb will even have properties in conflict with its basic energetics. Basil is a classic example. Though classified as heating, basil will bring down fever, which is usually caused by heat.

Special Potency

Properties not necessarily accounted for in the broader energetics - may even contradict the energetic use

Example: hawthorn (sour, warm)- special potency is cardiovascular

Example: dandelion (cold, bitter)- promotes and enriches breast milk

Areas to consider:

- Special biochemical constituents
- Special effect upon a particular area of the body
- Specific psychological or spiritual actions

Figure 22 Special Potency

Post-digestive Effect (Vipak)

Some herbs, after they are digested, have an effect in the distant tissues that is different than the effect in the digestive tract. Ayurveda considers the digestive tract of supreme important, so the vipak is usually not that critical to understand to apply herbal medicine.

Considering vipak is especially important especially in long term, when an herb will be acting on the body tissues for an extended period- several years, for example.

Three stages of digestion:

1. Alkaline secretions of mouth (sweet & salty) (kapha)
2. Acid secretions and enzymes of stomach (sour) (pitta)
3. Drying stage in large intestine (pungent, bitter, astringent) (vata)

Tastes	Vipak
Sweet & salty	Sweet (increase body substance)
Sour	Sour
Pungent, bitter, astringent	Pungent

Many exceptions exist (Vipak differs from primary taste of herb).

Example:

Gotu kola is mainly bitter, but has a sweet Vipak (special tonic for brain and nerves)

Vipak	Long term benefit	Long term negative
Sweet	Protect essence Regulate elimination Strengthen sexual potency	Mucus Arthritis Obesity
Sour	Promote secretions	Aggravate pitta Reduce sexual secretions
Pungent	Retain and reduce secretions	Gas, constipation Hypertension Skin- eruptions, dryness

Ayurvedic Dose and Preparations

Ayurvedic herbs are consumed in any number of ways.

The most common way of ingesting them is as powdered dry herb, stirred into something mushy, and swallowed. The material into which the herb is stirred is called the "vehicle" (*anupan*). The herb and vehicle are therefore intended to be tasted. The anupan is selected for its ability to pacify the dosha that the medicine is treating, and for its ability to "carry" the herb to the dosha being targeted. The most common vehicles are honey for kapha, ghee for pitta and warm milk for vata.

In India, medicine is often dispensed in single dose packets. Each tiny packet, called a *pudia*, is a hand folded square of paper containing a single dose of powder. Transfer the powder out of the paper into an anupan for swallowing.

Ayurveda has experimented with literally every substance in the natural world, many times over. The system ahs worked out ways to process herbs and minerals to modify their effects, positive and negative. Often, processing is necessary to concentrate active ingredients, or to reduce side effects or toxicity. These methods are low tech, simple, often laborious procedures using common plants or agricultural products, such as herb juice or goat milk, along with heat or fermentation.

A good example is Shudh kupilu (*Strychnos nux vomica*, "vomit nut," nux vomica), a very toxic herb that is widely used as medicine. It contains the toxic alkaloids strychnine and brucine. It is used as a tonic and energizer, cold and flu remedy, digestive aid and, with ghee, to reduce fevers. It is a vata medicine for nerve disorders.[89] For impotence is is taken with black pepper. It should never be taken with high blood pressure.

Here is how Baba Hari Dass detoxifies it: Put the fruit in cow dung for 7 days, then in whey for 7 days. Wash and roast it in ghee. On the night of the full moon grind it to a powder. The dose is strictly only one half the size or weight of a grain of rice.[90]

Tinctures are not traditional Ayurvedic preparations, although medicated wines are widely used. We do not yet recommend using Ayurvedic herbs in tincture form, as their utility has not been sufficiently proven. That does not mean that any given preparation will not work. Feel free to experiment with tinctures. They are just too new to draw conclusions.

Ayurveda uses a lot of herbs, but, on the whole tends to use medium strength medicines that combine well with food and are widely tolerated. The dose needs to be adequate to do the job. Compared to the drugs Americans are used to, Ayurvedic herb doses seem high. Use appropriate caution, but don't hesitate to use doses that will produce the desired effect.

I (Khalsa) had many experiences of Yogi Bhajan, in the early years after he arrived in the U.S., recommending herb doses that seemed impossible, or maybe even dangerous to the uninitiated. (Of course, they weren't. They were just normal Ayurvedic doses.) Once he presented a program that involved taking 30 large capsules of onion, garlic and ginger, with hot skim milk, for 10 days, four times per year, at each change of the season. For people used to taking 2 aspirin for a headache, that seemed ridiculous. But, for those brave enough to try, the results spoke for themselves. During the last century, published American herb doses became increasingly smaller. For example, today's average European dose is 7-15 times the typical American dose for a given herb. The average Chinese dose is 2 ounces (dry herb weight) per day, as tea. Ultimately, it's the amount of active compounds that get out of the herb and into you that's important.

VEHICLES

Dosha	Kapha	Pitta	Vata
Dosha Energetics	Dry, rough, warm	Sweet, cool	Warm, mucilage
Anupan	Honey	Ghee (May use medicated ghee, such as gotu kola ghee)	Oil (castor, sesame)

AYURVEDIC PREPARATION METHODS

Preparation	Ayurvedic Name	Description	Example
Powder	Churna	Ground, dry, herb powder	Triphala churna
Resin Tablet	Guggul	Sticky plant resin (guggul) mixed with dry herb powder and rolled into tablet	Triphala guggul
Tablet	Vati, Guti	Dry herbs pressed or rolled into a tablet	Agnitundi Vati
Tea Infusion (Hot)	Phant	Dry herb soaked in hot water to extract active ingredients	Yogi tea
Tea Infusion (Cold)	Hima	Dry herb soaked in cold water to extract active ingredients	Sevanti Hima
Tea Decoction	Kvath	Dry herb soaked in hot water to extract active ingredients	Dashmula Kvath
Medicated Wine	Arisht	Wine made from medicinal herbs, or "wine tincture" made from soaking herbs in wine (Arisht is fermented after decoction.)	Arjunarisht

Medicated wine	Asava	Wine made from medicinal herbs, or "wine tincture" made from soaking herbs in wine (Asava is fermented after decoction.)	Kumariasava
Infused oil	Taila	Herbal ingredients are extracted by cooking in oil, usually sesame	Dashmula oil
Medicated ghee	Ghrita	Herbal ingredients are extracted by cooking in ghee	Brahmi ghee
Jelly	Prash, Avaleha, Kalash	Fresh medicinal fruits, along with other herbal ingredients, are made into jelly by cooking and concentrating	Chyawanprash
Mineral ash	Bhasma	Minerals are incinerated in a complex process	Loha Bhasma
Ointment	Anjan	Herbs extracted into a semisolid fatty base for topical application	Sandalwood Ointment
Herbal Paste	Kalka	Fresh herbs are ground to paste consistency	Brahmi Kalka
Mineral Preparations made with Mercury	Rasa	Mercury is incinerated, almost always with sulfur	Makaradwaj
Fresh Herb Juice	Svarasa	Juice is expressed from fresh herb under pressure	Brahmi Svarasa

Figure 23 Ayurvedic Preparation Methods

Ajwain

Scientific Name: *Carum copticum*
Common Name: Wild Celery Seeds
Ayurvedic Name(s): Ajwain, Ajmoda
English Name: Bishop's Weed
Family: Apiaceae (Umbelliferae)
Part Used: Seed
Temperature: Hot
Tastes: Pungent
Dosha Effects: KV-P+
Tissues: Plasma, marrow, nerve
Actions: Antimicrobial, carminative, antispasmodic, diaphoretic, diuretic energizer, expectorant, lithotriptic,
Uses: Colds, flu, cough, colic, indigestion, edema, arthritis, laryngitis, bronchitis
Cautions: Hyperacidity, high pitta
Preparation and dose: Infusion, powder 250-500 mg

(Note: *Apium graveolens* is sometimes given as the Latin name for ajwain. That is the scientific name for the modern vegetable we know as celery, which is not used in India. The classification of the parsley family, *Apiaceae,* is complex and confusing. There are many medicinal and food plants in this family, and many varieties of each plant. They have different names and uses in different cultures. Yogi Bhajan referred to ajwain as "oregano seed," another, not quite scientific, description of this unique Asian seed. Older names, including *Trachyspermum ammi*, *Trachyspermum copticum* and *Bunim copticum*, may still be seen.)

A member of the parsley family, ajwain seed is crescent shaped (like dill or fennel, also from this family). Ajwain seeds are used as a spice. The taste is like that of caraway, but stronger, tasting bitingly hot and bitter, leaving the tongue numb for a while. They have a strong and distinctive thyme-like fragrance. The seeds are a staple in India- Indian restaurants often serve a mound of rice with ajwain seed added to enhance digestion.

Ajwain excels in relieving gas, and many folks say that a tea made from ajwain and fennel seeds is among the best carminative remedies.[91]

This herb promotes kidney function and generally benefits the nerves. It is benefits the respiratory system. As is generally true of the umbellifer seeds, it powerfully detoxifying.

The seeds are immune enhancing and antimicrobial, according to folk use in India.[92] It makes sense that ajwain would be antimicrobial, as the essential oil of the seed contains about 50% thymol, a well known antiseptic compound.[93] Ajwain has relatively high calcium and iron content.

Brew ajwain seed in tea formulas for an immune boost. During the flu season, add powdered ajwain seed to parantha filling.

Finally, ajwain is mildly aphrodisiac. Yogi Bhajan included it in his formulas for male sexual function, often combined with hing.[94]

Aloe

SCIENTIFIC NAME: *Aloe vera, Aloe barbadensis and other species*
COMMON NAME: Aloe
AYURVEDIC NAME(S): Kumari (maiden), ghrit kumari
ENGLISH NAME: Aloe
FAMILY: Liliaceae
PART USED: Whole leaf and inner leaf gel, dried latex
TEMPERATURE: Cooling
TASTES: Bitter, astringent, pungent, sweet
DOSHA EFFECTS: VPK = as gel or powder, except in very large doses will aggravate vata
TISSUES: All tissues
ACTIONS: Laxative (in latex), emollient, female tonic, antitumor, cholagogue, bitter, rejuvenative, emmenagogue, vulnerary, alterative, immunostimulating
USES: Amenorrhea, bursitis, conjunctivitis, constipation, inflammatory skin conditions, obesity, fever, jaundice, hepatitis, herpes diseases, dysmenorrhea, menopause, vaginitis, tumors, intestinal worms, enlarged liver or spleen venereal diseases
CAUTIONS: Ulcerative colitis, Crohn's disease, inflamed hemorrhoids, children under 12, pregnancy, uterine bleeding. Chronic internal use may promote excessive stool loss, and may deplete electrolytes. Potassium loss may potentiate cardiac glycoside toxicity. Use in high dose as laxative for no more than 8-10 consecutive days.
PREPARATION AND DOSE: Whole fresh aloe-small pieces of 1 square cm; powder-300 mg (larger doses as laxative); juice or gel-30 ml

You might think of aloe as a remedy for sunburn, but Ayurveda takes a different approach. Called "kumari" ("virgin"), this herb is said to restore the energy of youth and to renew the female nature. It is a main tonic for the female reproductive system, and it also nourishes the liver, spleen and blood.

The benefits of the plant have been known to many great civilizations, and it is widely known in Asia and the Pacific. One of its earliest advocates was the Greek physician Dioscorides.

Aloe vera is a one to two foot tall member of the lily family, though it looks very cactus-like. Its leaves are succulent, broad at the base and pointed at the tips, with spiny edges. These turgid leaves contain the clear healing gel.

Aloe can be used by anyone, as it balances all three doshas. Since it is sweet, bitter and cooling, it especially benefits pitta and combines well with shatavari.

Three distinct preparations are made from different parts of the plant. The inner gel, the sap and the skin- each has its own uses.

The inner leaf gel, which contains 96% water, is anti-inflammatory, antipruritic, vulnerary, and hypocholesterolemic. It is drunk as a liquid. A cooling medicine, it soothing nature coats the digestive tract, so it is used to treat ulcers and gastritis.

British herbalist and Bastyr University faculty member Rowan Hamilton commends the clear, mucilaginous gel collected from the fleshy part of the leaf, taken internally, for its purported antioxidant, immune stimulant, anti-cancer and anti-viral effects.[95] Acemannan, a carbohydrate fraction obtained from the gel, acetylated polymannose, a long chain sugar, support the immune functions.

Ayurveda particularly values this gel as a general detoxifier. Aloe helps clear the toxins out of the digestive system, facilitating digestion. The cooling nature of the gel reduces acidity. Kumari purifies the body and aids liver function, so it is helpful for the skin when taken internally. Consume 1-2 teaspoons of fresh gel daily for young and healthy skin. Many people tolerate several ounces per day of gel for acute needs. Aloe is the basis for the famous digestive herbal wine, Kumariasava. This medicine is used for anemia, liver inflammation, asthma and constipation.

Aloe balances blood sugar and fats[96] and promotes digestion. You may use aloe to encourage a menstrual period and balance the menstrual cycle.

The juice of the roasted leaf can be taken with honey for cold and flu.

The fresh skin contains yellow latex, sometimes called aloin, in which we find the laxative anthraquinone constituents. The skin, after the gel has been scraped out, is usually dried and powdered. Even a 500 mg dose can be quite stool loosening.

If the leaf is slit, a yellow latex exudes and dries to form a crusty material, which Hamilton says is traditionally called bitter aloe (or "bitter aloes"). ("Bitter Aloe" is also the common name for a specific species of aloe, also called Tap Aloe or Cape aloe. The scientific name is *Aloe ferox*.) This concentrated material is profoundly purgative and extremely bitter. Bitter aloe is typically dried to a brown resinous powder before use.

Aloe leaf is a popular remedy for skin healing. This remarkable plant gel is applied directly to the damaged skin. Hamilton says aloe has been found to be effective in treating cosmetic dermabrasion, frostbite, psoriasis and eczema. The juicy aloe plant is famous as a folk treatment for burns and minor wounds. It stimulates collagen synthesis and maturation during granulation in the wound-healing process. Studies also suggest that topical aloe for herpes lesions.[97]

Aloe also influences inflammation, fibrous tissue formation and wound contraction. It has been successfully used in tandem with hydrocortisone, helping reduce inflammation while suppressing hydrocortisone's inhibitory effect on wound healing, Hamilton mentions. Aloe also seems to inhibit free radicals, reducing damage at the site of inflammation. It appears that the aloe compounds emodin, aloe-emodin, and aloin produce anti-inflammatory salicylates when metabolized.

Amla

SCIENTIFIC NAME: *Emblica officinalis* (previously *Phyllanthus emblica*)
COMMON NAME: Amla
AYURVEDIC NAME(S): Amla (sour) or Amlaki
ENGLISH NAME: Indian Gooseberry
FAMILY: Euphorbiaceae
PART USED: Fruit
TEMPERATURE: Cooling
TASTES: Sweet, sour, pungent, bitter, astringent
DOSHA EFFECTS: PV-K+
TISSUES: Affects all tissues, elements, and increases Ojas
ACTIONS: Aphrodisiac, rejuvenative, nutritive tonic, laxative, refrigerant, stomachic, hemostatic, astringent
USES: Bleeding disorders, anemia, diabetes, hemorrhoids, diabetes, gout, vertigo, constipation, gastritis, colitis, hepatitis, osteoporosis, liver or spleen disorders, premature graying, hair loss, general debility and tissue deficiency, mental disorder, palpitation
CAUTIONS: Diarrhea
PREPARATION AND DOSE: Capsules or powder, long term, 1-2 grams per day. Acute uses, 6-8 grams per day

Amla is a small, very sour fruit that is the most widely used general rejuvenative. The bright green fruits have a sour, sweet, bitter, and astringent taste, with a cooling energy. It is especially beneficial for the heart of the body and the emotional heart, while it also promotes longevity, good fortune and love.

This fruit is a spectacular source of vitamin C, with 20-30 times the amount, pound for pound, of oranges. No wonder it is such a well know rejuvenator. Due to its vitamin C content, amla is a superbly powerful antioxidant. It is a superb tonic for the eyes, having been shown to improve nearsightedness significantly in recent studies.

Amla is a tonic for the blood, bones, liver, and heart. It enhances production of red blood cells and strengthens the teeth, hair, and nails, as well as improving eyesight and regulating blood sugar. Recent scientific evidence shows that amla prevents lipid peroxidation in cell membranes.

Traditionally, Amla fruit is used in the treatment of erysipelas, dyspepsia, gastritis, biliousness, hyperacidity, hepatitis, constipation, flatulent colic, colitis, hemorrhoids, bleeding disorders, alcoholism, menorrhagia, anemia, diabetes, gout, osteoporosis, premature graying, alopecia, fever, asthenia, mental disorders, vertigo, palpitations, inflammation, cough, and asthma.[98] [99] [100] [101]

Amla is tridoshic, and the best single herb for generally controlling pitta.

Amla fruit is commonly added to formulas for sensitive and weakened patients, where a gentle cleansing action is indicated.

Amla is the frontline anti-inflammatory herb, and is used for a wide variety of inflammatory conditions, including hemorrhoids, gastritis, and colitis. Underscoring its traditional designation as a "cooling" herb, amla fruit was found to be anti-inflammatory in carrageenan and dextran-induced rat paw edema in recent studies.[102]

It is the prime general herb for the eyes, and is said to treat premature gray hair, especially if inflammation is present, as it lowers pitta without disrupting the other two *doshas.* Having been shown to improve nearsightedness significantly in recent studies, amla is the most frequently used cataract medicine. Amla is a potent inhibitor of free radicals, which are one cause of cataracts. The herb improves eyesight generally, but acts slowly, possibly reaching its peak action over a period of several years.

Extracts of amla demonstrate liver protective benefit. In a carbon tetrachloride induced liver injury model in rats, the extracts inhibited the hepatotoxicity. The herbs promoted decreased levels of serum and liver lipid peroxides, glutamate-pyruvate transaminase, and alkaline phosphatase. In addition, the extracts were found to reduce elevated levels of collagen-hydroxyproline significantly, indicating that the extract can inhibit the induction of fibrosis.[103]

Due to its vitamin C content, amla is a superbly powerful antioxidant.[104] [105] [106] [107] [108] The fruit has been shown to increase levels of three important free radical scavenging enzymes in the brain.[109] The polyphenols (tannins) in amla are reported to exhibit antioxidant activity in the body and the test tube, and were found to inhibit acute iron overload hepatic lipid peroxidation.[110] [111] [112]

Researchers also recently confirmed the reputed cell protective effects of this valuable herb, as well as demonstrating protective effects against melanoma. Recent research shows that amla has anti-cancer properties, including its antioxidant and free radical squelching functions.[113] [114] [115] [116]

Studies have shown that amla protects against elevated cholesterol levels and the resultant arterial damage.[117] An animal study recently found that garlic, onion and amla, separately and together, reduced blood fats that had been pumped by feeding a diet of 21% butter and beef.[118] Amla does lower blood cholesterol, but, if nothing else is done for overall health, the effect is temporary. According to recent scientific investigation, the cholesterol level will rise again, when the herb is discontinued.[119]

The vitamin C found in amla is heat stable, bound to the tannins in the fruit, allowing it to be cooked into preparations like the famous "Chyavanprash," a rejuvenating herbal jelly.

The unripened amla fruits are prepared as digestive-enhancing pickles.[120] The dried fruit is made into infused oil for massage, particularly for the head. Amla oil adds luster and strength to the hair, and treats of premature graying and alopecia, all signs of exaggerated pitta.[121]

Angelica

SCIENTIFIC NAME: *Angelica glauca*
COMMON NAME: Angelica
AYURVEDIC NAME(S): Choraka
ENGLISH NAME: Angelica
FAMILY: Apiaceae (Umbelliferae)
PART USED: Root
TEMPERATURE: Heating, stimulating
TASTES: Pungent, sweet, bitter
DOSHA EFFECTS: VPK= P+ (in excess)
TISSUES: Blood, plasma, muscle, marrow, nerve, female reproductive
ACTIONS: Expectorant, diaphoretic, carminative, diuretic, anti-inflammatory, antimicrobial, antispasmodic, antiseptic, stimulates gastric and pancreatic secretions
USES: Cough, cold, flu, indigestion, colic with gas and eructation, arthritis, rheumatic pain, headaches, anemia, menstrual cramps, P.M.S., dysmenorrhea, amenorrhea
CAUTIONS: High pitta conditions, hypertension, concurrent use of UV-A light (may cause phototoxicity, increased risk of carcinogenesis and photodermatoses), blood thinning agent use, pregnancy
PREPARATION AND DOSE: Powdered root- 0.5 to 2 grams, 3-10 grams (Khalsa); root tincture- 2 to 4 ml; root infusion- 1 tsp/cup water (note possible discrepancies for doses of different preparations); milk decoction; paste

Angelica is a tall biennial, largest of the Apiaceae family, with large leaves and hollow stalks that can be eaten much like celery. It grows in temperate regions as far apart as Western Europe, the Himalayas, and Siberia. *Angelica archangelica*, the European species, is also used.

Choraka has a sweet pungent taste and a warming effect. Taken internally, it improves blood flow to the peripheral parts of the body. It has an overall strengthening nature and acts as a tonic to the nervous system. Like many other Angelicas, its ability to promote circulation lends it to migraine treatment.

It is an excellent remedy for a weak digestion that causes nausea, indigestion and gas. For this use, brew a tea and gradually increase the daily dose until the optimal program is determined.

Choraka has antibacterial and antifungal properties and a cleansing effect generally, so it detoxifies the body and enhances immunity. The herb improves blood flow and stimulates expectoration, so the warm, tonic properties bring relief from bronchitis, cough, asthma and respiratory mucus. As a hot diaphoretic tea, it will bring down fevers. Externally, the fresh leaves of the plant are crushed and applied as poultices in lung and chest diseases.

The mild warming and detoxifying tendencies of this herb support its use in osteoarthritis.

Like many other parsley family herbs, such as the famous Chinese dong quai, it helps to regulate the menstrual cycle and relieve period pain and pre-menstrual syndrome. Generally, it will promote menstruation, acting as an emmenagogue. For this purpose, choraka is often combined with hibiscus flower and rose petal.

Angelica finds its way into Ayurvedic formulas for emotional balance. It is sometimes combined with arjuna bark, rose petal, pearl bhasma and white sandalwood to balance Sadhaka Pitta. This combination balances the emotions and restores bliss and inner strength. Nutmeg, brahmi and zinc bhasma may be added to balance the connection between the heart and the mind.

Nancy Lonsdorf, M.D., Medical Director of The Raj Ayurveda Health Spa, recommends choraka for troublesome hot flashes. She suggests adding one quarter teaspoon of choraka powder to a basic female aging formula.[122]

Arjuna

SCIENTIFIC NAME: *Terminalia arjuna*
COMMON NAME: Arjuna
AYURVEDIC NAME(S): Arjuna
ENGLISH NAME: Arjuna
FAMILY: Combretaceae
PART USED: Bark
TEMPERATURE: Cooling
TASTES: Astringent, pungent
DOSHA EFFECTS: PK- V+
TISSUES: Blood, plasma, muscle, bone, nerve
ACTIONS: Heart tonic, circulatory stimulant, alterative, hemostatic, astringent
USES: Heart diseases of all types, angina, traumatic injury, broken bones, venereal diseases, diarrhea, malabsorption
CAUTIONS: None known
PREPARATION AND DOSE: Powder, medicated ghee, milk decoction. 1-3 grams per day, up to 30 grams per day in severe cases (Khalsa)

Mary was despondent. "I'll never have my life back," she sighed. At 72 years of age, Mary's heart problems were becoming unbearable. She would find herself at the hospital at least once a week with uncontrollable tachycardia (rapid heart beat). The drugs that would stabilize her heart rhythm left her feeling like she was wearing a lead blanket. And the merry-go-round continued.

Khalsa suggested that she try the famed Ayurvedic heart herb, arjuna. Mary never made that trip to the ER again.

Arjuna is one of our favorite herbs. We've seen it provide benefit countless times, in just about any type of cardiovascular disease. The medicine is comprised of the bark of a 60-90 foot deciduous tree found growing throughout India. Arjuna is a relative of the famous medicinal myrobalan trees *haritaki* and *bibitaki*, ingredients in the important medicine *triphala*. The thick, white-to-pinkish-gray bark is probably the most widely used cardiac herbal medicine.

Alan Keith Tillotson, Ph.D., author of *The One Earth Herbal Sourcebook,*, says "Arjuna bark is one of the most important heart tonics in Ayurvedic medicine, used to treat all forms of heart disease. It reduces the heart-damaging culprits of inflammation and mucus."This herb holds a position in Ayurveda very similar to that of hawthorn in European herbalism. Among the diseases for which it is prescribed in India are cardiac failure, hypertension, angina, endocarditis, pericarditis and edema.[123]

Herb McDonald, a veteran herbalist with a clinical practice in Albuquerque, New Mexico, shares this view. He calls arjuna "far and away the number one cardiovascular herb. It's the foundation of treatment for all cardiovascular diseases, especially arrhythmias. I use it with guggul for high cholesterol. Using arjuna in my practice has eliminated my use of hawthorn," says McDonald.

Herb mentions a case that he calls an "arjuna miracle." The patient was an 85 year-old woman with a history of circulatory disease, including two strokes. She was having regular episodes of rising heat sensations with palpitations, followed by a "crash" of feeling limp and heavy. When nothing could be discovered medically, she was brought to Herb and her daughter, a nurse, began taking hourly blood pressure readings. The blood pressure was alternating between 60/40 and 180/130! Herb gave arjuna at nine 730 mg capsules per day. Within 24 hours, the episodes ceased, never to return, and the blood pressure remained stable.

Modern clinicians here are beginning to use arjuna for coronary artery disease, heart failure and high cholesterol.[124] [125] Clinically, we have seen it benefit cholesterol countless times. Several studies over the last few years have shown that arjuna, at least in animals, reduces total cholesterol and increases HDL. [126] [127]

Arjuna's constituents include a variety of polyphenols, which probably account for much of its activity, including tannins, ellagic acid, gallic acid, proanthocyanidinic oligomers (PCOs) and flavonoids (arjunone, arjunolone, luteolin). It also contains triterpenoid saponins (arjunic acid, arjunolic acid, arjungenin, arjunglycosides), phytosterols, calcium, magnesium, zinc and copper.

Arjuna seems to primarily improve cardiac muscle function and pumping activity of the heart. The saponin glycosides might be accountable for the heart contracting benefits of arjuna, while the flavonoids and PCOs afford antioxidant action and vascular strengthening.

Scientific information about arjuna is beginning to accumulate. Angina pectoris, in particular, benefits from this medicine.[128] In a study from Delhi, India, patients with stable angina had a 50-percent reduction of angina after three months of therapy with arjuna alone. When looking at overall clinical condition, treadmill results and ejection fraction (heart strength), 66 percent showed improvement.[129] It is particularly effective for congestive heart failure.[130]

If that's not enough, arjuna also benefits cardiomyopathy and the treatment of heart attack (myocardial infarction) and protects the tissue of the heart from damage. [131] [132] Arjuna especially excels in treating disorders of heart rate, especially tachycardia.

Arjuna has noted antimutagenic and anticancer properties.[133] [134] [135] Known to be powerfully antioxidant, cxxxiii that stands to reason. Studies also show that arjuna is a powerful antibacterial.[136]

Historic Ayurvedic uses[137] include liver disease, including cirrhosis, urogenital disorders, diuresis and irregular menstruation. Furthermore, it can be used for hemorrhage, dysentery and diarrhea (all conditions for which the astringent polyphenols are appropriate).

Dr. Tillotson points out that "Looking at the traditional literature, we see that for more than 1,500 years Ayurvedic doctors have boiled arjuna bark in milk or ghee to make medicine, having patients ingest it daily for up to a year."A typical dose of dried arjuna bark is 1-3 grams per day, in powder. For congestive heart failure, 500 mg of extract four times per day has been used in studies. You may brew the bulk shredded bark into a tea with a pleasant red hue. In India, arjuna beverage tea formulas are commonly available, and they often include warming circulatory herbs like black pepper. It's a bit tart, so you may add other herbs, such as ginger, for flavor.

Asafoetida

SCIENTIFIC NAME: *Ferula asafoetida*
COMMON NAME: Hing
AYURVEDIC NAME(S): Hing
ENGLISH NAME: Devil's Dung, Asafoetida
FAMILY: Apiaceae (Umbelliferae)
PART USED: Dried sap (resin exudates from the root)
TEMPERATURE: Heating
TASTES: Pungent
DOSHA EFFECTS: VK- P+
TISSUES: Blood, muscle, plasma, bone, marrow, nerves
ACTIONS: Carminative, energizer, analgesic, antispasmodic, anthelmintic, antiseptic, aphrodisiac
USES: Indigestion, flatulence, intestinal colic, abdominal distention, constipation, arthritis, rheumatism, convulsions, whooping cough, epilepsy, palpitations, hysteria, asthma, worms, paralysis
CAUTIONS: high fever, rash, urticaria, pregnancy, hyperacidity
PREPARATION AND DOSE: Low dose powder, paste, 1 to 2.5 grams/day

Throughout central Asia, from Iran to Afghanistan and on through India, Ferula is an important spice in food and as an essential ingredient for home remedies. Indian asafoetida from Kashmir enjoys an exalted reputation in the international market.

Asafoetida gets its moniker from the Persian aza, for resin, and the Latin foetidus, for stinking. This dreadful smelling resinous sap exudate is from the living root of a perennial giant fennel plant we call hing.[138] With a strong, rotten sulfur smell, hing is several times more obnoxious smelling than the most rotten, funky garlic. The gum dries into "tears" as it exits the root. These tears are the best quality. It is also supplied as a mass or a paste with a gray to brown color with a consistency like shoe polish.

Hing is a powerful warming remedy for excess vata and pitta. As a carminative, it warms up the digestive tract and promotes proper digestion and circulation. As is the case with most smelly herbs, it nurtures the earth element, and therefore enhances stamina.

Hing promotes deeper assimilation of nutrients, particularly in the small intestine, that are associated with building of fat and muscle tissues.

Udavarta conditions involved the reverse in the proper directional flow of vata. Asafoetida is among the best remedies for udavarta, and for balancing heart problems caused by vata in general. A rectal suppository made from asafoetida, honey and rock salt, smeared with ghee for insertion, can be used. Others that work along with it include rock salt, cardamom, ginger, triphala, haritaki and calamus.[139]

It's critical to assure the proper function of the large intestine. Constipation can reduce sexual performance and prostate health, mainly by disrupting apana. Having clogged pipes can inhibit erectile capacity, ejaculation functions and semen production. For decades, I (Khalsa) have successfully used a formula taught by Yogi Bhajan for male urogenital health, based on these principles, that contains asafoetida gum, fennel seed, turmeric root, senna leaf and ajwain seed. The asafoetida promotes libido and increases agni. Fennel and ajwain, both parsley family herbs, are carminative and balance hormones, as they contain phytosterols. Turmeric tightens membrane tissue, while senna is laxative.

Asafoetida enhances singers' voices. In the days of the Mughals, the court singers would eat a spoonful of asafoetida with butter before singing practice.

The potent rotten smell of fresh asafetida resin does not seem to qualify it as a valuable food flavoring, but after frying and in small dosage the taste becomes pleasant, and can be added to foods for a pungent tone. For food use, powdered hing is usually diluted with a neutral powder, such as rice flower, and sold commercially in small tins.

Some folks do not eat garlic or onion for religious or lifestyle reasons. Hing is a good culinary substitute. It is commonly used in Indian cooking. A pea-sized amount is sufficient to add the asafoetida flavor to a large pot of food. The aroma of this spice is less when used in dilute powdered form. But the strongly scented resin must be fried shortly in hot oil before being added to the main pot of food. Hot oil simmering allows the flavor to disperse more evenly throughout the dish. Due to the incredibly strong odor, many people prefer to slip a little under the lid ten minutes before serving.

Do not use hing during pregnancy or in cases of high pitta.

Asana

SCIENTIFIC NAME: *Pterocarpus marsupium*
COMMON NAME: Kino
AYURVEDIC NAME(S): Asana
ENGLISH NAME: Indian Kino tree
FAMILY: Fabaceae
PART USED: Sap
TEMPERATURE: Cooling
TASTES: Astringent, bitter
DOSHA EFFECTS: VK+ P-
TISSUES: Blood, marrow
ACTIONS: Anti-diabetic, astringent, anti-inflammatory, anti-bacterial
USES: Blood sugar control, tightens mucous membranes of the gastro intestinal tract, chronic diarrhea, intestinal infection, colitis, mouthwash, gargle, douche for excessive vaginal discharge
CAUTIONS: None noted
PREPARATION AND DOSE: Cold infusion, juice, powder- 2-4 grams /day to control blood sugar

Asana's main claim to fame is in the treatment of diabetes.

Asana demonstrates some singular features, including beta cell protective and regenerative properties, as well as blood glucose lowering actions. In studies, the herb consistently was able to reverse the damage to the beta cells and actually repopulate the islets.[140] [141] [142] [143] Asana is capable of the almost complete restoration of normal insulin secretion. In scientific investigations, as compared to the control groups, asana groups had a significant percentage of subjects that did not become diabetic or hyperglycemic.

Furthermore, asana acts like insulin in the body, but lowers blood sugar through an unrelated pathway of that of insulin. There are different binding sites for insulin and asana, which means that blood sugar reduction can happen regardless of the availability of insulin.[144] [145]

The bark of this tree is one of the few remedies that is thought to have an effect on type I diabetes. Asana bark has been reported to regenerate the insulin producing cells of the pancreas, but only if the disease is of recent origin.[146] It acts in a protective manner, preventing beta cells from destruction by offsetting the effects of a toxic exposure.[147] This beta cell protection may be of particular benefit to newly diagnosed Type I diabetics that are still suffering from autoimmune activity.[148] [149] [150]

Asana is a rich source of epicatechin, the powerful antioxidant made famous in green tea.

Ashwaganda

SCIENTIFIC NAME: *Withania somnifera*
COMMON NAME: Ashwaganda
AYURVEDIC NAME(S): Ashwaganda ("smelling like a horse")
ENGLISH NAME: Winter Cherry
FAMILY: Solanaceae
PART USED: Root (sometimes leaves, fruit)
TEMPERATURE: Warming (very mildly)
TASTES: Bitter, astringent, sweet
DOSHA EFFECTS: VK- P and Ama + (in excess)
TISSUES: Muscle, fat, bone, marrow, nerve, reproductive
ACTIONS: Tonic, rejuvenative, nervine, aphrodisiac, astringent, sedative, anti-inflammatory,[151] antioxidant
USES: General debility, sexual debility, nerve exhaustion, problems of old age, loss of memory, loss of muscle energy, emaciation of children, insomnia, paralysis, multiple sclerosis, weak eyes, skin problems, rheumatism, cough, breathing difficulties, anemia, fatigue, glandular swelling, infertility
LEAVES: Fever, hemorrhoids (internally); wounds, hemorrhoids, tumors, sores, rashes (externally)
FRUIT: Ringworm (externally)
CAUTIONS: Severe congestion, high ama, lymph congestion, cold and flu
PREPARATION AND DOSE: Capsules or tea or milk decoction (cooked into hot milk) 1- 10 grams per day for acute conditions, 1 gram per day as a lifelong tonic (mainly men)

Walking down the sidewalk to pick up her mail so terrified Jodi that she would wind up collapsed and shaky. Only 22 years old, she had been trapped in her house for two years, petrified by panic. In total desperation, Jodi came to Khalsa for a consultation. Her friends rolled her in a blanket, carried her out the back door into the car and swept her off to the clinic. After two months using this renowned calming herb from India, Jodi drove herself to her next appointment. Another two months, and this once cowering young woman spent the afternoon shopping at the mall on her way to the next session. Jodi had conquered panic.

Ashwaganda, sometimes named "winter cherry," is the main tonic, especially for men. This rasayana is a nightshade plant- a relative of tomatoes and potatoes. Unlike ginseng, ashwaganda is not stimulating, but rather relaxing. That allows much higher doses to be taken, with no overstimulation. Ashwaganda is a superb remedy for nervous exhaustion.

The name ashwaganda means, "smelling like a horse." It is said to have a distinct odor of horse pee, but many people do not recognize the smell.

Ashwaganda is a noted sexual and stamina tonic. Studies show a testosterone-like effect.[152] In another double blind clinical trial, Withania (3 g/day for 1 year) was tested on the process of aging in 101 healthy male adults (50-59 years of age). Significant improvements in hemoglobin, red blood cells, hair pigment and seated stature were observed. Serum cholesterol decreased, nail calcium was preserved and 71.4% of those who received the herb reported improvement in sexual performance.[153] Ashwaganda is appropriate as a sexual tonic for women, as well, especially when combined with shatavari.

In addition to its sexual action, Ayurvedic herbalism uses ashwaganda for general debility and exhaustion, emaciation, memory loss, nerve diseases, cough, anemia, and insomnia. Modern clinicians are most likely to employ it for chronic fatigue, anxiety, insomnia and chronic heart and vascular disorders, where it is often combined with the famous arjuna bark.[154]

Study after study continues to confirm the stress tolerance, performance and endurance enhancing benefits of this herb.[155] [156] [157] One study indicated that the herb reduced brain damage caused by stress by 80%.[158] In another, ashwaganda was shown to increase physical working capacity, increase the size of the heart and the content of blood sugar fuel in the heart and liver.[159] [160] The medicine was tested in rats against chronic unpredictable stress behavior, depression, glucose metabolism, suppressed male sexual behavior, suppressed immune function and cognitive dysfunction. Stomach ulcer, adrenal gland atrophy, vitamin C level and levels of stress hormones were also measured. Surprisingly, the herb benefited them all.

Ayurveda considers it a "grounding" herb- one that nourishes and regulates metabolic processes and stabilizes mood. One study concluded, "The investigations support the use of Withania somnifera as a mood stabilizer in clinical conditions of anxiety and depression in Ayurveda."[161] Ashwaganda increases memory and maze test performance in animals.[162]

As well as being a slow-acting tonic herb, ashwaganda is, in our experience, a superb herb for treating chronic anxiety. It takes about a week to work up to the proper dose, and about another week for the herb to reach maximum effectiveness. Since ashwaganda is a slow-acting herb, you may take your daily dose at any time during the day. Used this way, ashwaganda prevents the onset of the anxiety episode.

Use this herb to reestablish long-term sleep rhythms. Rather than making you sleepy when you take the herb, this remedy seems to regulate sleep cycles over time, facilitating more refreshing sleep.

Ashwaganda is showing a variety of benefits for cardiovascular functions, including significant increase in coagulation time (blood thinning), which may also help impotence.[163] It also has anti-oxidant activity in the brain,[164] which may explain, at least in part, a host of its effects, including the reported antistress, immunomodulatory, cognition-facilitating, anti-inflammatory and anti-aging benefits. Recent studies show ashwaganda to have immune enhancing action and anti-tumor effects.[165] [166] [167]

A typical dose of ashwaganda is about a gram per day, taken over long periods, up to many years, as a rejuvenator, but, since ashwaganda is very safe, larger quantities are often used short term. In India, Withania is given with pungent, heating herbs (ginger, pepper, etc.) to increase its tonic effects.

For general rejuvenation, this is a good combination:

10 parts	*Ashwaganda*
1 part	*Pipali*
5 parts	*Ghee*
10 parts	*Honey*

Bala

SCIENTIFIC NAME: *Sida cordifolia*
COMMON NAME: Bala
AYURVEDIC NAME(S): Bala (strength), Khareti
ENGLISH NAME: Indian Country Mallow
FAMILY: Malvaceae
PART USED: Root (leaves, seeds and stems also used). Each part has a different therapeutic indication and must be prepared in its own way for maximum effect.
TEMPERATURE: Cooling
TASTES: Sweet
DOSHA EFFECTS: VPK= and Ama+ (in excess)
TISSUES: All tissues, especially marrow and nerve
ACTIONS: Tonic, rejuvenative, demulcent, diuretic, energizer, nervine, aphrodisiac, analgesic, vulnerary
USES: Heart disease, facial paralysis, neuralgia, rheumatism, asthma, sciatica, insanity, exhaustion, sexual debility, dysentery, leucorrhea, chronic fevers, cystitis, convalescence
CAUTIONS: Congestive disorders with high kapha or Ama, hypertension
PREPARATION AND DOSE: Decoction, milk decoction, paste, medicated oil, powder 250 mg to 1 gram

Bala is probably the most widely used rasayana tonic herb, after ashwaganda. The tridosha nature is rare in the herb world, so bala is widely applicable and, for that reason, quite worth noting. It is particularly tonic to vata. This is a sweet, cold, heavy herb that builds immune function. It is well tolerated in most patients. Bala contains five of the six tastes, a very rare property, so it is widely nourishing to all the body tissues.

Bala is soothing and mucilaginous, so it is particularly used for vata nerve disorders, and it is combined with other tonics for specific organs, such as with arjuna for the heart. This herb increases libido, and has a Vrishya effect, enhancing the quality and quantity of reproductive fluids (*shukra dhatu*) for healthy conception.

Bala is anti-inflammatory, [168] and generally benefits the lungs. **It contains a mild ephedrine-like compound, so it is a little energizing when**

administered.[169] For this reason, monitor it carefully in cases of hypertension. It therefore sees use as a mild bronchoconstrictor for asthma.[170 171]

In paralysis, bala is prepared as a milk decoction, along with ashwaganda and kapi kachu.

For external use, bala is prepared as a medicated oil for joint complaints, muscle cramps and nerve pain. This taila is applied in cases of frozen shoulder and similar debility. A liniment containing equal parts of the bala root and Dashmula may be applied in sciatica.[172]

A related herb, Mahabala *(Sida rhombifolia)*, is used in gas, colic, emaciation, impotence and diarrhea. Mahabala is also used as massage oil in the treatment of joint conditions.[173 174] *Atibala (Abutilon indicum)*, finds application in diseases of the genitourinary tract, including urethritis, cystitis and gonorrhea.[175]

Take 1 gram or up to several grams per day, as tolerated, as powder, decoction or milk decoction.

Barberry

SCIENTIFIC NAME: *Berberis aristata* and *Berberis vulgaris*
COMMON NAME: Indian barberry
AYURVEDIC NAME: Daru Haridra
ENGLISH NAME: Tree Turmeric
FAMILY: Berberidaceae
PART USED: Root, fruit, stem (typically bark of root)
TEMPERATURE: Cooling
TASTES: Bitter, astringent, pungent
DOSHA EFFECTS: PK- V+
TISSUES: Plasma, blood, fat
ACTIONS: Alterative, hepatic cleansing action, anti-hemorrhagic, anti-inflammatory, antiseptic, cholagogue, anti-emetic, stimulating hypotensive, increases platelet and white blood cell counts in leukocytopenia, sedative, antipyretic
USES: Bacterial infections, gall bladder inflammation or stones, hepatic congestion, jaundice, hepatitis, liver tumors, dysentery (amoebic, bacillary), diabetes, fever (remittent and intermittent), malaria, enlarged spleen, pyorrhea, conjunctivitis, acne, boils
CAUTIONS: Pregnancy (possibly), children under 2 years (possibly)
PREPARATION AND DOSE: 1-2 ml 3 times per day; decoction-1 heaping tsp boiled in 8 oz water for 10-15 min, 3 times per day (note possible discrepancies for doses of different preparations)

Indian barberry is a bitter detoxifying remedy that is primarily used for the liver. The main active constituent is berberine.

The plant alkaloid berberine has a long history of medicinal use in Ayurveda and Chinese medicine, as well as Native American herbalism. Berberine-containing herbal preparations have demonstrated significant antimicrobial activity against a variety of organisms including bacteria, viruses, fungi, protozoa, intestinal parasites and chlamydia. The principal clinical uses of berberine include bacterial diarrhea, intestinal parasite infections and ocular trachoma infections (a chronic contagious bacterial conjunctivitis, caused by a chlamydia).[176]

Evidence has accumulated that berberine might be quite valuable in the treatment of cancer cells of various types. A study from The University School of Medicine, in Ube, Japan, indicates that berberine might benefit esophageal cancer.[177] A similar study from from Taiwan revealed that berberine inhibited, and eventually, at higher doses, killed human colon tumor cells in laboratory culture experiments.[178] Another study, done in Italy, established that berberine inhibited the ability of infectious yeast to produce an enzyme it needed to colonize the skin and mucosal surfaces.[179]

The extract of the roots of Indian barberry showed hypoglycemic activity, and was found to have significant anti-inflammatory activity.[180] Berberine acted in severe diarrheas and cholera by reducing the increased capillary permeability.[181] Berberine has been found to be effective in controlling gastroenteritis in children. It was a good antidiarrheal agent and could be easily administered in children in the form of palatable suspension.

Betel

SCIENTIFIC NAME: *Areca catechu*
COMMON NAME: Betel nut
AYURVEDIC NAME(S): Sopari
ENGLISH NAME: Betel nut, Areca nut
FAMILY: Palmae
PART USED: Seeds
TEMPERATURE: Warm
TASTES: Acrid, bitter
DOSHA EFFECTS: VK – P+
TISSUES: Spleen, stomach, colon
ACTIONS: Anthelmintic, vermifuge, carminative, diuretic, astringent
USES: Eliminates worms, purgative with castor oil, gas, bloating, constipation, edema
CAUTIONS: Avoid while pregnant
PREPARATION AND DOSE: 6-12 grams in decoction, 30 grams for tapeworm

Betel nut is used in Asia as a mild social drug, like cigarettes and coffee in Europe, and it has therapeutic applications.

The tradition of chewing betel is age-old and deeply rooted in India. It is likely that the habit was originally developed in the Southeast Asian island tropics.

As a vice, it is somewhat frowned upon by certain segments of society.

We could say it's a "slightly naughty" habit, perhaps akin to chewing tobacco. Chewing the nut produces red saliva, which is often spit on the sidewalk. Not pretty.

Paan, as it is commonly known in Hindi, is a packet of herbal ingredients, including sliced betel nut, wrapped in a betel pepper leaf (hence the common name for the nut). The mildly narcotic sopari nut is the key ingredient in the paan packet. These mildly addictive chemicals reduce inner restlessness and tensions in habitual paan eaters. However, these ingredients can also cause nausea, dizziness, perspiration and initial symptoms of poisoning in those who are not used to paan. Paan chewers eventually lose their teeth.

Betel is chewed as a mouth freshener. The betel preparation is called tambula in Sanskrit, derived from the term *tamra,* meaning copper, indicating red color, the color of the Areca nut. According to Sushruta, paan keeps the mouth clean, strengthens the voice, tongue and teeth and guards against oral disease.

It also aids in digestion and purifies blood. Sopari is a general female reproductive remedy for conditions that include menstrual cramps and PMS.

Betel nut is a central nervous system stimulant, which makes the senses more vivid, because it affects one's perception of time, when taken in sufficient dose. Normal oral administration, in which powder is simply swallowed, without the lime, does not produce psychoactive effects.

For therapeutic purposes, use 6-15g (boiled in water for oral use).

Bhumy amalaki

SCIENTIFIC NAME: *Phyllanthus niruri, P. fraternus* or *P. amarus*
COMMON NAME: Phyllanthus
AYURVEDIC NAME(S): Bhumy amalaki
ENGLISH NAME: Phyllanthus
FAMILY: Euphorbiaceae
PART USED: Plant
TEMPERATURE: Cooling
TASTES: Bitter, astringent, sweet, pungent
DOSHA EFFECTS: VPK=
TISSUES: Bone, plasma, blood
ACTIONS: Alterative, vulnerary, anti-inflammatory, diuretic, cholagogue
USES: Hepatitis, jaundice, skin rashes, itch, venereal diseases, diabetes, anemia, liver and spleen disease
CAUTIONS: High vata
PREPARATION AND DOSE: Powder-250 mg to 1 gram, poultice externally

Bhumy amalaki is a common rainy season weed found in both cultivated fields and wastelands.

Essentially, bhumy ("earth") amalaki (same as amla, the famous tree fruit) is a dwarf version of the amla tree. They are closely related Euphorbias that, at one time, botanists had in the same genus. In this case, the entire plant is used. Bhumy amalaki is an annual herb. The height varies from 30 to 60 cm.

This remedy is the standby for liver problems. Use it whenever a general hepatic is indicated. In Khalsa's experience, it increases bile flow in a very mild way, so is well tolerated by people for whom a stronger cholagogue is contraindicated.

It can be used as a long term, non-flushing remedy for all liver conditions, including skin conditions like eczema and acne, and eye problems.

Bhumy amalaki has been used for secondary hepatitis and other pain, in Ayurvedic medicine, for over 2,000 years. It has use for jaundice, gonorrhea, frequent menstruation and diabetes. The young shoots of the plant are given as an infusion for the treatment of chronic dysentery.[182] **Topically, it is used as a poultice for skin ulcers, sores, swelling, and itch.**

Bhumy amalaki blocks DNA polymerase, the enzyme needed for the hepatitis B virus to replicate. In one study, 59% of those infected with chronic viral hepatitis B lost one of the major blood markers of infection (hepatitis B surface antigen) after using the herb for 30 days.[183] The herb has shown clinical efficacy in viral Hepatitis B. Other studies have failed to confirm this effect.

The root, leaves, fruits, milky juice, and whole plants are all used as medicine. It is useful in indigestion, thirst, bronchitis, leprosy, anemia, urinary discharge, anuria, biliousness, asthma, hiccups, and as a diuretic.

The fruits are used externally for ulcers, wounds, sores, scabies and ring worm.

In the "in case you ever need to know" department, in many parts of India, especially in deserts, the roots, mixed with guggul gum, are given to camels to cure indigestion.

Use up to 10g per day in capsules.

Bibitaki

SCIENTIFIC NAME: *Terminalia belerica*
COMMON NAME: Bibitaki
AYURVEDIC NAME(S): Bibitaki
ENGLISH NAME: Beleric Myrobalan
FAMILY: Combretaceae
PART USED: Fruit
TEMPERATURE: Hot
TASTES: Astringent, sweet
DOSHA EFFECTS: KP- V=
TISSUES: Plasma, muscle, bone
ACTIONS: Astringent, rejuvenative, expectorant, laxative, anthelmintic, antiseptic, lithotriptic
USES: Sore throat, cough, laryngitis, bronchitis, catarrh, stones, dysentery, parasites, eye disease, chronic diarrhea
CAUTIONS: High vata
PREPARATION AND DOSE: Infusion, decoction, powder- 1-5 grams per day

Another of the famous myrobalan fruits of Ayurveda, bibitaki fruit grows on a large deciduous tree growing to a height of 25-30 meters, occurring throughout India up to 1000 meters in elevation, except in the dry regions of western India.

The fruit has an astringent and sour taste, and a warming energy, making it the best single herb for generally controlling kapha. It is a powerful rejuvenative herb that nourishes the lungs, throat, voice, eyes, and hair. It excels at removing stones and accumulations of toxins (mucus, cholesterol, mineral deposits) in the digestive, urinary, and respiratory tracts. It is unusual in being both laxative and astringent, so it purges the intestines, while simultaneously toning the tissues of the digestive tract.

The fresh ripe fruit has a stronger laxative property, while the sun-dried fruit is less laxative. The cooked or steamed fruit loses its laxative activity and becomes more astringent and constipating.

Bibitaki has diuretic, anodyne, styptic, digestive, antihelminthic, expectorant, antipyretic, and antiemetic properties. Presumably, the high level of tannins (17%) in the fruit accounts for its healing actions.[184]

The medicine combines rasayana properties with a mild laxative activity. It reduces inflammation and fever (pitta), and treats cough and respiratory congestion (kapha). It is used in a broad selection of digestive disorders, including gastric ulcers, gallstones, chronic diarrhea, parasites and hemorrhoids.

Since Ayurveda considers bibitaki to be anti-kapha, we would expect that it would reduce fats in the body. Science now shows that, in fact, at least in experimental animals, the herb reduces atherosclerosis, fat in the heart and fat in the liver.[185] [186] Bibitaki has been shown in recent studies to protect the liver from damage.

It is also applied in topical preparations in the treatment of rheumatism and wounds.

Bilwa

SCIENTIFIC NAME: *Aegle marmelos*
COMMON NAME: Bilwa, Bael
AYURVEDIC NAME(S): Bilwa
ENGLISH NAME: Stone apple tree
FAMILY: Rutaceae
PART USED: Fruit, immature
TEMPERATURE: Cooling
TASTES: Astringent, sweet
DOSHA EFFECTS: K- V+, increases Agni
TISSUES: Plasma, blood, fat, nerve
ACTIONS: Astringent, digestive energizer, stomachic
USES: Diabetes (leaves), chronic diarrhea (esp. children), malabsorption, colic, bleeding, cough, insomnia, amoebic dysentery
CAUTIONS: Do not use in acute fevers, chronic fevers ok

PREPARATION AND DOSE: Decoction, confection, powder- 250 mg to 1 gram

Bilwa fruit is from a woody tree. It is a sweet, cooling, aromatic, alterative, nutritive medicine. It is symbolic of riches and fertility. The tree is called *Shivadurme*, the tree of Shiva, and is considered sacred.

The unripe fruit is astringent, and is used in the treatment of diarrhea, chronic and amoebic dysentery, dyspepsia and dysentery. The astringency benefits intestinal ulcers. When fresh, the fruit is a laxative, useful in constipation. Preparations of the fresh fruit have found their way to Europe at times, where they were used as laxatives. These properties lend it to treatment of irritable bowel syndrome, as it tends to normalize overall bowel function. The fruit has carminative properties, and is antimicrobial, so is used for intestinal infection. It also treats melancholia, heart palpitations and fever.[187]

The ripe fruit is nutritious and is used in food and candy.

The leaves of bilwa stimulate the pancreas to secrete insulin. One teaspoon of fresh leaf juice per day is the typical dose. The dried leaves may be substituted. Bilwa, at the appropriate dose, is quite useful at controlling blood sugar, and can be a valuable part of a well crafted diabetes program. The leaves also treat fever, asthma and jaundice.

The roots are also used, mainly for diarrhea.

This herb is common in India, but is difficult to find in America.

Black Pepper

SCIENTIFIC NAME: Piper nigrum
COMMON NAME: Black pepper
AYURVEDIC NAME(S): Kali Mirch, Kali Maricha
ENGLISH NAME: Black pepper
FAMILY: Piperaceae
PART USED: Fruit (peppercorn)
TEMPERATURE: Hot
TASTES: Pungent
DOSHA EFFECTS: KV- P+
TISSUES: Plasma, blood, fat, marrow, nerve
ACTIONS: <u>Alterative</u>, <u>expectorant</u>, energizer, anthelmintic, febrifuge, carminative, analgesic, antiseptic, increases agni
USES: Chronic indigestion, sinus congestion, obesity, toxins in colon, fever, intermittent fever, cold extremities, suppressed metabolism
CAUTIONS: Inflammatory conditions of the digestive organs, urticaria, skin rash, high pitta
PREPARATION AND DOSE: Infusion, milk decoction, medicated ghee, gargle for sore throat, powder 250 mg to 1 g

In Asia, black pepper is the foremost detoxifier and anti-aging herb. It is a warming, carminative digestive remedy that increases circulation, lowers blood pressure and contains compounds that prevent osteoporosis.

Pepper seems to increase release of carcinogens through the liver, reducing cancer. Piperine, a main active ingredient, protects against liver damage almost as well as milk thistle. Piperine is also getting a reputation for increasing bioavailability and absorption of nutrients. For example, in one recent study, scientists measured the absorption of turmeric active ingredients. Administering the turmeric along with piperine increased bioavailability by 154%, and reduced the time for absorption by half.

Black pepper reduces free radicals. It is antioxidant, and prevents the depletion of glutathione. It also prevents the destruction of other antioxidants, such as vitamin A. [188] [189] [190]

Pepper is an anti-kapha herb that burns up ama, particularly to release sinus congestion. Its warming nature balances cold herbs in formulas. It is ideal for kapha conditions such as glaucoma and kaphaja epilepsy.

Pungent herbs usually increase libido in the short term, and so does black pepper. Kali mirch, though, is extremely drying in nature. It is so drying, in fact, that celibate yogis use it to reduce sexual secretions, decreasing sexual desire over the long term. Khalsa has used up to 4 Tbs. per day as powder to treat extreme pitting edema, such as after heart surgery.

An excellent Ayurvedic preparation for sinus congestion is to boil 10 peppercorns in milk, strain, and drink. Use kali mirch with honey early in the morning to clear ama from the system.

For a tasty nerve and eye tonic, mix 50 peppercorns (white or black), 50 almonds, and 25 grams of anise seeds. Grind all ingredients and mix. Add raw sugar if desired. Take one teaspoonful twice daily in warm milk.

Black tea

Scientific Name: *Camellia sinensis*
Common Name: Tea
Ayurvedic Name(s): (Chai, a generic term for tea, which usually refers to black tea with flavorful spices)
English Name: Black tea
Family: Theaceae
Part Used: Leaves and buds
Temperature: Warming
Tastes: Astringent
Dosha Effects: K-VP+
Tissues: Plasma, nerve, blood
Actions: Nervine, antioxidant, antibacterial, astringent, digestive aid, anti-inflammatory
Uses: Tighten mucous membranes, sooth irritated eyelids, insect stings, swellings, sunburns, headaches, nerve tonic, hepatitis, weight loss, tooth

decay
CAUTIONS: None known
PREPARATION AND DOSE: Specific beverage tea doses

This herb was introduced into common use in India in the last century. From that time, we all know what happened. India and black tea became synonymous. Today, it is the national drink, and India made tea famous in England.

This herb in its "black" form, is the basis for what we know as chai, which simply means "tea." In India, it connotes a brew with added warming and flavor spices, such as clove and cardamom, and milk. Each region has its favorite recipe, and each Grandma has her special twist. This gets confusing, of course, because "tea" is simply a word that describes an herbal water extraction.

Tea, black or green, has taken the scientific community by storm, with a wide range of applications in food and medicine. First and foremost, tea fights free radicals, the chemicals now thought to be the most important cause of cell damage and aging.

Much of the research on tea has centered on the active ingredients called polyphenols, powerful antioxidant chemicals. Tannins, large polyphenol molecules, form the bulk of the actives in tea, with catechins the dominant category, comprising about 90%. One catechin in particular stands out. Epigallo-catechin- 3 gallate (EGCG), which typically makes up about 50% of the catechin content, appears to be the most beneficial ingredient. EGCG is about 100 times more potent than vitamin C and 25 times more potent than vitamin E.

Tea brims with cancer-fighters. Tea antioxidants block cancer by preventing damage to cell DNA, and studies are revealing that tea has powerful effects in reducing the rate and severity of many types of cancer, including breast, skin, stomach, lung, colon, prostate, and possibly even skin cancer. In addition, it prevents metastasis from an original site in the skin, stomach, small intestine, liver or lung.

In particular, tea may benefit prostate cancer.[191] [192] The prostate cancer mortality rate among Japanese men, who habitually drink four to six cups of tea a day, is considerably lower than that for Western men. A study from Kobe University in Japan found that mice fed tea extract and subjected to prostate cancer were less likely to develop the disease. A recent report from the Mayo Clinic stated that tea even kills some prostate cancer cells.[193]

In the test tube, EGCG has powerful anticancer effects on human lung cancer cells.[194]

Tea benefits oral health and reduces cavities in at least five ways. It kills the bacteria that cause cavities. Research from the past decade has identified a number of substances in tea that can weaken the cavity-causing effects of bacteria, including Streptococcus mutans.[195] [196] It blocks the attachment of the bacteria associated with dental caries to the teeth. It inhibits the collagenase activity of the bacteria that live below the gum line. The polyphenols in tea are anti-inflammatory, so they reduce gum disease (gingivitis). Finally, it increases the resistance of tooth enamel to acid induced erosion.[197]

For the cardiovascular system, tea has been shown to reduce total cholesterol and LDL, as well as triglycerides, and to improve the ratio of LDL cholesterol to HDL cholesterol.[198]

Tea lowers blood pressure.[199] Since many cases of high blood pressure are essentially caused by high blood fats, it is likely that this is the mechanism by which tea brings down the blood pressure. EGCG also reduces platelet aggregation, about as much as aspirin or Ginkgo biloba extract, thinning the blood, and reducing the chance of stroke.

Along with lowering fats in the blood, tea appears to enhance weight loss.[200] Researchers at the University of Geneva, publishing in the American Journal of Clinical Nutrition,[201] indicate that, compared to placebo, tea extract caused a appreciably greater increase than pure caffeine in 24-hour energy expenditure (thermogenesis) and the portion of fat calories burned. The scientists concluded, "The tea extract may play a role in the control of body composition via sympathetic activation of thermogenesis, fat oxidation or both." Results indicated that 266 extra calories were burned per day while taking the tea product, and it only takes the burning of a small amount of extra calories every day to promote serious weight loss over time.

Several studies have also shown that tea can lower blood fats, including cholesterol.[202]

Tea enhances immune function.[203] It fights infection from many different pathogens, including protozoa, viruses,[204] [205] including HIV,[206] and bacteria. The tea polyphenols (particularly EGCG) were found to have bactericidal properties, and are believed to damage bacterial membranes. The active ingredients inhibit pathogenic bacteria that cause food poisoning.[207] [208]

In the the skin, the active polyphenols may protect against sunburn. Green and black tea extracts were rubbed on areas of the skin of human volunteers, to test the ability to protect against sun damage from relatively low levels of ultraviolet (UV) radiation aimed at the subjects' forearms. The subjects had less acute redness formation after exposure to UV light than untreated areas.

Scientists at Rutgers University, in New Brunswick, NJ, tested tea, applying the polyphenol (epicatechin) containing portion, topically and also as a beverage, on the effects of cancer causing chemicals and UV light. External use reduced cancerous skin tumors by 94 percent, while drinking tea for two weeks before and during exposure diminished sunburn as well as malignancy.[209]

Recently there has been some suggestion that tea is able to block certain undesirable male hormones in the body. In some studies tea extract has been shown to inhibit male hormones, the underlying cause of male pattern baldness (androgenic alopecia).[210] [211]

Tea helps to regulate bowel function and regularity. One study showed a significant improvement with a daily dose of 500 mg of total polyphenols. People who drink tea have less constipation.

Tea may promote longevity. At least, Japanese females who are traditional practitioners of the tea ceremony have particularly low mortality rates. Considering all the other benefits of this herb, though, this seems logical.[212]

Much of the science on the health benefits of tea is based on the amount of green tea typically consumed in Asian countries- about three cups per day (providing 240-320 mg of polyphenols). An equivalent dose would be a good target for those wishing to reap the benefits of tea.

Brahmi

SCIENTIFIC NAME: *Bacopa monniera*
COMMON NAME: Bacopa
AYURVEDIC NAME(S): Brahmi
ENGLISH NAME: Water hyssop
FAMILY: Scrophulariaceae
PART USED: Aerial parts, root
TEMPERATURE: Cold
TASTES: Bitter, astringent, sweet
DOSHA EFFECTS: VPK=
TISSUES: Nerves, digestive, reproductive, respiratory
ACTIONS: Tonic, purgative, diuretic, anthelmintic, analgesic
USES: Neuralgia, epilepsy, mental illness, indigestion, ulcers, gas, constipation, asthma, bronchitis, infertility, rheumatic conditions, tonic for impotence and premature ejaculation, improves mental function, memory, and reduces learning time
CAUTIONS: None noted
PREPARATION AND DOSE: Powder with warm water. 2 grams per day.

Note: In India, gotu kola (*Centella asiatica*) is often used interchangeably with another similar herb, Bacopa (*Bacopa monniera*). Both are called "brahmi." Bacopa can also be called water hyssop. Centella can also be called gotu kola (the Sinhala name) or mandukaparni ("frog leaved").

These plants are not very well distinguished in the old Ayurvedic texts.There is some discussion about how interchangeable they really are. But a careful look at the texts pretty clearly indicates that two different plants are being discussed.

Centella is a sweeter, slightly heavier plant, with more tonic qualities. Bacopa is a colder, bitterer plant, with slightly more detoxifying qualities. Both target the brain and nerves.

Baba Hari Dass differentiates Centella as the "weaker brahmi" and Bacopa as the "stronger brahmi." Charaka recognizes both as being supporters of mental faculties, but maintains that brahmi has a more specific role in treating mental diseases (insanity, anxiety, depression, epilepsy), while mandukaparni advances mental function through a more general rasayana effect. Charaka classified Centella as an intellect promoting or nervine tonic and as a "divine great drug."

Do you ever find yourself in the kitchen without a clue about why you came in there? No, not you. Whatever it was, it must have been important, for here you are. Maybe if you go back out into the living room, you'll magically remember why you traipsed to the kitchen. Or, just maybe, some herbal medicine can jog that aging memory.

This herb, Bacpoa, is more used in South India, whereas gotu kola is used as brahmi in north India. Many authorities consider them to be functionally identical, although their energetics vary somewhat.

Bacopa, also called brahmi, or water hyssop, has been a part of traditional Ayurvedic medicine since at least the sixth century A.D. An indication of the respect for this herb is the name: "brahmi" means "god-like." It's used in Asia for nerve diseases, mental exhaustion and to improve memory- it's a powerful brain food. Meditators use it to increase comprehension, concentration and recollection. Because it increases the ability to solve problems effectively, it is often found in Ayurvedic formulas to prevent stress.

This powerhouse also does double duty as a nerve tissue builder, diuretic, sedative and tonic for the heart. More recent investigations are showing it to have anti-stress benefits.[213, 214]

And if that's not enough, it's also employed in asthma, hoarseness, anxiety, epilepsy, neurasthenia, emotional stress, bronchitis, cough, water retention and joint pain.

Bacopa is a nervine tonic, diuretic, and sedative. The sedative and cardiotonic effects are due to the presence of hersaponin, one of four saponins isolated from the plant. Other active principles of brahmi, contained in the leaves, are steroidal saponins, including *bacosides*. These compounds provide the capability to enhance nerve impulse transmission and thereby strengthen memory and general cognition.[215 216 217]Scientific literature is pointing to some good uses for brahmi in the treatment of cognitive and behavioral disorders.[218 219]

Numerous studies of people with impaired mental abilities have shown impressive results.[220 221]

Brahmi is safe and effective for children. Indian schoolchildren take it at home. Indian scientists gave brahmi to 40 schoolchildren aged 6-8 in a single-blind trial. The tots improved in maze learning, immediate memory and perception. Their reaction/performance times all improved. The dose was 1 gram per day for three months, of the dried plant extracted into a syrup form.[222] Children with ADHD also get benefit from Bacopa. **In a double-blind, placebo-controlled, randomized trial, Bacopa improved virtually every measure of children's ADHD symptoms.**[223]

Bacopa is a traditional treatment for epilepsy and similar convulsive disorders. Preliminary scientific information finds that perhaps 50% of patients will have lowered occurrence of seizures.[224 225]

Recent research is revealing that brahmi is a potent antioxidant with powerful free radical scavenging capacity, which may account for many of its effects.[226 227]

The typical dose is two grams of the whole herb twice a day with warm water.

Bringraj

SCIENTIFIC NAME: *Eclipta alba*
COMMON NAME: Bringraj, Bhangra
AYURVEDIC NAME(S): Bhringaraj, Kesharaja (Ruler of the hair)
ENGLISH NAME: Thistles (in India)
FAMILY: Asteraceae (Compositae)
PART USED: Herb (whole plant, including leaves and root)
TEMPERATURE: Heating
TASTES: Bitter, pungent
DOSHA EFFECTS: VK- and increases P in excess
TISSUES: Plasma, blood, bone, marrow, reproductive
ACTIONS: Rejuvenative, alterative, hemostatic, tonic, antipyretic, nervine, laxative, vulnerary
USES: Balding, premature hair graying, alopecia, enlargement of liver and spleen, cirrhosis, chronic hepatitis, bleeding, dysentery, skin diseases, mental disorders, anemia
CAUTIONS: Very cold conditions
PREPARATION AND DOSE: Hot or cold infusion, decoction, medicated oil, medicated ghee, powder 6 g to 10 g

Bringraj is the main herb used for the hair, with an affinity for the head. It is fundamentally a cooling herb that, in general, controls pitta, which is the dosha that causes balding and prematurely graying of the hair.

As a rasayana for pitta, it is, in many ways, similar to other cooling hepatic remedies, such as dandelion.[228] *It is hepatoprotective*[229 230] *and cooling to the mind and senses.*[231] *The actions are similar to another cooling rasayana, mandukaparni. The liver affinity and cooling nature makes it suitable for inflammatory skin diseases and hot conditions of the eyes and head.*[232 233] *Bringraj lowers blood lipids.*[234]

Ayurveda also uses *Eclipta erecta*. *Eclipta prostata* is used in Chinese medicine for essentially the same indications, and is basically interchangeable.

The dose is up to 4 grams per day for chronic conditions. Higher doses can be used as tolerated. The herb is quite cooling. The response is dose dependent.

Eclipta infused oil is used for abhyanga, especially for application to the head. It is used, as well, for inflammatory skin disease. Sometimes amla, which is also anti-pitta, is added to the oil.

Calamus

SCIENTIFIC NAME: *Acorus calamus*
COMMON NAME: Calamus Root
AYURVEDIC NAME(S): Vacha –"speaking" (more clearly)
ENGLISH NAME: Sweet flag
FAMILY: Araceae
PART USED: Rhizome
TEMPERATURE: Warming
TASTES: Pungent, bitter, astringent
DOSHA EFFECTS: VK- P+
TISSUES: Plasma, muscle, fat, nerve, reproductive, marrow
ACTIONS: Energizer, mentally rejuvenative, decongestant, expectorant, nervine, antispasmodic, emetic
Uses: Colds, cough, asthma, sinusitis, arthritis, epilepsy, shock, coma, deafness, loss of memory, hysteria, neuralgia, seizures, increasing mental cognition in thinking better and learning easier
CAUTIONS: Bleeding disorders including epitaxis, bleeding hemorrhoids
PREPARATION AND DOSE: Medicated ghee, medicated oil, milk decoction, paste, powder 1-4 grams/day

Vacha is a major herb for the mind. It is said to stimulate the power of self-expression and to enhance intelligence. Ancient yogis and seers used this herb. Calamus promotes circulation to the brain, sharpens memory, enhances awareness and increases communication and self-expression.

It is a bitter herb that acts as a carminative and mucolytic. These qualities, taken together, obviously suggest vacha as a superior remedy to pacify vata.

The warming respiratory and digestive functions are well known on European herbalism, but the mind applications are unique to Ayurveda.

This herb is very popular among Khalsa's students. When he teaches about it in classes at Bastyr University, where he instructs future physicians and herb professionals, it always becomes popular within a small cadre of those in the know. For burned out medical students, especially cold, scattered vata types, finals week becomes a much easier proposition.

This herb is often combined with gotu kola, which is cooling and mild. The complementary energetics makes the combination suitable for a wide variety of people.

For attention deficit disorders, it combines well with brahmi, jatamamsi, shankpushpi and licorice. For vata insomnia, calamus will warm and pacify the errant dosha. Use a daily dose taken with meals, to have a gradual effect.

The Charaka Samhita lists vacha medicated ghee for epilepsy involving vata and kapha. It is prepared by decocting one part of vacha in four parts ghee and eight parts water.

Khalsa has had extensive experience with using vacha to treat epilepsy, especially juvenile petit mal (absence) seizures. It is dramatically effective. It can often completely replace antiseizure medication. (Caution: do not treat epilepsy casually. It is a serious and complicated condition, with many causes, and a collection of associated family and social issues.) Cross taper the dose of vacha with the medication, with close monitoring. Always consult a qualified professional. Sarpaganda combines well with vacha for epilepsy.

For epilepsy, use the vacha in ghee, along with aragvadha, kaitarya, brahmi, hing, choraka (Angelica glauca) and jatamansi.[235]

Like epilepsy, Ayurveda recommends vacha and sarpaganda for a category vaguely called "insanity." Khalsa, who has a specialty in autism spectrum disorders, uses both these medicines extensively for this condition.

Vacha is combined with triphala as a general rasayana that bestows intelligence, longevity and good memory.[236]

Calamus is quite emetic in doses not much larger than the suggested dose. Higher doses also may stimulate "weird thoughts"- not quite hallucinations, but unusual mental experiences- that are not necessarily pleasant. Based on these issues, it may not be compatible for coadministration with other psychoactive drugs, although little is known about these concerns.

It seems almost a shame to use such a powerful and valuable herb on common stomach and lung problems, but vacha is quite serviceable for dyspepsia. For cough, combine it with licorice root.

Chanchal Cabrera says that, in the British herbal tradition, calamus root is thought to be a stomach acid balancer. A dose of up to 5 ml of tincture per day will reduce acid, while higher doses stimulate acid production.[237]

Vacha is used for balancing heart problems caused by kapha in general, along with neem, and pipali.

Calamus contains asarone and beta-asarone, constituents of the essential oil that are known carcinogens. and liver toxins. Use caution with the Asian genetic varieties of Acorus calamus in those with liver dysfunction.[238] The European variety does not have this effect, but also does not seem to have the psychoactive characteristics. The North American species has no asarone. Asarone has a sedative effect.[239] The Chinese species, used essentially the same, is Acorus gramineus.

The mind activating properties of vacha have been credited to the asarones. They are precursors to 1,2, 4-trimethory-5-propenylbenzene, a phenyethylamine that is thought to be ten times as potent as mescaline.[240]

There has been much hand wringing about the potential problems with calamus, but remember that it has been used for millennia by peoples on several continents, as medicine and food. Prashanti de Jager calls it, "Another case of an uninformed witch hunt, similar to the recent fate of ephedra and bala."[241]

Past concerns have limited the use of vacha in America. This is a truly useful and valuable herb. Many people could benefit from calamus if they became aware of it. According to Prashanti de Jager, "Don't be fooled, the calamus from India is safe and endlessly useful."[242]

Vacha is a potent herb, so the effective dose is quite reasonable, which increases compliance.

Use 1 to 4 grams per day. Work up gradually to the effective dose.

Apply vacha as a medicated ghee in the nostril for general brain and mind benefit, or sniff the milk decoction our infused oil for the same purpose. It is used to restore consciousness in extreme conditions.

The nasya is applied for sinus congestion. Calamus decoction is used in a neti pot as a general remedy for brain conditions.

The pathological dose of calamus is supposedly about 30 grams of the fresh herb. Frankly, you would be vomiting long before you ever ingested that much. Believe us, people have tried, and were sorry they had.

Camphor

SCIENTIFIC NAME: *Cinnamomum camphora*
COMMON NAME: Camphor
AYURVEDIC NAME(S): Karpura
ENGLISH NAME: Camphor
FAMILY: Lauraceae
PART USED: Crystallized distilled oil
TEMPERATURE: Slightly warming
TASTES: Pungent, bitter
DOSHA EFFECTS: KV- P+ (in excess)
TISSUES: Plasma, blood, fat, nerve, marrow
ACTIONS: Expectorant, decongestant, energizer, bronchodilator, nervine, analgesic, antiseptic
USES: Asthma, whooping cough, bronchitis, pulmonary congestion, hysteria, delirium, insomnia, epilepsy, gout, rheumatism, nasal congestion, tooth decay, eye problems
CAUTIONS: Use only in monitored low doses because in excess camphor acts as a narcotic poison and aggravates pitta and vata
PREPARATION AND DOSE: Cold infusion with ½ oz crystals to 1 gallon water (dosage 2 oz), medicated oil, powder 1 to 2.5 grams

The large, handsome evergreen camphor tree is the natural source of camphor gum.

Camphor has a wide range of medicinal uses. Typically, it is applied externally to the skin, where it acts as a rubefacient, counterirritant and local anodyne. It is also a mild antiseptic. The gum is a favored ingredient in liniments and medicinal oils, as it liquefies obstinate toxic deposits and causes them to flow.

Camphor is sometimes used internally as a very powerful detoxifier. It is a powerful stimulant for digestive, circulatory and nervous systems.

Traditionally, the tilak (forehead marking) is often made from camphor and saffron. This combination cools the head and frontal lobes and promotes cool thinking and meditation.

For external application, in a glass bottle, put 100 ml of coconut oil and add 5 grams of camphor. Close the bottle tightly with a cap. Put the bottle in sunlight for two hours. Apply this oil on the affected area.

Camphor, as a massage medium, is used for muscular pain and dysmenorrhea.

Yogi Bhajan recommended camphor gum as a first rate blood cleanser. He concocted a tincture of saffron and camphor which he called "blood of Christ", and recommended it for extreme cases in need of detoxification, taken internally.

The strong taste of camphor finds its way into tooth brushing mixtures.

Ghee and camphor drops are administered through the nose for sinus pain. Camphor preparations may be applied to the chest to ease congestion.

Burning camphor purifies the atmosphere. It is somewhat germicidal in this form, and is widely used in India as a ritual practice.

Cooling Oily Skin Cleanser

1 cup fresh mint leaves
1 quart pure water
5 g camphor powder

Boil the mint leaves in the water until it reduces to half. Strain. Let stand until cool and then add the camphor powder. Refrigerate. Treat the skin regularly with this cleansing rinse. It leaves your face wonderfully cold and clean.

Cardamom

SCIENTIFIC NAME: *Elettaria cardamomum*
COMMON NAME: Cardamom
AYURVEDIC NAME(S): Ela
ENGLISH NAME: Cardamon
FAMILY: Zingiberaceae (related to ginger)
PART USED: Fruits, seeds (seeds are medicinal- grow in fruit "pod")
TEMPERATURE: Hot
TASTES: Pungent, sweet
DOSHA EFFECTS: VK- P+ (in excess)
TISSUES: Plasma, blood, marrow, nerve
ACTIONS: Carminative, stomachic, energizer, antispasmodic, expectorant, diaphoretic
USES: Colic, flatulence, flavoring in foods, colds, coughs, bronchitis, hoarse voice, loss of taste, poor absorption, indigestion, asthma
CAUTIONS: Ulcers and high pitta
PREPARATION AND DOSE: Powdered fruit- 0.5 to 10 g; milk decoction; infusion (do not boil)

Cardamom is an ancient spice, native to India. It is the seed of a perennial tropical vine, related to ginger. It is an excellent digestive enhancer, especially for cold and sweet food. Banana, especially, is traditionally taken with cardamom, according to Baba Hari Dass.[243] Yogi Bhajan taught a fascinating antianxiety recipe that combined banana, milk, cardamom and nutmeg.[244]

Since it is widely consumed as a food, it is regarded as being quite safe. It is used in herbal medicine to treat gastralgia, enuresis (involuntary urination), spermatorrhea, phlegm, indigestion and gas.

This herb has a warming, anti-mucus action, so is particularly appropriate in lung formulas and to rejuvenate the spleen. It removes kapha from the stomach and lungs, as well as being good for reducing high vata generally.

One compound in cardamom oil, terpinen-4-ol, appears to suggest that cardamom can be effective in treating yeast vaginitis. Studies have shown that preparations containing high amounts of terpinen-4-ol have been as effective against yeast infections as the pharmaceutical antifungals nystatin and clotrimazole. Cardamom may have twice as much terpinen-4-ol as tea tree oil.

Studies have shown that cardamom has pain-relieving, anti-inflammatory, and antispasmodic effects.[245]

Ayurveda uses another variety, black cardamom (*Amomum subulatum Roxb.*), native to the Eastern Himalayas.[246] These pods are dark brown and 1 inch long. Black cardamom has a fresh and aromatic scent, with camphor easily discernible. Traditionally, the drying procedure is over open flames, so the herb acquires a strong smoky flavor. The taste is very woody, robust and intense. It combines well with savory flavors, but is not used in sweet dishes.

Medicinally, it is essentially equivalent to green cardamom. Black cardamom is tonic for the heart and liver. It is an appetizer and cholgogue.

Castor

SCIENTIFIC NAME: *Ricinus communis*
COMMON NAME: Castor oil
AYURVEDIC NAME(S): Erand
ENGLISH NAME: Castor oil
FAMILY: Euphorbiaceae
PART USED: Expressed oil from the seed
TEMPERATURE: Heating
TASTES: Pungent, sweet
DOSHA EFFECTS: V- PK+
TISSUES: Liver, spleen, nerves, digestion
ACTIONS: Cathartic, demulcent, analgesic, nervine
USES: Constipation, epilepsy, paralysis, insanity, nervous disorders, liver disorders, warts, cysts; anti-inflammatory when externally applied to bruises, injuries, and stiffness; reduce benign masses like breast and ovarian cysts, promote childbirth
CAUTIONS: Castor bean seed internally are deadly poisonous but oil is not

PREPARATION AND DOSE: 1 to 2 tablespoons (4-6 hours before purgative); external preps like castor oil packs and massage oil (great massage vehicle for vata)

Marsha Akers is a colleague of Khalsa. Some time ago, her feet hurt so bad, she said it felt like she had "pieces of glass cutting into my feet." Barely into middle age, Marsha, a massage therapist, who had to stand on those feet all day long, thought her career was over. Finally, she was diagnosed medically as having bone spurs.

Desperate to try anything, Marsha soaked her feet in a warm salve of castor oil each night for 30 minutes. The relief was immediate, and continued to increase each night. Two weeks later, she was pain free for the first time in months. Marsha's pain has never returned. She feels great, and best of all, she still keeps going full time in her busy Gresham, Oregon, massage practice, where she's known for her liberal use of- you guessed it- castor oil salve!

The evergreen castor plant is native to tropical Africa and India, where it may grow to a 40-foot tree. The beans contain an extremely deadly toxin, which must be removes by special processing before the oil is usable.

Castor is a wonderful panacea for a large number of health concerns.[247] ***It is pungent and sweet with heating energy. Applied externally, it is analgesic and nervine, so it is the main treatment for nerve conditions.***[248]

Castor oil is the main treatment for vata dosha. Tierra uses it for all vata derangements, including pains, constipation and arthritis.[249] Following the vata idea, ***this very special oil is used in the treatment of epilepsy, paralysis, insanity and many other nervous system disorders***. Castor oil supports joint, muscle, connective tissue and skin health. It is used for wounds, trauma and minor pain.

Castor oil is the "arnica of Ayurveda," and treats damaged structural and connective tissue and prevents bruising. It is not designed for acute pain relief, although chronic pain can often be prevented or relieved. Use on area of chronic joint pain, including fibromyalgia or osteoarthritis.

Castor oil is astringent and helps to stabilize hypermobile joints, such as neck subluxations. It is used in to reduce benign masses and swellings, including ovarian cysts, breast cysts, varicose veins, swollen lymph glands, enlarged liver or spleen and lipomas. Gentle castor oil massage to the lactating mother's breasts improves the secretion of milk.

Apply castor oil to large areas of nerve involvement or organ dysfunction such as an involved leg or as an abdominal pack for an affected liver, menstrual pain, constipation or general abdominal discomfort. Use it on burns, bedsores, rashes, skin itch, cracked heels, torn cuticles and minor cuts or wounds.[250]

The leaves are poisonous, but they may be steamed and directly applied externally to relieve pains from bruises, injuries and stiffness, aches and pains, rheumatism, arthritis, lumbago and bursitis.

Also, apply it to infected skin, including warts and fungus, pimples or stretch marks. Castor oil is used in the treatment of disorders of the nervous system, including epilepsy and paralysis. Also apply it to neuralgia, foot neuropathy and sciatica.

Castor oil is extremely messy, so compliance becomes a big problem. Traditionally, it is applied as a moist pack. A castor oil ointment is available as a water-soluble gel. It penetrates completely, leaving no residue.

Use castor oil ointment on bruises, sprains, strains, hemorrhoids, anal fissures, cracked heels and other traumatized tissue. Apply the ointment or pure castor oil to skin as desired over area of discomfort. Rub it in completely. Alternatively, apply a ½ inch thick layer. Cover with dressing, such as plastic sheet. Allow to remain on skin, covered, for several hours, or overnight.

Use it on specific areas of trauma (anal irritation, etc.). Allow it to remain and soak in as long as possible. Apply it an abdominal pack for ovarian cysts or liver detoxification. Use it as a breast pack for benign breast cysts. To prevent bruising, apply it immediately after trauma and allowing it to remain overnight, or for several hours.

The energetic characteristics of castor oil are a good match with the typical fibromyalgia patient. The treatment tends to be a little on the slow side in fibromyalgia, but, in the Khalsa's experience, long term use can be very effective.

Swallow 1 teaspoon honey with 1 teaspoon castor oil for hiccups.[251, 252]

Michelle Bennett is a professional herbalist practicing in Seattle, Washington, who had received some bad news from her dentist. Her mouth was full of gum disease, with a full set of pockets that averaged 9.5 mm. Resolving to forgo periodontal treatment and bone grafting, Michelle set out on an intensive natural regime, using gotu kola mixed with castor oil as a daily gum pack. Her dentist eventually retracted the recommendation for periodontal procedures. In fact, he was so encouraged that he asked her to consult with him on gum disease cases in his practice.

Castor oil, taken internally, treats "udavarta" conditions, in which vata in the digestive tract has become reversed. Bowel loosening castor oil will normalizing the vata of the large intestine.

Ayurveda sometimes uses castor oil as a medicinal ingredient in an antivata food recipe. Khalsa's wife, Jagdish Kaur, about as vata as they come, once used mung beans with castor oil for two weeks, on the suggestion of Yogi Bhajan. She found it to be very effective for a collection of vata issues, but don't ask her to describe the taste. She still remembers the recipe with, er, affection.

Chiretta

SCIENTIFIC NAME: *Swertia chiratata*
COMMON NAME: Chiretta
AYURVEDIC NAME(S): Kirata tikta, Chiretta
ENGLISH NAME: Chiretta
FAMILY: Gentianiaceae
PART USED: Whole herb
TEMPERATURE: Cooling
TASTES: Bitter
DOSHA EFFECTS: P- KV+
TISSUES: Blood, plasma, nerve
ACTIONS: Very cooling, bitter digestive, antibacterial, diaphoretic
USES: Fevers, malaria, nausea, indigestion, bloating, improve appetite and digestion, hiccups, tuberculosis, liver problems, gallstones
CAUTIONS: Avoid in digestive hyperacidity
PREPARATION AND DOSE: Powder- 250 mg to 1 gram

This plant grows above 4,000 ft. It is sometimes known as Nepalanimba (Nepalese bitter).

Chiretta is a close relative of European gentian, in the same botanical family. It is used similarly to gentian, as a very general, very cold bitter. It is also similar in action, bitterness and use to kalmegh.

Chiretta is a popular digestive bitter that clears amapitta from the intestines. Unlike other bitters, which, as a rule, tend to be constipating, as it acts as a mild laxative. It balances the liver, so it can stimulate the appetite.

The bitter medicine is anti-inflammatory, so it alleviates asthma, lowers fever, removes impurities from the blood and is used in skin diseases. It is also anthelmintic.

Mahasudarshan (literally "the great formula for good vision") contains bitter herbs that cool and cleanse the eyes, and is the main Ayurvedic eye remedy.[253] The formula contains chiretta, guduchi, barberry, black pepper, long pepper, ginger root and the triphala combination.

Chiretta is used with cardamom, turmeric and kutki for gastrointestinal tract inflammation. It is combined with neem, manjishta and gotu kola for inflamed skin.

Yogi Bhajan had this to say, "There is a kind of dried long grass in India called chiretta, which is very bitter but highly purifying to the blood. Soak a handful in water at night. In the morning pour the water off and drink one cup. But it is very, very bitter. The next day put another handful in water and make into tea. You will never have any skin problems. You must take ghee or almond oil in milk along with this, because it is very drying."[254]

Chrysanthemum

Scientific Name: *Chrysanthemum morifolium*
Common Name: Chrysanthemum
Ayurvedic Name(s): Sevanti
English Name: Chrysanthenum
Family: Asteraceae (Compositae)
Part Used: Flower
Temperature: Cold
Tastes: Sweet, slightly bitter
Dosha Effects: -PK +V
Tissues: Lung, liver
Actions: Carminative, alterative, tonic, febrifuge, antispasmodic, antibacterial
Uses: Inflammation, colds, flu, headaches, rejuvenative, conjunctivitis (as eyewash), dry eyes, dizziness, vision, hypertension
Cautions: Unknown
Preparation and dose: Standard infusion; powder- 3 to 9 grams

Of course we think of this plant as a pleasant decorative flower, but did you ever think it would have medicinal properties? Chrysanthemum flower is a cooling anti-pitta remedy with an affinity for the head. It cools pitta in the eyes, and helps vision.

Chrysanthemum is an immune booster, especially effective for feverish conditions of the upper respiratory tract. This medicine has a history of in vitro effect against several bacteria, including strep, staph, and shigella.[255]

Studies have shown that acacetin-7-O-beta-D-galactopyranoside, a compound in chrysanthemum, inhibits HIV in vitro. Several chrysanthemum compounds had similar effects.[256 257]

Chrysanthemum flower, a cooling diaphoretics, is used to reduce fever and inflammation. Chamomile flowers and rose petals combine well with it to reduce inflammation. Chrysanthemum is very cooling to the mind, as well. It helps to surrender the egoistic will and also soothes anger.

Chrysanthemum tastes good as tea, so drink up.

Cinnamon

Scientific Name: *Cinnamomum cassia*
Common Name: Cinnamon
Ayurvedic Name(s): Twak
English Name: Cinnamon
Family: Lauraceae
Part Used: Inner bark
Temperature: Heating, drying
Tastes: Sweet, spicy, astringent
Dosha Effects: VK- P+

TISSUES: Plasma, blood, muscles, marrow, nerves
ACTIONS: Carminative, diaphoretic, astringent, energizer, aromatic, antibacterial, menstrual cramps (Khalsa), antihemorrhagic (Khalsa)
USES: Dysmenorrhea, nausea and vomiting, hypertension, pulmonary, gastric, intestinal, and renal bleeding; onset of cold or flu, oral candida, diabetes
CAUTIONS: Contraindicated in large doses; extended periods of time; cinnamon allergy; pregnancy large amounts can cause digestive irritation; doses over 2 g have caused convulsions, delirium hallucinations, and death (exceedingly rare)
PREPARATION AND DOSE: Powdered bark- 0.3 to1.2 g per day; oil- 0.05 to 0.2 ml; tincture- 2 to 4 ml per day (note possible discrepancies for doses of different preparations)

Cinnamon is a very mild herb that is well tolerated by a broad variety of people. It is a pungent, sweet and hot tonic. It increases general vitality, warms and energizes the body as a whole, counteracts congestion, stops diarrhea, improves digestion, relieves abdominal spasms, is antirheumatic and aids the peripheral blood circulation. [258 259 260]

An evergreen tree native to Sri Lanka and India produces cinnamon bark (*Cinnamomum verum, C. zeylanicum*).[261] For spice and medicine use, cinnamon trees are cultivated on plantations in tropical regions, including Indonesia. The outer bark is stripped, leaving the inner bark, which is the harvested spice. The strips of dried bark curl up into the familiar sticks, or "quills."

Cinnamon use dates back thousands of years. Egyptians added it to their embalming mixtures around 500 B.C. Hebrews, Greeks, and Romans utilized it as a spice, perfume, and medicine. By the seventeenth century, Europeans regarded cinnamon as a culinary spice. Nineteenth century Western doctors recommended cinnamon as a digestive remedy for stomach cramps, nausea, diarrhea and colic. Cinnamon bark is a familiar ingredient in many products-toothpaste, mouthwash, perfume, soap, lipstick, gum, nasal spray and colas.

The bark contains *cinnzelanin* and *cinnzelanol*, both known insecticides. Cinnamon is an ingredient in many herbal formulas for lice, scabies, and other skin parasites.[262]

Medicinally, cinnamon is largely known for being a muscle relaxant, so it can be employed for menstrual cramps, for which it excels.[263] Many American women have found it to be a dramatic remedy, often giving relief on the first try, after years of monthly pain.

Cinnamon is a warming herb. This property also makes it a very good choice to promote menstruation. Cinnamon enhances circulation to the uterus, so the warm relaxing blood can relieve the cramps. As you would imagine, cinnamon is often used together with other warming herbs, like ginger, for this symptom.

Cinnamon has a long reputation for killing bacteria. It may safeguard against E. coli, a bacterium that causes food-borne diseases in 10,000 to 20,000

Americans each year. Microbiologists at Kansas State University tested batches of apple juice that contained 100 times the number of bugs typically found in contaminated food. At room temperature, one teaspoon of cinnamon killed 99.5 percent of the bacteria in three days.[264] Since cinnamon is such a strong inhibitor of bacteria, add it liberally to your food while traveling to stave off food poisoning. A 2001 study found that cinnamon oil killed a wide variety of respiratory disease causing organisms.[265] Another investigation from done in Taiwan indicated that constituents from cinnamon had an "excellent inhibitory effect" on nine species of pathogenic bacteria.[266]

Cinnamon is one of the most widely used natural ingredients in oral care products. With its antibiotic, anti-viral and analgesic properties, it's tailor made for toothpaste and mouthwash.

Cinnamon bark might control blood sugar levels in diabetics. United States Department of Agriculture (USDA) scientists discovered that cinnamon reduces the amount of insulin required for glucose metabolism. The spice made fat cells much more responsive to insulin. Researchers found that the most active compound -- methylhydroxy chalcone polymer (MHCP) -- upped glucose metabolism roughly 20-fold in a laboratory assay of fat cells. A dose of 1/8 to 1/4 tsp of ground cinnamon per meal for diabetic patients may help to regulate their blood sugar levels.[267]

A recent study found that vegetarians have high blood levels of salicylic acid, the anti-inflammatory ingredient in aspirin. Scientists suggest that this may partly explain why people who eat a diet rich in fruits and vegetables generally have a lower incidence of heart disease and cancer.[268] Cinnamon has one of the highest concentrations of salicylic acid.

Cinnamaldehyde, one of the constituents, is sedative and analgesic. Eugenol, another compound in the essential oil, relieves pain. This herb excels in treating flu. It supports immune functions and cuts mucus.

For athlete's foot, the essential oil of cinnamon is quite reliable. This oil is *HOT*, though, so you need to be cautious in applying it. Dilute the essential oil with any vegetable oil, such as almond, or hand lotion, or even rubbing alcohol. Start with a 10% solution and work up to a strength that is effective. Infected toenails will often tolerate applications of pure cinnamon oil. The thin oil penetrates very well into the tissues under the nail. Apply the oil once or twice daily.

Strangely enough, cinnamon enhances the flow of blood through the body, but, paradoxically, herbalists revere it for its ability to stop excessive bleeding. Speaking of blood flow, a study of scents that would cause sexual stimulation found that the smell of baked cinnamon buns had the greatest effect on men. The odor that enhanced penile blood flow the most was, surprisingly, a combination of lavender and strong cinnamon.[269 270]

The classic patient who can benefit from cinnamon is cold, dry and frail, and often has osteoarthritis, shortness of breath and digestive problems.

Since cinnamon is common as a culinary herb, it is necessary to be a selective shopper to get good quality. You will find medicinal quality cinnamon in your health food store, herb pharmacy, or from a top quality medicinal tea manufacturer.

Clove

SCIENTIFIC NAME: *Eugenia caryophyllata*
COMMON NAME: Cloves
AYURVEDIC NAME(S): Lavanga
ENGLISH NAME: Cloves
FAMILY: Myrtaceae
PART USED: Dried flower buds
TEMPERATURE: Hot
TASTES: Pungent
DOSHA EFFECTS: VK- P+
TISSUES: Plasma, muscle, marrow, reproductive, nerve
ACTIONS: Energizer, carminative, expectorant, analgesic, aphrodisiac
USES: Colds, cough, asthma, indigestion, vomiting, toothache, laryngitis, pharyngitis, low blood pressure, impotence
CAUTIONS: Inflammatory conditions, hypertension, high Pitta
PREPARATION AND DOSE: Powder- 2.5 to 5 grams; infusion (do not boil); milk decoction[271]

Clove is an evergreen tree that grows to about 30 feet. It is native of Indonesia and the Malacca Islands. It has bright green leaves and nail-shaped rose-peach flower buds. Upon drying, the buds turn a deep red brown. These are beaten from the tree and dried. The Latin word 'Clavus' means nail shaped, referring to the bud.

Clove is an important commodity in the spice trade. It is still much used in perfumes, mulled wines and liqueurs, love potions, dental products and, stuck in an orange as pomade, an insect repellent.

Cloves are widely used medicine in Asian herbalism. They promote circulation in the lungs and the stomach. Clearly, they are warming. They treat cough, and enhance digestion. Herbalists use cloves to promote fluid flow in the lymph system.

The volatile oil is a powerful analgesic. The main chemical constituent is eugenol. Eugenol facilitates the contraction of muscle fibers. As a pain reliever it helps with muscle pain, rheumatism and arthritis. It is a very warming substance and a powerful rubefacient. Clove oil is valuable for relieving bronchitis and asthma as an inhalant. Historically, it has been used for "muscular numbness." Clove has special benefit for nerve function, which means it balances vata. It is included in Yogi Tea largely for that reason.

Clove oil is very potent oil and should be used with care. Do not use it undiluted in massage, or in baths, as it may irritate the skin and mucous membranes and can cause dermatitis. It is best avoided during pregnancy.

One of the lesser known benefits of clove oil is in combating athlete's foot and similar skin fungus.

In animal experiments, clove lowers triglycerides and blood sugar.[272]

Coleus

SCIENTIFIC NAME: *Coleus forskohlii* syn. *Plectranthus barbatus*
COMMON NAME: Patharchur
AYURVEDIC NAME(S): Coleus
ENGLISH NAME: Coleus
FAMILY: Lamiaceae
PART USED: Leaves and root
TEMPERATURE: Standardized extract- not specified
TASTES: Aromatic
DOSHA EFFECTS: Standardized extract- not specified
TISSUES: Plasma, muscle, blood, nerve
ACTIONS: Antispasmodic, heart tonic, lowers blood pressure, dilator of bronchioles and blood vessels, carminative, anti-inflammatory
USES: Asthma, bronchitis, glaucoma, congestive heart failure, improve circulation, increase blood flow to brain, relieve gas, bloating, abdominal discomfort, thyroid support, diabetes
CAUTIONS: None known
PREPARATION AND DOSE: Decoction – 15 g root to 2 cups (500 ml) water; 50 mg extract standardized to contain 18% (9mg) forskolin bid to 3 times per day.

Coleus is in the mint family. It has long been used in India, Thailand and parts of South East Asia as a pickle and spice. It is an ingredient in various minor medicine concoctions for heart disease and stomach cramps, as well as lung disorders, insomnia and convulsions.[273]

This herb did not get much attention until standardized extracts began to appear in recent years. It is really much more of a contemporary phenomenon as an herbal medicine. It contains a constituent, forskolin, which activates the enzyme adenylate cyclase, which is a turnkey compound that starts a cascade of critical events within every cell of the body.

This herb increases cyclic adenosine monophospate (cAMP) in cells. This action has far reaching application in healing.[274] Increase in cAMP results in inhibition of platelet activation and degranulation, inhibition of mast cell degranulation and histamine release, increased force of contraction of the heart muscle, relaxation of the arteries and other smooth muscles, increased insulin secretion, increased thyroid function, and increased lipolysis, all of which benefit hypertension and diabetes. Coleus is quite effective in glaucoma.

Many of these same properties make it suitable for a general cardiovascular remedy, and for hypertension and cardiomyopathy.[275]

Coleus is now being used for asthma, intestinal colic, uterine cramps and painful urination.

Extracts of coleus have been investigated for weight loss. Initial, very preliminary, reports indicate that it increases lean mass. Cyclic AMP facilitates hormonal action, and may regulate the body's thermogenic response, increasing the basic metabolic rate, upping utilization of body fat. One small, uncontrolled, human trial with 50 mg per day of forskolin reduced body weight substantially.[276] An early animal study found antiobesity effects, as well.[277]

Coriander

SCIENTIFIC NAME: *Coriandrum sativum*
COMMON NAME: Coriander, Dhania
AYURVEDIC NAME(S): Dhanyaka, Kottamalli
ENGLISH NAME: Coriander
FAMILY: Apiaceae (Umbelliferae)
PART USED: Seeds, leaves, fruit- fresh plant (cilantro, Chinese parsley)
TEMPERATURE: Cold
TASTES: Bitter, pungent
DOSHA EFFECTS: PKV=
TISSUES: Plasma, blood, muscle, cardiovascular
ACTIONS: Carminative, alterative, diaphoretic, diuretic, energizer
USES: Burning urethra, cystitis, urinary tract infection, rash, burns, urticaria, sore throat, vomiting, hay fever, allergies, indigestion
CAUTIONS: High vata with nerve tissue deficiency
PREPARATION AND DOSE: Hot or cold infusion; fresh juice of (cilantro); powder –2.5 to 5 grams

Coriander is a culinary spice that does double duty as a mild warming carminative. Ayurveda considers coriander specific for strengthening the urinary tract. Both the seeds and the leaves may be used in infusion for urinary tract infections. It also is used for stomach upset, indigestion and gas. The pungent taste and digestion aiding property is suitable for kapha. The seeds are ground into a paste and applied to skin and mouth ulcers.

Coriander is diaphoretic and diuretic. It has a mild blood sugar improving action, so it could be part of a diabetes dietetuic program. It is widely used, along with dry ginger as a folk remedy for cold and flu.

A poultice of the seed can be applied for headache or arthritic joints.

New research shows that coriander has antioxidant effects in fats.[278]

The leaf, which we call cilantro, has bitter and astringent taste. Cilantro has a cooling energy, and enhances digestion without upping pitta. Cilantro juice is used as acute medicine for allergy. It is applied to skin rashes as a wash.

Cumin

SCIENTIFIC NAME: *Cuminum cyminum*
COMMON NAME: Cumin, Jira
AYURVEDIC NAME(S): Jiraka
ENGLISH NAME: Cumin seed
FAMILY: Apiaceae (Umbelliferae)
PART USED: Seeds
TEMPERATURE: Cold
TASTES: Pungent, bitter, spicy
DOSHA EFFECTS: PKV=
TISSUES: Liver, spleen
ACTIONS: Carminative, antispasmodic, energizer
USES: Digestive weakness with accompanying gas, bloat, colic, headache, fomentation for healing painful bruises and injuries
CAUTIONS: Unknown
PREPARATION AND DOSE: Powder- 3 to 9 grams

Cumin is in the parsley family. There is great confusion and a multitude of opinions about the botany of the parsleys- the Apiaceae. This family is used by the hundreds of species around the world, for food and medicine. There are 3,000 species of Apiaceae around the world. They have been crossbred and hybridized over and over, until the species have blended almost beyond distinction. And the wild varieties often look much different from the modern culinary varieties.

Ayurveda distinguishes two varieties. Common, or green cumin, is widely available in America. It is the milder tasting and acting.

Cumin seed is an anti-gas remedy with actions very similar to fennel, coriander, dill and anise, to which it is closely related. Taken internally, it is mildly diuretic and emmenagogue, and treats hemorrhoids. It encourages lactation and reduces nausea.[279] Ayurveda considers cumin to be a particularly good antidote to pungent foods like tomato and chili.

Cumin is used in mild insomnia and the common cold. Like most Apiaceae, it kills worms.

As a poultice, it treats breast or testicles swelling. Smoked in a pipe with ghee, it relieves hiccups.

Cumin decoction is called *jaljira* (water of cumin). Drink it during hot weather to stay cool. It has very mild weight loss properties.

Black cumin (kala jira, Krishna jeeraka, Sushava) is *Bunium persicum* (previously often *Carum bulbocastanum* or *Cuminum nigrum*). It is sometimes called *shahi jeera* "Imperial cumin." Black cumin was apparently more commonly used in India before the introduction of caraway from Europe. It is typically smaller and finer than green cumin.

It has similar medicinal properties, but with a stronger, earthy, nutty taste. Do not confuse this with Black seed, sometimes called onion seed, or kalonji (*Nigella sativa*).

Cumin and caraway have different modern scientific names, but are closely related, and have similar energetic properties and tastes. Cumin and caraway (*Carum carvi*) are both called jira.

Caraway apparently originated from Central Europe to Asia. It is not completely definitive, however, that caraway is truly indigenous to Europe. It is mainly cultivated in Finland, the Netherlands, Eastern Europe and Germany today. The Latin term carum is apparently a corruption of the Greek word for cumin. *Carum carvi*, the true caraway, is found wild wild in the northern Himalayas. Its actions are essentially the same as cumion and other similar parsley family seeds.

Dandelion

SCIENTIFIC NAME: *Taraxacum officinale*
COMMON NAME: Dandelion
AYURVEDIC NAME(S): Dughdapheni
ENGLISH NAME: Dandelion
FAMILY: Asteraceae (Compositae)
PART USED: Root, leaf
TEMPERATURE: Cold
TASTES: Bitter, sweet
DOSHA EFFECTS: PK- V+
TISSUES: Plasma, blood
ACTIONS: Cholagogue (root), diuretic (leaf), antirheumatic, stomachic, choleretic, mild aperient, antitumor, mild laxative, alterative, bitter digestive
USES: Kidney and liver disorders, rheumatism, gout, abnormal blood sugar, allergies, hypertension, hypercholesterolemia, edema, skin diseases, congested lymphatics, gall stones, breast sores, breast cancer, edema, ulcers
CAUTIONS: Contact with fresh latex may cause contact dermatitis; bile obstruction, acute gall bladder infection, acute gastrointestinal inflammation, intestinal blockage
PREPARATION AND DOSE: Tincture (1:1)—2 to 8ml per day-4 times per day; decoction- 1 tsp root/cup water; infusion- 1 Tbsp leaf/cup water (note possible discrepancies for doses of different preparations)

The little dandelion is a significant herbal medicine in three of the world's largest and oldest systems of herbalism- Traditional Chinese Medicine, Ayurveda, and European. While not a standout in any of these systems, it is a respected member of the materia medica of each. Mainly it benefits the liver.[280]

The leaf is a powerful diuretic, which of course also detoxifies through the kidneys. The root, though, is the celebrated liver cleanser.

Dandelion tastes bitter, and due to its high mineral content, making it effective for conditions of pitta, such as eczema, acne, boils, and jaundice. Dandelion contains bitter glycosides, the bitter resin taraxacerin, phytosterols (including sitosterol), tannins, triterpenes, a wide variety of minerals, most notably potassium and calcium, and several vitamins, including A and C.

It's startling that dandelion is higher in nutrient content than many other foods we consume as vegetables. For example, while carrot has 11,000 I.U. of vitamin A per 100 grams, dandelion has a colossal 14,000 I.U.[281]

Dandelion has been shown, in human and animal studies, to increase bile flow, an action that benefits liver congestion, bile duct inflammation, and gallstones.

Oddly enough though, one of its best applications is largely unknown here in North America. Dandelion is a very good herb for the prevention and treatment of breast disease of various types.

Benign cysts, such as those that form in the breast, are the result of kapha dosha. They tend to accumulate in fatty tissue. Since the breast is a fatty organ, it is particularly susceptible to these cysts.[282]

Dandelion is a detoxifying herb, especially for conditions involving heat, such as an inflamed breast cyst. This herb especially promotes detoxification of the lymph system. Mammary glands are lymph tissues, so dandelion benefits in this way, too.

These qualities give dandelion the reputation in Ayurveda and Chinese medicine for being useful in breast cancer, mammary gland inflammation,[283] sore breasts, breast tumors of various types, cysts, suppressed lactation,[284] and swollen breast lymph glands. This herb is also indicated for reducing abscesses and dissipating nodules, particularly of the breast, and particularly if they are firm and hard. For these uses, dandelion is taken internally and applied externally over the nodule as a poultice.[285] Seeing as dandelion is diuretic, it also improves water retention, a frequent factor in breast tenderness.

Dandelion has been shown in research to have action against tumors.[286] One recent Chinese medicine journal article called dandelion "the main treatment in gynecological recalcitrant, difficult conditions."[287]

Fibrocystic breast disease is a common, uncomfortable disease that affects 20-40 percent of premenopausal women. This disease is thought to be due to an increased estrogen to progesterone ratio. Since the liver is the primary site for estrogen clearance, dandelion benefits this disease. The herb has also been found to possess phytosterols, the plant building blocks of hormones, but it is not known if these play a role in dandelion's benefit for breast tissue. [288] Also, it helps water retention, a common factor in breast tenderness.

So, this little lawn pest is good medicine. Women of all ages can profit from using it. Try it out.

Methods to use dandelion:

- Dandelion root in capsules – 3,000 mg per day
- Tincture – 1 tsp. per day
- Tea- ¼ oz. by dry weight of herb, brewed, per day

- Roasted dandelion root-
- brew like coffee
- mix ½ and ½ with coffee, brew

Mix with chicory root and/or burdock root- ¼ oz. of each herb, simmer for twenty minutes- take three times per day with meals

Fennel

SCIENTIFIC NAME: *Foeniculum vulgare*
COMMON NAME: Fennel
AYURVEDIC NAME(S): Sampf, Methica
ENGLISH NAME: Fennel
FAMILY: Apiaceae (Umbelliferae)
PART USED: Seed (also stem as vegetable)
TEMPERATURE: Slightly warming (disputed)
TASTES: Sweet, pungent
DOSHA EFFECTS: VPK=
TISSUES: Plasma, blood, muscle, marrow
ACTIONS: Carminative, antispasmodic, anti-inflammatory, galactagogue, stomachic, phytoestrogenic, mild expectorant, emmenagogue
USES: Flatulence and colic in adults and infants, indigestion, coughs
CAUTIONS: Pregnancy (possible), overdose of essential oil can cause nausea, vomiting, seizures, and pulmonary edema
PREPARATION AND DOSE: Tea, powder, Acute- up to 12 grams per day. Chronic- 1-2 grams per day; infusion- 1 tsp crushed seeds/cup water; 1:4 tincture-10 to 60 gtt per day-4 times per day

Khalsa would pick fennel seed as the premiere carminative in the world, especially for adults. Literally, he has never seen a case of painful gas that was not relieved by fennel seeds, provided of course, that the dose was high enough.

Fennel increases digestive fire without aggravating pitta. Fennel is a cooling spice that calms the nerves and promotes mental alertness. The temperature energetics of fennel are in dispute. Clearly, it must not be very far from neutral, if there is any variation in classification. Generally, the seeds of the parsley family are mildly warming. Carminatives are typically warming, and fennel is a prime carminative. However, some authorities maintain that fennel is slightly cooling. We could compromise and say that the digestive effects are slightly warming, and the mental effects are slightly cooling. Fennel is widely said to be the most sattvic spice.

Anise (*mishraya*) has similar properties and may often be substituted. In fact, the main ingredient in fennel is anethole.

Fennel contains creosol and alpha- pinene, substances that loosen lung mucus and help clear the chest, benefiting asthma. Recent research shows that this spice also lowers blood pressure. [289 290 291]

This herb has been used for centuries to promote lactation, which makes sense, from what we now know about its hormonal action. It will also hasten a period. As a bonus, it increases libido.

To increase the flow of mother's milk (galactagogue) fennel seed is the standout. It's beginning to show up in commercial lactation tea recipes in America.[292 293] Use this herb as a delicious tea, and increase the dose until the desired effect is achieved.

For gas, try chewing 1 tablespoon of the tasty seeds, or brew a tea with 1 tablespoon seeds in a cup of water. You may use the powdered seeds as a seasoning, or in capsules. The expectorant properties lend fennel to use in cold and flu remedies, often with raw sugar to thin mucus.

Of course, you can also steam the stalk as a delicious celery-like vegetable. The properties are similar, but milder than the seed.

Fenugreek

SCIENTIFIC NAME: *Trigonella foenum-graecum* ("Greek hay")
COMMON NAME: Fenugreek
AYURVEDIC NAME(S): Methi, Medhika
ENGLISH NAME: Fenugreek
FAMILY: Leguminosae
PART USED: Seed (also stem and greens as vegetable)
TEMPERATURE: Hot
TASTES: Bitter, pungent, sweet
DOSHA EFFECTS: VK- P+
TISSUES: Plasma, blood, marrow, reproductive
ACTIONS: Tonic, hypoglycemic, expectorant, aphrodisiac,
USES: Diabetes cough, high cholesterol
CAUTIONS: Pregnancy (phytohormone source)
PREPARATION AND DOSE: Powder or in food- up to 4 ounces, dry seed weight, per day, as desired.

An ancient herbal medicine has been showing some remarkable benefits in treating the worst health epidemic in twenty first century America- diabetes. The more we study this outstanding remedy scientifically, the more startling the benefits seem to be in many areas of health and disease.

Fenugreek seed is native to southeastern Europe, northern Africa and western Asia. This legume has become widely cultivated in other parts of the world. Fenugreek is used as a seasoning in foods, especially in Egypt, India and the Middle East. The spice has a maple smell and flavor that leads to its use as a spice in foods, beverages, confections, tobacco, and as an imitation maple syrup flavor.

The seeds may also be eaten raw or boiled, or the greens consumed fresh in salad. Some cosmetic products also contain extracts of fenugreek.

Historically, fenugreek has been for a collection of digestive complaints, including gastritis, gas and ulcers.[294] It increases the production of pancreas enzymes.[295] Studies that show the newly discovered anti-inflammatory effects make this more likely. Traditional indications for this herb include arthritis, bronchitis and fevers.[296]

It is also reputedly useful for inducing labor, as it is known to stimulate uterine contractions.

Gargling with fenugreek may relieve sore throats and sooth coughs. It is thought to be a general male reproductive tonic. With its anti-inflammatory effect this remedy has been used topically for abscesses, boils, wounds, burns, eczema, gout, and skin ulceration.

Fenugreek may stimulate a flagging appetite, as other bitter herbs traditionally do, and may be given in times of convalescence to improve food intake, weight gain and speed of recuperation.

Fenugreek seeds contain iron, vitamin A, vitamin B1, vitamin C and phosphates. The seed is also high in fiber and protein.

Cyclic terpenoids are important plant constituents are among the most significant in herbal medicines. The key cyclic terpenoids, *sapogenins* and *phytosterols*, have structures similar to plant and animal steroid hormones, accounting for their potent actions in human metabolism. The best-known sterol is cholesterol, which, despite its negative reputation, is a critical component of cell membranes, organs, the brain and the nervous system. Cholesterol is the building block for all steroid hormones, such as cortisol, estrogen, progesterone and testosterone.

Some plant sapogenins can mimic or regulate human steroid hormones or hormone precursors. A constituent, *diosgenin,* abundant in yams (*Dioscorea* spp.), can be converted into steroid hormones in the laboratory, but the body cannot convert it into steroid hormones. Fenugreek is richer in diosgenin and other saponins than yams. As a legume, it shares the trait of being rich in these plant sterols with other better-known legumes, such as alfalfa.[297 298] Traditionally, fenugreek was prescribed to increase breast milk production and breast size, so this may account for some of its ethnic uses.

The best-documented medical application for of fenugreek is blood sugar control. Studies demonstrate benefit in both insulin-dependent (type 1) and noninsulin-dependent (type 2) diabetics.[299] Doses as low as 15 g per day may bring about beneficial outcomes in fasting blood sugar, after meal blood sugar elevation, and overall glycemic control. [300 301] ccxciv Though 15 grams is a stiff dose of this bitter spice, it is actually possible to ingest this dose with a little culinary ingenuity.

Keep in mind that 100 grams fills a cereal bowl. In our clinical experience, this treatment works remarkably well for drug free blood sugar reduction, but Americans have a hard time consuming this amount. In spite of the taste, diligence pays off, though. Asian experiments often prepare the fenugreek dose in a flatbread or other such consumable.

Soluble fiber reduces cholesterol and blood sugar, so it has long been assumed that fenugreek assisted diabetes through that mechanism. In addition, new evidence supports the role of a novel compound from fenugreek. Not found in any mammal tissue, the peculiar amino acid, *4-hydroxyisoleucine*, increases insulin production.[302] Studies in rats and dogs indicate that the effect is at least in part from a direct pancreatic B cell stimulation.[303] Test tube studies demonstrate the effect in humans, also.[304]

Fenugreek reduces serum cholesterol levels, especially in diabetics. Although few studies support these indications, fenugreek saponins can lower cholesterol and other blood lipids.[305 306] The soluble fiber enhances these results.[307 308]

With their fiber and mucilage content, the seeds can act as a bulk laxative. These seed fibers swell up in contact with water, expanding the bowel contents and stimulating peristaltic activity. Fenugreek seed in capsules are sometimes recommended as a *galactagogue* to increase breast milk production.

There is some evidence that fenugreek can decrease some stone-forming substances in the kidney, particularly calcium oxalate.[309]

Recent evidence seems to indicate that fenugreek has antioxidant benefits, and that it increases enzyme activity in the liver.[310]

Very preliminary research indicates an anticancer activity.[311]

Fenugreek is available as bulk seeds, capsules, tinctures, or in tea formulas. Embittered and defatted preparations are accessible. The only familiar side effect is mild digestive distress when it is taken in high doses. Recommended doses can vary rather widely.

For topical use, powder and water are formed as a paste.

For laxative purposes, 0.5-1 tsp of freshly powdered herb, followed by additional 8 oz. of water, is used one to three times daily.

Flaxseed

SCIENTIFIC NAME: *Linum usitatissimum*
COMMON NAME: Flax
AYURVEDIC NAME(S): Uma
ENGLISH NAME: Flaxseed
FAMILY: Linaceae
PART USED: Seed
TEMPERATURE: Heating
TASTES: Sweet, astringent, pungent
DOSHA EFFECTS: V- PK+
TISSUES: Plasma, blood, muscle, bone
ACTIONS: Laxative, demulcent, emollient, expectorant, nutritive tonic
USES: Chronic bronchitis, asthma, pneumonia, chronic constipation, diarrhea, convalescence
CAUTIONS: May aggravate congestion in the colon and may not be strong enough for severe constipation
PREPARATION AND DOSE: Infusion, milk decoction, paste, powder- 2.5 to 1 gram

Flax seed is a rich source of soluble fiber, insoluble fiber and edible oil. It is a nutrition packed grain, with a dense caloric content.

Essential fatty acids (EFAs) are building blocks for hormone-like prostaglandins. Some prostaglandins are beneficial, and yet others provoke damaging responses, including inflammation. The "series-one" prostaglandin PGE prevents inflammation, reducing the symptoms of arthritis.

Fatty acids are incorporated into cartilage and bone. They make up the main structural component of all cell membranes. Your brain, nerves, retina, adrenal glands, skin and mucous membranes particularly need EFAs. In fact, your brain is made of more than 60% fats. They contribute to the level of the anti-inflammatory prostaglandins, helping to reverse the inflammatory damage caused by pitta excess.[312]

Whole, unrefined foods generally contain some EFAs. Whole grains and seeds are especially rich sources. Dietary supplement sources of EFAs include flax seed oil.

Plant estrogens, including daidzein, equol, and enterolactone, which are found in soy beans, whole wheat, berries, and flax seed, may help reduce the risk for certain hormone-stimulated cancers, such as breast and prostate, by replacing human estrogen with the benign plant estrogens they contain.

Add powdered flax seed, daily, to your diet, as necessary to create a soft, spongy stool.

Garlic

SCIENTIFIC NAME: *Allium sativa*
COMMON NAME: Garlic
AYURVEDIC NAME(S): Rasoon (lacking one taste), Lasunam
ENGLISH NAME: Garlic
FAMILY: Liliaceae
PART USED: Rhizome
TEMPERATURE: Hot, drying
TASTES: Pungent (add remainder- describe "lacks one") possesses all tastes except it lacks sour taste
DOSHA EFFECTS: VK- P+
TISSUES: Works on all tissues
ACTIONS: Antibacterial, antifungal, antiparasitic, carminative, anticoagulant, antithrombotic, hypotensive, hypocholesterolemic, antidiabetic
USES: Bacterial infection, hypertension, atherosclerosis, dysentery, diabetes, colds, flu, asthma, bronchitis
CAUTIONS: Patients with hot constitutions; acute inflammation, insomnia, dehydration, hypoglycemia, pemphigus, impending surgery (possible), organ transplants, concomitant use of anticoagulants; large amounts can inhibit iodine uptake by thyroid, may cause GI upset in sensitive individuals.

PREPARATION AND DOSE: tincture 1:1 , 120-250 drops ; fresh clove with food

In American culture, garlic is mainly known for reducing cholesterol, but it does so much more.

Overall, according to published research, garlic appears to reduce blood pressure levels by about 5 to 10%. This may not seem like much, but every bit counts when you are reducing the total chronic damage from hypertension. Clinical herbalists using garlic usually claim to see larger reductions with higher doses. Many studies have researched the effects of garlic on blood pressure.[313]

Perhaps the best of these trials looked at 47 subjects with mild hypertension. For 12 weeks, half were given placebo and the other half received a daily dose of 600 mg of garlic powder, standardized to 1.3% alliin. Garlic reduced systolic blood pressure by 6% and diastolic pressure by 9%.[314] Another study done in a Rhode Island hospital achieved a reduction of about 5.5% in systolic blood pressure.[315] Cholesterol was reduced by about 7%.

Historically, garlic has been a very popular herb in Ayurveda, where it is used to pick up sluggish digestion, care for diarrhea associated with intestinal infection, and to treat malabsorption. Strangely, Ayurveda suggests garlic for stomach ulcer. This is starting to look more reasonable, as recent test tube evidence from the Netherlands has confirmed that garlic is able to kill a bacterium associated with ulcer, Helicobacter pylori.[316]

Moreover, it is employed in asthma, ear infection, edema, and as a general stamina-enhancing tonic. Garlic substantially increases libido. Ayurveda recommends garlic for diabetes, a benefit now being born out by modern research.[317]A study from India done in 1999, for instance, showed that garlic given to diabetic mice caused a significant progressive reduction in the serum glucose levels.[318]

Modern naturopathic physicians use garlic for bronchitis, yeast infection, cough, athlete's foot and acne. A peeled clove, possibly wrapped in gauze, can be inserted as a vaginal suppository and retained overnight for vaginal yeast infection. Garlic is more potent against yeast than the popular drug, nystatin, according to modern research.[319]

Garlic supports immune function in patients with AIDS.[320 321]

Herbalists consider this herb to be a detoxifier. A 1999 study has shown that, in rats, garlic juice prevents the toxic effects of mercury on the fetus.[322] Garlic is a powerful antioxidant,[323]a characteristic that, among others, allows it to have anticancer effects.[324] Research has recently shown garlic to benefit cancerous human bladder cells.[325]

The herb affects rheumatoid arthritis, says a controlled Russian study. Of fifteen patients who received garlic, 86.5% showed good response with no side effects.[326]

Yogi Bhajan was asked about treatments for cancer. "Actually, I don't want to claim anything, but this garlic pudding has reversed somebody's irreversible cancer. That's the gift of it. I don't know what it is, I never named it. I can just tell you. Take milk and garlic and make a pudding of it. Lots of garlic! And sometimes people use a little rice. As you make rice pudding, instead of making rice pudding, make a garlic pudding with the least rice in it. And instead of sugar, they use maple syrup. That guy took it for five days to seven days, and when he went for a check up, they found it is receding. For a terminal cancer patient, yes, it is a monodiet."[327]

A relatively new modern use is the treatment of cataracts. Garlic constituents recently prevented them.[328]

Garlic is essentially a food. Two cloves per day is a common dose. Larger doses should not hurt, and you might experience better results if you are willing to include more in your diet or use a higher dose as a supplement.

Gentian

SCIENTIFIC NAME: *Gentiana lutea, G. kurroo*
COMMON NAME: Gentian
AYURVEDIC NAME(S): Kirata, Katuki, Trayamana
ENGLISH NAME: Gentian
FAMILY: Gentianaceae
PART USED: Root
TEMPERATURE: Cooling, drying
TASTES: Bitter, pungent
DOSHA EFFECTS: PK- V+
TISSUES: Plasma, blood, muscle, fat
ACTIONS: Bitter digestive, antipyretic, antibacterial, anthelmintic, alterative, laxative, gastric stimulant, peristaltic, cholagogue, anti-inflammatory
USES: Dyspepsia, gastritis, heartburn, lazy digestion, fevers, jaundice, hepatitis, enlargement of liver or spleen, genital herpes, atonic and sub-acid states
CAUTIONS: Pregnancy (possible); acute gastric inflammation and irritation; large doses for extended periods can harm digestion and induce frontal headaches
PREPARATION AND DOSE: Decoction-- ¼ tsp/cup water; 1:4 tincture- 1 to 30 gtt per day-4 times per day; bitter aperitif--30 ml; powder in capsules- 5 grams (Khalsa)

The general benefit of gentian lies in its bitter taste. Bitter taste cleanses the liver and stimulates digestive secretions. Several species may be used interchangeably.

Gentian root, an anti-inflammatory and fever remedy, form the basis of a well known European herb combination for sinus infection.[329]

Anti-inflammatories are necessary in colitis and other hot digestive conditions, and can be dramatically beneficial. These include gentian root and licorice root.

In formulas, bitter gentian may be substituted by other bitters, such as chiretta (also in the Gentian family) or kutki.

Gentian might be a bitter pill to swallow, but it is renowned for getting your digestion going.

Ginger

SCIENTIFIC NAME: *Zingiber officinale*
COMMON NAME: Ginger
AYURVEDIC NAME(S): Sunthi, Nagara (dry), Ardraka (fresh)
ENGLISH NAME: Ginger
FAMILY: Zingiberaceae
PART USED: Root (rhizome)
TEMPERATURE: Hot
TASTES: Pungent, sweet
DOSHA EFFECTS: VK- P+
TISSUES: Works on all tissues
ACTIONS: Carminative, antiflatulent, antitussive, antimicrobial, hypolipidemic, antioxidant, antiemetic, spasmolytic, antiatherosclerotic, cardiotonic
USES: Digestive disturbances involving flatulence, burping, and colic, circulatory sluggishness, motion sickness, nausea, burns (fresh juice), migraine headaches, lumbago, pyrexia
CAUTIONS: Pregnancy (large doses) (Concern in pregnancy was possible abortifacient effect, based on animal studies with extreme doses. No longer thought to be contraindicated in pregnancy.) Central Nervous System (CMS) depression and cardiac arrhythmias (animal studies only).
PREPARATION AND DOSE: Capsule, tea, juice, or in food. 500 mg per day

This herb almost needs no introduction. Called "the universal medicine,"[330] ginger is truly a medicine chest in a jar. It can be given to almost anyone, and will almost always have at least some benefit.

No one quite knows how old ginger is, as it has never been found growing in the wild. It is presumed to have originated in tropical India, but it is also an ancient part of Chinese food and medicine. As one of the important spices to open of the spice trade routes, it became popular in Europe. In fact, one of the most popular ginger uses started there. It was popular to keep a jar of ginger on the counter in 19th century English pubs so the clientele could add it to their drinks. Ginger ale was born.

This hot herb increases circulation, promotes digestion, and reduces phlegm in the lungs. Ginger is used to treat, among other diseases, colds, indigestion, arthritis, hemorrhoids, and menstrual cramps.

Ginger supports heart health and generally benefits the cardiovascular system. A recent animal study showed significant improvements in glucose, serum total cholesterol, serum alkaline phosphatase, serum triglycerides, HDL-cholesterol, VLDL-cholesterol and atherogenic index. The effects of the ginger were enhanced by the use of garlic.[331]

Tasty, aromatic ginger is a time-tested remedy for stomach upset. Ginger's effect on motion sickness and nausea has been thoroughly proven, [332] so it's not surprising that Europeans practitioners use ginger in tea for indigestion. It reduces spasm, absorbs and neutralizes toxins in the gastrointestinal tract and increases the secretion of digestive juices, including bile and saliva.[333] Ginger contains ingredients that soothe the gut and aid digestion by increasing peristalsis that moves food through the intestine.[334] A study from India demonstrated that ginger speeds up the time it takes the stomach to empty, a benefit for feelings of abdominal discomfort and bloating.[335]

A study recently reported in *Obstetrics and Gynecology* looked at seventy pregnant women with morning sickness. After using just 1 gram of dry ginger per day, for only four days, 87.5% of the ginger-takers reported improvement, compared with 28% who took a placebo.[336] Another study found that women taking ginger syrup achieved great benefit with nausea. Of the women in the ginger group, 67% who had been vomiting daily stopped vomiting within 6 days, compared to only 20% who took a placebo.[337]

European authorities at one time suggested that ginger be avoided in pregnancy on theoretical grounds, but ginger toxicity has yet been reported in humans. Considering that it has been used very effectively for millennia by pregnant women, it's probably acceptable in normal doses.[338]

Among its many uses, ginger treats diabetes, lowering blood sugar and treats closely related cardiovascular conditions. Ginger lowers blood fats, including triglycerides, reduces oxidation of LDL and prevents arterial plaque.[339] [340] [341] Published research found that a higher dose of ginger (500 mg/kg, about an ounce for an average adult) produced a significant lowering of blood cholesterol.[342]

Compounds in ginger have shown benefit in the prevention of cancer.[343] [344] [345]

Widely used for arthritis, especially osteoarthritis, in Asian herbalism, ginger is especially appropriate for cold, non-lubricated joints. There is some preliminary scientific information on ginger for this purpose.[346] [347] Traditional herbalists use it for promoting menstruation and relieving menstrual cramps. Ginger increases peripheral circulation, so is used clinically for cold hands and feet. Being diaphoretic, it treats cold and flu.

In our personal experience, ginger works well for carpal tunnel wrist pain. Slice the fresh roots lengthwise in thin, flat strips. Wrap the wrist with the strips, cover with a bandage and leave overnight. Norma Pasekoff Weinberg, in *Natural and Herbal Remedies for Carpal Tunnel Syndrome*, recommends a compress made from cooked, fresh grated ginger.[348]

Asian medicine uses ginger for migraine.[349] In my (Khalsa's) observation, **ginger** is absolutely the best thing for treating a migraine at the time that it develops, one of the few things that will work at the time. Stir two tablespoons of ginger powder into water and drink it at the onset of visual disturbances- the "aura"- before the pain starts. Usually that will knock it cold. The migraine may try to restart in about four hours, in which case you have to do this again.

Fresh ginger root is tan and knobby, with a thick skin. Good quality pieces are firm and plump, with an unwrinkled, smooth skin. Ginger is a multipurpose spice, equally delicious in both sweet and savory dishes.[350] This spice has a somewhat biting and hot note, with a rich, sweet, warm, and woody aroma.[351]

Use ginger fresh, as dried powder or "crystallized" with sugar. Use it in gingerbread, ginger ale, gingersnaps, and Indian or Chinese dishes. Try ginger chunks in a stir fry, or mixed in honey or with a little molasses as a glaze, perhaps for carrots.[352] Even add fresh juice to a fresh juice mix, perhaps apple, to add some snap. In my home, my family likes to dice peeled fresh ginger root, sauté it until crunchy, and use the crispy bits as a condiment. Prepared this way, ginger will last about a week in the refrigerator. Herbs and spices are typically not significant sources of nutrients in the diet, but ginger has relatively high calcium and iron content.[353]

Ginger is very safe, so consume it as desired in food, or use up to 3 grams per day in capsules. Use 1 tsp. chopped fresh root, brewed as tea, 3 times a day.

Gokshura

Scientific Name: *Tribulis terrestris*
Common Name: Gokshura, Gokharu
Ayurvedic Name(s): Gokshura, Shvadamstra
English Name: Caltrops, Puncture vine
Family: Zygophyllaceae
Part Used: Fruit
Temperature: Cooling
Tastes: Sweet, bitter
Dosha Effects: VPK=
Tissues: Plasma, blood, marrow, nerve, reproductive
Actions: Tonic, diuretic, lithotriptic, aphrodisiac, nervine, analgesic
Uses: Difficult or painful urination, edema, chronic cystitis, nephritis, kidney or bladder stones, gout, rheumatism, sciatica, impotence, infertility, venereal diseases, cough, dyspnea, hemorrhoids, diabetes
Cautions: Dehydation
Preparation and dose: Decoction, medicated oil, milk decoction, powder- 3 to 9 grams per day

This well known Ayurvedic herb is standout for sexual building. It has a particular affinity for the urogenital tract. The name literally means "cow scratcher," a reference to its fruit (a prickly seed case).

Gokshura is highly esteemed as a vajikarana and rasayana medicine. It is sweet and cold, so it is appropriate for pitta conditions. As a tonic, it balances vata.

Gokshura is an exceptional remedy in urogenital conditions. It promotes urine flow and soothes the membranes. It pacifies vata and will not promote secondary excess dryness, as other diuretics do. Gokshura is renowned for prostate support. The plant and seeds are used in the treatment of spermatorrhea, impotence, dysuria, gonorrhea, incontinence, gout and infertility.

This herb is sometimes combined with guggul, triphala and trikatu in a traditional Ayurvedic tridoshic compound formula called gokshuradi guggul, used to support the proper function of the genitourinary tract.

Gokshura is also used in cough and asthma.

The seed pod is cardioactive. It dilates the coronary artery and improves coronary circulation, as well as lowering blood pressure.[354]

Gokshura is also highly esteemed as a vajikarana. It is a common ingredient in aphrodisiac formulas. One contemporary product combines 22 other multipurpose herbs, many of which actually are herbs with targeted aphrodisiac effects, including saffron, shankpushpi, jyotishmati, jatamansi, ashwaganda and nutmeg.[355] Animal studies confirm the effect of increasing sexual functions.[356] In the treatment of spermatorrhea and impotence, equal parts of gokshura, sesame seed, kapikachu and ashwaganda may be consumed with honey, ghee and goat's milk, 3 grams total, on an empty stomach, twice daily.

One proprietary combination for premature ejaculation includes the herbs gokshura, shatavari, trikatu, ashwaganda, and musali, along with an assortment of minor ingredients.

Gokshura promotes mental clarity, and in fact, Khalsa recommends it for its exceptional clinical effect in depression. This herb contains harmine alkaloids, which may explain its sedative properties. It may be taken with ashwaganda as a tonic nervine in nervous disorders.

Guduchi

SCIENTIFIC NAME: *Tinospora cordifolia*
COMMON NAME: Guduchi, Gilo
AYURVEDIC NAME(S): Guduchi, Amrita, Ambrosia
ENGLISH NAME: Amrit, Heart-leaved Moonseed
FAMILY: Menispermaceae
PART USED: Stem (mainly) and root, powdered bitter starchy extract
TEMPERATURE: Hot
TASTES: Bitter, astringent, sweet
DOSHA EFFECTS: VPK=
TISSUES: Blood, fat, reproductive
ACTIONS: Bitter digestive, febrifuge, diuretic, aphrodisiac, rejuvenative
USES: Fever, malaria, convalescence from febrile diseases, hyperacidity, hepatitis, jaundice, diabetes, heart disease, arthritis, hemorrhoids, gout, skin disease, tuberculosis
CAUTIONS: Use with care during pregnancy
PREPARATION AND DOSE: Powder- 3-10 grams per day

Guduchi is a viney plant from the Moonseed (Menispermaceae) family. It is often found climbing neem trees throughout tropical India and Southeast Asia.

As medicine, it has a broad spectrum antimicrobial and immunostimulating activity. It is a source of berberine. This herb is primarily used in acute infection, at rather high dose, but also sees some application in chronic immune support.

It is said by some to be the best herb for clearing the srotas. It is a potent, yet well tolerated, detoxifier that is found in many Ayurvedic formulas. Because of this ability, it is included in formulas to assist the delivery of herbs to the tissues. Guduchi aids all aspects of healthy metabolism (the 13 agnis). It particularly clears the srotas in the brain, facilitating mental activity (medhya rasayana). It supports proper function of shleshaka kapha, so it also aids proper communication and coordination between all the various cells and their many related functions, promoting better overall health.

Guduchi balances and purifies fat tissue and assists in the breakdown of fat. According to Ayurvedic philosophy, fat is an important raw material for building healthy bones.

Yogi Bhajan was fond of this medicine and often recommended it for acute respiratory infection.

Tridoshic guduchi is commonly used for fevers, infectious skin diseases, tuberculosis, bronchitis, syphilis, cancers and malaria. Researchers have confirmed the antipyretic activity of guduchi.[357] Bitter herbs with hot temperature are rare. This combination of energetics is specific for detoxification while still promoting circulation of the body's fluids.

As a bitter, it finds application for gastrointestinal disturbances. Its detoxifying nature lends it to uses in ama inflammatory conditions, such as rheumatoid arthritis, hepatitis and jaundice.

Other uses include impotence, spermatorrhea, and general debility. One herbal combination for BPH includes guduchi, along with shilajit, purified zinc mineral ash, kachnar, turmeric, punarnava, sandalwood and sarsaparilla.

Guduchi directly nourishes the hair for better quality and strength (Keshya effect).

The juice is diuretic and a snakebite antidote.

Guduchi lowers blood sugar, so shows promise in treating diabetes.[358] It is also prepared as a sedimented extract that is predominantly starchy in nature (guduchi satwa, gulwelsatva or Indian quinine). The satwa is produced by crushing the stems and roots in water, removing the fibrous material and decanting, followed by sun drying the sediment.[359] It treats chronic dysentery, fever, headache, urinary diseases and malabsorption.[360]

Guggul

SCIENTIFIC NAME: *Commiphora mukul*
COMMON NAME: Guggul
AYURVEDIC NAME(S): Guggulu
ENGLISH NAME: Indian Bedellium
FAMILY: Burseaceae
PART USED: Resin
TEMPERATURE: Heating
TASTES: Bitter, pungent, astringent, sweet
DOSHA EFFECTS: KV- P+ (in excess)
TISSUES: Works on all tissues
ACTIONS: Soth har (anti-inflammatory), vedana sthapak (pain killer or analgesic), medohar (reduces weight), rasayana (rejuvenation), hridhya (heart tonic), energizer, rejuvenative, alterative, nervine, antispasmodic, analgesic, astringent, antiseptic, expectorant
USES: Arthritis, rheumatism, gout, nervous disorders, diabetes, obesity, bronchitis, whopping cough, hemorrhoids, skin disease, sore/ulcers, cystitis, endometritis, tumors
CAUTIONS: Acute kidney infection, acute stage of rashes
Preparation and dose: Pill, paste, powder- 250 to 500 mg

Guggul scrapes the channels. It is a powerful, deep acting detoxifier. It treats cold and congealing kapha and vata disorders. These qualities lend it to uses with other herbs in the treatment of skin diseases and arthritis, especially amavata (osteoarthritis) and gout.

Secondarily, it is used for nerve pain, obesity, digestive insufficiency, oral infections and menstrual problems.

This resin is a standby for the management of lipids. Particularly valuable in lowering cholesterol, guggul rivals any natural substance. Without dietary adjustments, guggul has lowered total cholesterol by over 20 percent, while increasing good HDL cholesterol by 36 percent.[361] It also sees use in coronary thrombosis.

Jeff Pyatt, now 44, is an associate of Khalsa's. Says Pyatt, "I've really appreciated having access to this approach. It's helped in so many ways. My father died of heart disease at 42, and a while back a test showed that my cholesterol, which has always been low, had jumped to 214, with the HDL down. The doctor said not to worry, but I learned about the Ayurvedic herb guggul from K.P., and began to use that. When I saw my doctor again 6 months later, my total cholesterol was back down to 150 and my HDL was up. The doctor was amazed."

"The results I got were phenomenal. I tell everybody I talk to about the great effect." says Guruchander Singh Khalsa, D.C., of Espanola, N.M. (no relation).

Dr. Khalsa, a successful chiropractic physician, has had total cholesterol numbers of over 300 for 20 years. He comes from a family with genetically high cholesterol. On his mother's side, one brother died at age 42 of a massive heart attack, and all the remaining siblings have had quadruple bypass surgery, along with heart attacks. Dr. Khalsa has managed to avoid serious disease with diet and yoga, but the cholesterol numbers were becoming seriously worrisome. His thyroid function was depressed, as well, with the thyroid stimulating hormone reading at triple the normal value. After a bit of professional consultation, we settled on having him try guggul gum at 6 grams per day, to quickly lower blood fats, and a combination of gotu kola leaf, saw palmetto berry, scullcap leaf, elder berry, and willow bark, to increase thyroid function. Four months later, the cholesterol had dropped a whopping 180 points, and the thyroid blood test was exactly normal.

Like its effect on blood lipids, guggul can assist in managing overall body fat. Guggul (*Commiphora mukul*) seems to exert its effect at least partially through the thyroid, which could account for its fat loss benefit.[362 363 364]

The combination of guggul and triphala recently showed a surprising effect in controlling body fat. When 48 obese subjects took these Ayurvedic combinations three times a day for three months, with no attempt to control their food intake, the resulting weight loss averaged almost 18 pounds, along with a drop in total cholesterol of 18 points. The dose used in the study was only 500 mg of the combination, three times per day. [365]

Another placebo-controlled study combined guggul extract with *Garcinia cambogia* extract and tyrosine. Over six weeks, twenty obese persons had a significant decrease in body fat mass and average body weight. The subjects lost body fat, but not lean mass. Fatigue went down, and there were no adverse effects.[366]

Guggul can be taken in a dose of 1,500 mg, three times daily.

Gurmar

Scientific Name: *Gymnema sylvestre*
Common Name: Gurmar
Ayurvedic Name(s): Meshasringi, Shardunika, Madhunashini
English Name: Gurmar
Family: Asclepiadaceae
Part Used: Leaves
Temperature: Heating
Tastes: Astringent, pungent
Dosha Effects: K- VP=
Tissues: Blood, plasma
Actions: Digestive stimulant, diuretic, astringent
Uses: Diabetes, obesity, hypoglycemia, kidney stones, enlargement of liver and spleen
Cautions: None known

PREPARATION AND DOSE: Powder - 1 gram to 5 grams per day

An exciting herb, gurmar leaf, well known in Ayurvedic medicine, is just beginning to get serious attention here. It is particularly appropriate for American audiences, because it represents a serious chance of treating diabetes, which is increasing in epidemic proportions in the U.S.

Gymnema sylvestre is a woody climbing plant that grows in the tropical forests of central and southern India. The leaves, when chewed, interfere with the ability to taste sweetness, which explains the Hindi name, gurmar, "destroyer of sugar." Gurmar disables the tongue's ability to taste sweet taste for about 4 hours when a leaf or a pinch of powder is chewed.

Gurmar carries astringent and pungent tastes, with a net heating effect. It is balances Kapha and essentially neutral to pitta and vata.

Gymnema certainly could be the backbone of a natural diabetes program. This herb has been used in India for the treatment of diabetes (madhu meha, or "honey urine") for over 2,000 years. Used primarily for adult-onset diabetes (NIDDM), it continues to be recommended today in India.

Gurmar leaves raise insulin levels, when administered to healthy volunteers.[367] The leaves are also noted for lowering serum cholesterol and triglycerides.[368] Gurmar tends to be a blood sugar normalizer, lowering glucose significantly only in hyperglycemic people. It significantly improves cholesterol and triglyceride levels, as well. It is not yet clear what specific constituent in the leaves is responsible for sugar and blood fat lowering action. Some researchers have suggested gymnemic acid as one possible candidate.

Traditionally, 6-12 grams of the powdered leaf per day is used.[369] Studies recently performed in India have used 400 mg per day of an extract of the gymnema leaves. In adult-onset diabetics, ongoing use for periods as long as eighteen to twenty-four months has been successful.[370] In juvenile onset diabetic patients, a similar amount has been used as an adjunct to ongoing use of insulin.

In one recent study at the University of Madras, gurmar showed the potential for pancreas repair, raising the output of insulin to normal levels.[371] Another Indian study reported that 25% of the participants were able to discontinue all diabetes medication with the use of gurmar alone.[372]

Gymnema's antidiabetic action appears to be due to a combination of mechanisms. Two animal studies with diabetic rats indicate that Gymnema extracts doubled the number of insulin-secreting beta cells in the pancreas and returned blood sugars to almost normal.[373 374] Gymnema upgrades the activity of enzymes responsible for glucose uptake and utilization and suppresses peripheral utilization of glucose by somatotrophin and corticotrophin. Plant extracts have also been found to inhibit epinephrine-induced hyperglycemia.

In addition, gurmar has also been used in the treatment of upper respiratory infections and fevers. Applied topically to the skin, a paste of gurmar draws out infections.

Khalsa's experience shows that gurmar will reduce sugar cravings over the long haul if taken daily. Use it in capsules- it's extremely bitter. This precludes the sugar numbing capability, but few real world patients are inclined toward that, anyway.

The typical therapeutic dose of an extract, standardized to contain 24-percent gymnemic acids, is 400-600 mg daily, but very broad variations exist. It is better to start with a very small amount and titrate the dose, based on blood sugar monitoring.

Haritaki

SCIENTIFIC NAME: *Terminalia chebula*
COMMON NAME: Haritaki
AYURVEDIC NAME(S): Haritaki, Abhaya
ENGLISH NAME: Chebulic Myrobalan
FAMILY: Combretaceae
PART USED: Fruit
TEMPERATURE: Heating
TASTES: All tastes but salty, but especially astringent and sweet
DOSHA EFFECTS: VPK=
TISSUES: Works on all tissues
ACTIONS: Tonic, astringent, laxative, nervine, expectorant, anthelmintic, rejuvenative
USES: Cough, asthma, hoarse voice, vomiting, hemorrhoids, malabsorption, diarrhea, abdominal distention, parasitic infection, jaundice, spleen disease, tumors, heart disease, itching, edema, nervous disorders
CAUTIONS: Pregnancy, dehydration, severe emaciation or exhaustion, in excess high Pitta
PREPARATION AND DOSE: Decoction, powder- 250 to 500 mg

Haritaki fruit comes from a medium to large-sized tree distributed throughout tropical and sub tropical Asia, including China and Tibet. Found growing wild in the forests of Northern India, Uttar Pradesh and Bengal, and is also common in Tamil Nadu, Karnataka, and in Southern Maharashtra. The dried fruit was also known as the black myrobalan of ancient commerce. At one time, it was exported to Europe for the production of ink.

Ripe haritaki fruits are harvested during the autumn season, to assure the strongest medicinal and laxative effect. Tediously drying the fruit properly in the sun reduces the laxative effect slightly. Cooking or steaming, which is more efficient than drying, reduces it even further, due to oxidation of the laxative constituents.

Named after the Hindu god Hara (Shiva), it brings fearlessness in the face of death and disease, and purifies the mind of its attachments.

Haritaki contains every taste except salty, and has a warming energy. It is a rasayana for vata, but balances all three doshas. Haritaki is the best single herb for generally controlling vata, and is considered by some to be the single most important Ayurvedic herb. Widely used in Tibetan medicine, it is called the "king of herbs" there. Since vata promotes constipation, the gentle laxative qualities of haritaki are perfect for balancing that dosha. The vipak of haritaki fruit is very strongly sweet, making it an excellent choice as a laxative in weak or elderly patients. It nourishes the brain and nerves.

Haritaki enhances digestion and is a medhya treatment that sharpens the senses. It displays alterative, astringent, expectorant, anti-inflammatory, anodyne, cardiotonic, laxative, antiseptic, and antiemetic properties.

It is strongly astringent, contracting tissues, and is therefore used for various ulcers, prolapses, and fluid discharges.

Haritaki fruit contains anthraquinone laxative constituents, as well as astringent tannins.[375] To bring out these opposing actions of these constituents, physicians administer the powder with warm water to strengthen the laxative action, or with ice-cold water to promote the astringent action. A decoction of the dried crushed fruits is highly astringent and an effective, albeit, traditional remedy for diarrhea.

Haritaki's astringent and antimicrobial properties also make it an effective tooth powder or mouthwash in periodontal disease, or even for daily use.[376]

Haritaki is called "the mother," and is thought to increase mental/spiritual awareness. It is given to children upon the premature loss of a parent.

According to recent scientific reports, haritaki prevents cancer[377] and helps wounds heal faster.[378]

Hibiscus

Scientific Name: *Hibiscus rosa-sinensis*
Common Name: Hibiscus
Ayurvedic Name(s): Japa
English Name: Hibiscus
Family: Malvaceae
Part Used: Flower
Temperature: Cooling
Tastes: Astringent, sweet
Dosha Effects: PK- V+
Tissues: Blood, plasma, muscles, marrow, nerve, reproductive
Actions: Alterative, hemostatic, emmenagogue, demulcent, antispasmodic, refrigerant
Uses: Dysmenorrhea, menorrhagia, painful urination, cystitis, cough, toxins in blood, venereal disease, fever
Cautions: Severe chills, high vata
Preparation and dose: Beverage tea, infusion hot or cold, powder- 250 to 1 gram

The name for this beautiful deep red herb is *japa*, because it strengthens devotion in meditation with a mantra (japa). Hibiscus flowers are used to destroy all life obstacles, spiritual and material, and to assist in realization of all goals. They are said to purify the physical and spiritual heart, and to promote wisdom.

A cooling herb, it makes a good beverage for reducing the effects of summer heat and for treating fever. It is astringent and sweet.

In the body, hibiscus is a blood cleanser, and is generally beneficial for kidneys and reproduction (first and second chakra disorders), especially those due to heat and congestion. Japa flowers nourish the skin and hair.

Hibiscus has detoxifying actions in the body. It is used to improve the complexion and to enhance normal hair growth. Ayurvedic practitioners use it to normalize menstruation.

Ayurveda says that hibiscus flower increases devotion, promotes wisdom and aids in meditation. It purifies the heart.

For the physical heart, hibiscus normalizes blood pressure. Several scientific studies, including a 2003 study in the *Journal of Ethnopharmacology*, found that a tea of hibiscus flower benefited blood pressure and had a protective effect on the heart.[379 380 381]

A growing collection of recent research shows that hibiscus protects against liver damage. New research is also underscoring the possibility of hibiscus in normalizing blood sugar.

Brew a delicious tea and drink throughout the day as desired.

Jambul

Scientific Name: *Syzygium cumini; Eugenia jambolanum*
Common Name: Jambul
Ayurvedic Name(s): Jamun
English Name: Jambul
Family: Myrtaceae
Part Used: Fruits, seeds
Temperature: Neutral
Tastes: Bitter, astringent
Dosha Effects: KP- V+
Tissues: Spleen, stomach
Actions: Astringent, carminative, antidiabetic
Uses: Diabetes, diarrhea, colic
Cautions: None known
Preparation and dose: 0.3 to 2 grams of dried fruit 3 times daily

This native of India now grows throughout the tropics. Jambul is also called jamun, rose apple, or java plum.

It is a tasty fruit that is eaten as food.[382] Mature fruits are eaten raw and made into tarts, sauces and jam. Their juice is much like grape juice Astringent fruits are pickled in brine.

Jambul fruit, or seeds alone, is used in Ayurvedic medicine as one of the most powerful hypoglycemic herbs.[383] Doses of as little as one gram of powdered dry herb per day can be effective. Jambul is thought to be particularly synergistic with okra. Sri Chakravarti explicitly recommends this combination, mentioning that you should be able to see large blood sugar reductions in ten days.[384]

The juicy fruit-pulp contains astringent gallic acid and tannins. The astringency is used for medicinal effect. Powdered jambul seeds, leaf juice and fruit jam treat diarrhea. Their astringency is used to control bedwetting, at a dose of one teaspoon at bedtime, and excessive bleeding. The fruit is eaten with salt or honey for hemorrhoids.

The leaves kill bacteria. A paste of leaves is applied to wounds.

The bark is a sweet and sour diuretic, digestive and antiparasitic for worms.[385]

Juniper

SCIENTIFIC NAME: *Juniperus spp.*
COMMON NAME: Juniper
AYURVEDIC NAME(S): Hapusha
ENGLISH NAME: Juniper berries
FAMILY: Coniferae
PART USED: Berries
TEMPERATURE: Hot
TASTES: Pungent, bitter, sweet
DOSHA EFFECTS: KV- P+
TISSUES: Blood, plasma, muscle, fat, bone, marrow, nerves
ACTIONS: Diuretic, diaphoretic, energizer, analgesic, disinfectant, bactericidal, carminative
USES: Edema, dropsy, sciatica, lumbago, rheumatism, swollen joints, diabetes, arthritis, weak digestion, dysmenorrhea, weakened immune system
CAUTIONS: Acute nephritis, cystitis, pregnancy
PREPARATION AND DOSE: Infusion, paste, powder- 250 to 500 mg

Juniper has analgesic actions, and increases circulation to joints, so it seen as a rheumatic remedy. Herbalists use juniper as a respiratory remedy. In addition, it treats cystitis and similar urinary complaints.

The berry of the juniper tree is one of the best diuretics in Western herbalism. It also provokes sweating (diaphoretic), for which it is particularly good for vata.

Recent scientific information shows that juniper prevents liver injury.[386]

Juniper infused oil is appropriate for kapha massage.

Kalmegh

SCIENTIFIC NAME: *Andrographis paniculata*
COMMON NAME: Kalmegh
AYURVEDIC NAME(S): Bhuinimb, Kirata, Mahateet
ENGLISH NAME: Creat, Green Chirayta, King of bitters
FAMILY: Acanthaceae
PART USED: Leaf and root
TEMPERATURE: Cooling
TASTES: Bitter, acrid
DOSHA EFFECTS: PK-V+
TISSUES: Plasma, blood, muscle
ACTIONS: Laxative, vulnerary, antipyretic, antiperiodic, anti-inflammatory, expectorant, depurative, soporific, anthelmintic, antibacterial, hepatoprotective
USES: Hyperdispsia, burning sensation, wounds, ulcers, chronic fever, malarial and intermittent fevers, inflammations, cough, bronchitis, skin diseases, leprosy, colic, flatulence, diarrhea, dysentery, hemorrhoids
CAUTIONS: High doses may cause anorexia, emesis, and gastric discomfort; pregnancy
PREPARATION AND DOSE: 1.5-6 g/day dried herb ; 3-12 mL/day of 1:2 fluid extract

This herb is a very widely used medicine in both Ayurveda and Chinese medicine. It is a wild annual shrub from the plains of Asia that is also cultivated in the gardens of North India. It's been a household remedy in Asia for many centuries. In Ayurveda, which calls it "kalmegh" ("king of the bitters"), it is used for upper respiratory infection (flu, bronchitis). Chinese medicine utilizes Andrographis for fever and headache of colds and flu, tonsillitis, larynopharyngitis, bronchitis and inflammation. Andrographis has been used for more than 12 years in Scandinavia for reducing the symptoms and duration of colds.

This herb has been widely studied by scientists, with dozens of studies in the literature. Historically, this medicine has also been used as a digestive aid, gallbladder remedy and treatment for fever and worms. The bulk of the evidence points to its traditional actions as an immune booster, but Andrographis has been studied for male birth control, diabetes, cardiovascular benefit and as an antioxidant. The most significant action seems to be as a hepatoprotectant.

A study from Chile showed very great benefit for people with colds. A group of 158 people took Andrographis and measured their symptoms of headache, tiredness, earache, sleeplessness, sore throat, nasal secretion, phlegm, frequency and intensity of cough. At day 4, a significant decrease in the intensity of all symptoms was observed for the Andrographis paniculata group.[387]

A double blind placebo controlled study performed in Sweden treated 50 patients in the early stages of a cold with an herbal preparation containing 85 mg of Andrographis paniculata extract three times daily. After five days, 68 percent reported complete recovery, compared to only 36 percent of the controls. In the treated group, 55 percent called their colds unusually mild. These patients also took less sick leave from work.[388]

Based on the historical and scientific evidence for kalmegh's effect on the immune system, it seems like this herb might have some benefit for HIV. A test tube study from The University of California at Davis found that a compound, dehydroandrographolide succinic acid monoester (DASM), made from Andrographis, inhibited HIV.[389]

An initial study was undertaken to investigate this possibility. Researchers from Bastyr University in Seattle, Washington gave the herb to HIV infected patients. Andrographis produced a significant rise in the mean CD4(+) lymphocyte level in their blood, a sign of increased immune function.[390]

The main constituent responsible for these actions seems to be andrographolide, a bitter diterpenoid lactone. This compound and similar related structures have cooling (antipyretic) and anti-inflammatory effects.

Andrographis is sometimes now being manufactured in a combination with the immune enhancing echinacea, lemon balm, slippery elm bark, cinnamon bark and Chinese frittillaria bulb.

Kapi Kachu

Scientific Name: *Mucuna pruriens*
Common Name: Kapikacchu
Ayurvedic Name(s): Atmagupta, Vanari
English Name: Velvet bean
Family: Fabaceae
Part Used: Seed
Temperature: Warm
Tastes: Bitter, sweet
Dosha Effects: KV- P=
Tissues: Reproductive, nerve
Actions: Tonic, aphrodisiac, astringent, rejuvenative
Uses: General debility, sexual debility, infertility, asthma, nervous debility, paralysis, Parkinson's disease, leucorrhea, spermatorrhea
Cautions: Menstrual bleeding, menorrhagia
Preparation and dose: Milk decoctions, confections, powder- 250 mg to 1 gram

Kapi kachu is one of the popular medicinals of India. It is a constituent of more than 200 indigenous herb formulations. All parts of kapi kachu posses valuable medicinal properties. After the discovery that the seeds contain l-dopa, a Parkinson's disease drug, its demand increased many fold and demand has motivated Indian farmers to start commercial cultivation.

The roots are bitter, warming, anthelmintic, diuretic, aphrodisiac, purgative, febrifuge and tonic. It is useful to relieve constipation, dysmenorrhea, neuropathy ulcers and fever.

Kapi kachu has recently been getting attention for increasing libido, for which it works well for some people.

Kokum

Scientific Name: *Garcinia cambogia*
Common Name: Garcinia
Ayurvedic Name(s): Kokum
English Name: Garcinia
Family: Guttiferae
Part Used: Root, fruit
Temperature: Cooling
Tastes: Pungent, bitter
Dosha Effects: PK- V+
Tissues: Fat, nerve
Actions: Sedative, antispasmodic, cholagogue, cooling, demulcent, emollient, antiseptic
Uses: Obesity, anxiety, nerve pain, muscle spasms, insomnia
Cautions: High vata conditions
Preparation and dose: Extract, powder- 250 to 500 mg

Malabar tamarind (*Garcinia cambogia*) is a small fruit that grows in South Asia, where the fruit is called "kokum." Though used in native cuisine to prepare sour condiments, this herb has only recently drawn the attention of modern researchers as a fat-loss remedy.[391]

Garcinia is a medium to large evergreen tree. The fruit resembles a small yellow or reddish pumpkin, with a distinctive sweet, acidic taste. When completely ripe, it is too sour to eat fresh. It contains 16-30% hydroxycitric acid by dry weight, along with other fruit acids. Sprinkled over food, or dried and used in curries, it is used as a spice as one would use limes or tamarinds. With kokum, the food is said to be more "filling and satisfying."

Traditionally, a tea of the fruit rind is given in rheumatism and bowel complaints. In the Ayurvedic system of medicine, sour flavor is said to activate digestion. Kokum fruits are used as purgatives, in the treatment of worms and parasites, tumors and dysentery.

Another noteworthy common use of Garcinia is for food preservation. "Colombo curing" of perishable foods is a commercial enterprise typical of South India, which makes use of the antibacterial qualities of the acid in the fruits.

The oil is used as an emollient.

Hydroxycitric acid

The rind of Garcinia contains hydroxycitric acid (HCA), which promises to be a dramatic addition to the field with an impressive array of benefits. When extracted from the fruit, HCA increases energy, lowers appetite, and inhibits the conversion of sugars in to fat, and it does all this without stimulating the central nervous system, according to Terry Willard, Ph.D.[392]

While human scientific studies done with HCA are relatively recent, animal studies look very promising. HCA is widely available in health food stores, and practitioners report good clinical success.

HCA inhibits the creation of fat, lowers the production of cholesterol and fatty acids, increases the production of glycogen in the liver, suppresses appetite and increases the body's production of heat by activating the process of thermogenesis.

Significant research has been done on the effects of the purified active ingredient, HCA. In its sodium salt form, is considerably more powerful than the crude fruit powder. Calcium salts of HCA are also used. HCA has been shown in animal experiments to suppress appetite and to reduce the formation of fats and cholesterol in the liver. In addition, it pulls LDL cholesterol out of circulation. Furthermore, there is an increase in glycogen production, which may be the cause of the perceived energy increase people experience when they take HCA. Fortunately, HCA does not speed up metabolism. In animal studies, HCA retained its full effectiveness in reducing food intake for one month of sustained use. It's not known just how HCA reduces appetite.

HCA does not prevent hunger, but causes early satiation, and therefore the early and more satisfying conclusion of meals. The desire for sweets also is diminished. Unlike caffeine and other energizing weight loss products, HCA is not a stimulant, although some users report improved energy levels.

A placebo-controlled study from 1999 combined guggul gum extract (another Ayurvedic herb) with *Garcinia cambogia* extract and tyrosine. Over six weeks, twenty obese persons had a significant decrease in body fat mass and average body weight. The subjects lost body fat, but not lean mass. People had more energy, and there were no adverse effects.

High-fat diets (more than 30% of calories from fats) and high levels of alcohol consumption may interfere with the effects of HCA. Additional fluid and fiber intake. along with moderate exercise, should improve its effects. For some people, HCA may have a "loading period" of several days before it reaches full benefit.

Kokum has been used safely as a food for centuries in many areas of tropical Asia. They continue to be consumed in large amounts. Neither acute nor chronic toxicity is reported with regular consumption of Garcinia products as either food or tonics. The scientific study of its action finds that it is extremely safe.

Willard suggests a dose of 500 to 1,000 mg of HCA, three times daily. More recent research suggests that doses of up to 6,000 mg per day may be more effective. Some users may do better with even higher doses.

Kutaj

Scientific Name: *Holarrhena antidysenterica*
Common Name: Kutaj, C
Ayurvedic Name(s): Kutaja
English Name: Kurchi, Coneru, Tellicherry bark
Family: Apocynaceae
Part Used: Bark, root, seed
Temperature: Cold
Tastes: Bitter, astringent, pungent
Dosha Effects: PK-V+
Tissues: Blood, muscle
Actions: Astringent, anthelmintic, amoebicidal
Uses: Colitis, parasites, malabsorption, hemorrhoids, menorrhagia, both acute and chronic diarrhea and dysentery
Cautions: Constipation, vertigo, sleeplessness, agitation, anxiety in very high doses
Preparation and dose: Decoction, herbal wine, powder- 2-6 grams per day

Kutaj is an effective remedy for amoeba infection and the accompanying diarrhea.[393 394]

Amoeba infection is very serious, and can be life threatening. It is common in the tropics, and travelers sometimes become infected from unclean water. Modern antiamoeba drugs are quite effective, but have very serious side effects. People taking these drugs are often quite uncomfortable, experiencing nausea and fever.

Treating such a serious infection with natural medicines is a personal choice. We encourage you to act responsibly.

Kutaj is astringent, so it will also treat non-amoeba diarrhea and hemorrhoids, but there might be more effective astringents available.

It kills other bugs, too, as well as worms. Animal studies show that alkaloids from kutaj rediuces diarrhea and kills E.coli.[395] Test tube science finds effect against Staph, as well.[396]

Kutki

Scientific Name: *Picrorrhiza kurroa*
Common Name: Katuka
Ayurvedic Name(s): Katuka
English Name: Kutki
Family: Scrofulariaceae
Part Used: Root
Temperature: Cold
Tastes: Bitter, pungent
Dosha Effects: KP-V=

TISSUES: Plasma, blood, fat
ACTIONS: Bitter digestive, laxative, alterative, antibiotic, antipyretic
USES: Fever, cough, asthma, bronchitis, hepatitis, parasites, eye inflammation, toxic blood conditions, obesity, diabetes
CAUTIONS: High vata conditions, severe debility, hypoglycemia
PREPARATION AND DOSE: Tincture, ghee, decoction, powder- 250 to 500 mg

Kutki is a cold, bitter, detoxifying herb. It is a digestive bitter, and its cooling quality lends it to liver therapy.

Kutki contains a wealth of medicines for diabetes. The main properties stimulate digestive secretions, which in turn stimulate pancreatic insulin secretion.[397] Kutki also enhances immune functions.

A unique action of this herb is to normalize the function of the liver, which is obviously a key to proper healthy living. Kutki assists the liver in storing blood sugar in the form of glycogen, which is essential in diabetes management. It is sometimes used to protect the liver from the toxic effects of anti-diabetic drugs.

Contemporary herbalists use it for hepatitis, and the anti-inflammatory effects benefit asthma.

Licorice

SCIENTIFIC NAME: *Glycyrrhiza glabra*
COMMON NAME: Licorice
AYURVEDIC NAME(S): Yashtimadhu (sweet stick)
ENGLISH NAME: Licorice
FAMILY: Fabaceae (Leguminosae)
PART USED: Root
TEMPERATURE: Cold
TASTES: Sweet, bitter
DOSHA EFFECTS: VP- K+
TISSUES: Works on all tissues
ACTIONS: Expectorant, tonic, demulcent, rejuvenative, laxative, sedative, emetic
USES: Coughs, colds, bronchitis, hyperacidity, ulcers, painful urination, sore throat, laryngitis, abdominal pain, general debility
CAUTIONS: High kapha; edema; hypertension; inhibits absorption of calcium and potassium
PREPARATION AND DOSE: Milk decoction, medicated ghee, powder- 250 to 500 mg

Although thought of more primarily as an adrenal herb, licorice is a strong liver protector and detoxifier. It protects liver cell membranes and reduces liver inflammation, making it useful in hepatitis. Licorice also suppresses free radicals in liver cells, preventing damage. Since licorice is a strong anti-inflammatory, it has value in skin toxicity disorders. Studies, primarily from Japan, show that active ingredients in licorice, glycyrrhizin, a triterpene glylcoside, and glycyrrhetinic acid, are strongly liver protective. Glycyrrhizin is prescribed widely in Japan for hepatitis.

Licorice protects and detoxifies the liver through diverse means. It is antioxidant, antiviral, and increases interferon and antibody production. Studies demonstrate that licorice will help the liver to detoxify even powerful poisons like carbon tetrachloride, a common industrial chemical. The root of licorice is extremely sweet, so small amounts in tea are delicious. Therapeutic doses may be overwhelmingly sweet. In capsules, the usual dose is 1-8 per day. Licorice is a light laxative, so work up slowly to a comfortable dose. Licorice may occasionally increase blood pressure in susceptible people, so those with a history of hypertension should avoid this herb.

Licorice is used to improve eyesight, strength, sexual potency and libido. It is considered, as tonics generally do, to enhance the effects of other herbs in a formula, so it is widely used.

Licorice root is probably the most extensively studied adrenal herb in the world. Rich in both saponins and flavonoids, licorice root is anti-inflammatory. The structure of the saponins resembles adrenal hormones. Many studies have proved its anti-inflammatory and anti-allergy properties. Licorice preserves the effect of the body's hormone, cortisol, allowing it to maintain longer anti-inflammatory action.

Licorice root is a highly regarded remedy in the major herbal traditions of the world. Although mainly a hormonal, digestive, or respiratory remedy, licorice is now emerging as a quality liver botanical.

Research over the last two decades in China and Japan has revealed that licorice is an herb with solid hepatoprotective features. According to Paul Bergner, clinical director for the Rocky Mountain School of Botanical Studies, licorice is "as significant a hepatoprotectant as the better-known milk thistle seed, and acts through separate mechanisms from that herb."

A 1996 study of licorice for Hepatitis B, done in Japan, revealed that the herb had positive actions in that disease, as well.

A 1993 study of licorice extract, done in India, on patients with liver failure due to hepatitis, produced a 72.2% survival rate, compared to the control group, of whom only 31.1% survived.

Licorice is a medicine cabinet in a bottle for the liver. Its actions are numerous. In protecting the liver, it acts as an antioxidant, an antiviral, enhances interferon and antibody production, promotes T-Cell activity in the liver, and protects the liver from autoimmune liver injury. Several animal studies have shown glycyrrhizin to protect liver cells from damage from chemicals.

Licorice benefits patients receiving chemotherapy for cancer, preventing the hepatic side effect from the drugs.

Licorice root reduces inflammation in the skin. This herb contains steroid-like substances, which, taken internally, or even applied topically, rapidly provide relief.

A study done in 1994 reinforced the excellent reputation of this herb in atopic dermatitis. Thirty-seven children were given a Chinese herbal medicine containing licorice. After twelve months, 18 of the children had experienced at least a 90% reduction in their disease symptoms. [398]

Licorice root, while not specifically demonstrated to treat FMS, is probably the most studied herb for CFS. Sharol Tilgner, N.D., recommends it highly. She points out that licorice is anti-inflammatory, anti-viral, protects the liver, and supports the immune system. CFS patients show a deficiency of glucocorticoid hormones, produced in the adrenal glands, which is improved with licorice root.[399 400]

Licorice is a delicious, sweet tasting herb, and so can be used as a tea. Taken as capsules, the typical dose would be about 4000- 5000 mg per day.

Lotus

SCIENTIFIC NAME: *Nelumbo nucifera*
COMMON NAME: Lotus
AYURVEDIC NAME(S): Padma, Kamala, Pushkara
ENGLISH NAME: Lotus
FAMILY: Nymphaceae
PART USED: Root and seed
TEMPERATURE: Cooling
TASTES: Sweet, astringent
DOSHA EFFECTS: PV-K+ (in excess)
TISSUES: Plasma, blood, marrow, reproductive, nerve
ACTIONS: Rejuvenative, aphrodisiac, astringent, hemostatic, nervine
USES: Bleeding disorders, diarrhea, menorrhagia, leucorrhea, impotence, spermatorrhea, heart weakness, venereal disease
CAUTIONS: Indigestion, food stagnation, constipation
PREPARATION AND DOSE: Decoction, powder- 250 mg to 1 gram

Lotus seed and root

Lotus brings material and spiritual abundance to the life. This herbal food relaxes the mind and opens the heart chakra and the root chakra. The seeds, especially, assist devotion and spiritual aspirations. Of course, the beautiful flower, with its roots in the mud and its petals thrusting toward heaven, has been a symbol of spiritual renewal for millennia.

Lotus is a rejuvenating tonic, especially for the heart and reproductive system. Both the seed and the root can be prepared as food. The root is a common ingredient in Chinese stir fried dishes. Peel and slice the root and use it somewhat like potato. Use the seeds the way you would use Garbanzo beans. You may also take the powdered herb in capsules, or brew as a tea.

Mandukaparni

SCIENTIFIC NAME: Centella asiatica
COMMON NAME: Gotu kola
AYURVEDIC NAME(S): Brahmi, Mandukaparni
ENGLISH NAME: Indian Pennywort
FAMILY: Umbelliferae, Apiaceae
PART USED: Herb
TEMPERATURE: Cold
TASTES: Bitter, sweet
DOSHA EFFECTS: VPK=
TISSUES: Reproductive, blood, marrow, nerve
ACTIONS: Nervine, rejuvenative, alterative, diuretic, febrifuge
USES: Nerve disorders, chronic skin conditions and many other connective tissue diseases, epilepsy, senility, memory loss, anxiety, hair loss, premature aging, venereal diseases
CAUTIONS: Itching aggravation, and headaches or temporary loss of consciousness in large doses possible
PREPARATION AND DOSE: Chronic, powder 1-2 grams per day. Acute, tea, 30-90 grams per day (Khalsa)

Note: In India, gotu kola (*Centella asiatica*) is often used interchangeably with another similar herb, Bacopa (*Bacopa monniera*). Both are called "brahmi." Bacopa can also be called water hyssop. Centella can also be called gotu kola (the Sihnala name) or mandukaparni ("frog leaved").

There is some discussion about how interchangeable they really are.

Centella is a sweeter, slightly heavier plant, with more tonic qualities. Bacopa is a colder, more bitter plant, with slightly more detoxifying qualities. Both target the brain and nerves.

Baba Hari Dass differentiates Centella as the "weaker brahmi" and Bacopa as the "stronger brahmi." Charaka classified Centella as an intellect promoting or nervine tonic and as a "divine great drug."

Thinking about thinking? Feel like you're about to max out your personal hard drive? Here's an herb with a long history of brain building.

Mandukaparni is a mainstay of herbal medicine in Ayurveda, although this herb has been around the fringes of European herbalism for many years. In fact, it was used in France in the 1880's. A superior herb for the nervous system, gotu kola has a host of benefits.[401]

It is a jungle creeper that grows in hot moist climates in the South and Southeast Asian tropics, from India to the Philippines. It is a common green vegetable, eaten raw with many different kinds of foods, much like a salad. This food is exceptionally high in B-complex vitamins, especially in B1, B2 and B6, all of which are essential nutrients for the nervous system.

And street vendors sell the freshly squeezed juice as a tropical energizing, brain boosting cocktail. A glass of that gives you some zip! After all, it's the jungle food of the elephants, especially in Sri Lanka, and we all know about their memories! Fresh, it's a delicious salad vegetable. The juice of the fresh leaves is available at some juice bars.

Brahmi, which means "godlike," is a reference to its anti-aging properties and to its use as an aid to meditation. It has a bitter taste and is cooling to the body. It is used to promote circulation, especially to the blood vessels of the skin and mucous membranes, and is a rejuvenator for the nerves and brain.

Gotu kola balances all three doshas. It is a bitter/cold/sweet herb, and an excellent nerve nutrient. As the main herb for the nervous system, it is used in the repair of nerve tissues from crushing trauma, such as spinal injury, neuromuscular disorders, and to increase general brain function, memory, concentration, and mental acuity. These qualities support gotu kola as the most used herb in enhancing meditation.

Gotu kola strengthens memory, concentration and intelligence, promotes longevity, improves the voice, physical strength and the complexion.[402] This medicine is used to treat diseases as diverse as epilepsy, senility, hair loss and psoriasis.

A study in rats showed an impressive improvement in memory. The treated rats were able to retain learned behavior 3 to 60 times better than the control rats.[403]

More recently, a new study out of Korea shows that constituents in gotu kola show potential for treating Alzheimer's disease.[404] Follow up animal research from India used gotu kola tea to improve cognitive behavior in two different types of experiments in a laboratory model of Alzheimer's.[405]

Known for centuries in Asia for its treatment of leprosy, gotu kola heals a host of corrupt skin conditions, including wounds, cellulite, varicose veins, and dermatitis. This herb stimulates the growth of hair and nails, increases blood supply to connective tissue, enhances the formation of structural constituents in connective tissue, promotes the tensile integrity of the skin, and increases protein growth (keratinization) in the skin.

These qualities give gotu kola the ability to actually heal and re-grow new skin, gently closing and repairing even long-standing, painful lesions and skin ulcers, and it even heals scars. Several studies have shown impressive results in the treatment of even the most dramatically scarred skin.

Gotu kola is anti-inflammatory and antioxidant.[406] [407] Evidence of this continues to pour in. In 1999, European and Indian researchers, in several new studies, confirmed that gotu kola compounds promote rapid healing of wounds. Internal wounds and intestinal ulcers also respond to gotu kola.[408]

Gotu kola may be used externally, in salves, to treat insect bites, herpes blisters, seborrheic dermatitis and chapped hands and lips and stings.

The active substances in gotu kola are thought to be triterpenes (steroid-like compounds), which have a balancing effect on connective tissues. These triterpenes improve the function and integrity of the collagen matrix and support the "ground substance," the basic "glue" that holds the cells of our bodies together.

Since gotu kola is basically a mild salad vegetable, the dose can be very high. Try one to four teaspoonfuls of fresh juice every morning. For acute skin disease, use one to two ounces of dry herb, by weight, as a tea, per day. Many people use a modest dose of 1 gram per day in capsules for daily rejuvenation. It is often taken with ghee, clarified butter. Try a cup of gotu kola tea with honey before meditation.

For inflammatory skin disorders, gotu kola works much better, and faster, when the dose is very high. One could consume from 1 to 3 ounces of dried herb per day. This can be accomplished as tea, but gotu kola also makes a tasty cooked green vegetable. Carefully clean the dried herb, removing the stems. Rehydrate the herb. Cook it much like spinach. It's a little bitter, but quite palatable. It goes well, mixed half and half with spinach. Use the mix to prepare saag or korma. Gotu kola and spinach saag has become a favorite dish for students to share in Khalsa's clinical herb classes.

Use brahmi ghee as nasya for nervous disorders. Take 2 drops in to each nostril up to several times per day.

Brahmi oil is used for abhyanga to treat the nervous system. As a body wrap, it enhances blood circulation, clears the skin, improves memory, and increases jatharagni.[409]

Manjishta

SCIENTIFIC NAME: *Rubia cordifolia*
COMMON NAME: Manjishta
AYURVEDIC NAME(S): Manjishta
ENGLISH NAME: Indian Madder, Bengal Madder
FAMILY: Rubiaceae
PART USED: Root
TEMPERATURE: Cooling
TASTES: Bitter, sweet, pungent
DOSHA EFFECTS: PK-V+
TISSUES: Plasma, blood, muscles
ACTIONS: Alterative, hemostatic, emmenagogue, astringent, antitumor, lithotriptic, diuretic
USES: Amenorrhea, dysmenorrhea, menorrhagia, menopause, bleeding disorders, gall stones, jaundice, hepatitis, diarrhea, dysentery, broken bones, traumatic injuries, cancer, heart disease, skin problems, paralysis, rickets, dropsy, herpes
CAUTIONS: Severe chills, high vata
PREPARATION AND DOSE: Decoction, powder- 250 to 1 gram, paste, medicated

ghee

This climbing plant is found at hill stations and in the Himalayas up to 8000 feet in India.

Manjistha supports the formation of quality nutrient plasma (Rasa Dhatu), blood (Rakta Dhatu), and fat (Meda Dhatu).

It is anti-inflammatory, wound healing and blood purifying, so it finds use in chronic arthritis, while increasing appetite.[410]

Manjishta induces menstrual bleeding and stimulates and contracts the uterus, so is used for amenorrhea, and to clean the uterus after delivery.

It is used to treat kapha and pitta disorders, including herpes, acne, psoriasis, eczema and dermatitis.

Mugwort

SCIENTIFIC NAME: *Artemisia vulgaris*
COMMON NAME: Mugwort, Damanaka
AYURVEDIC NAME(S): Nagadamani
ENGLISH NAME: Mugwort
FAMILY: Asteraceae (Compositae)
PART USED: Flowering tops
TEMPERATURE: Heating
TASTES: Bitter, spicy
DOSHA EFFECTS: VK-P+ (in excess)
TISSUES: Skin, blood, muscles, marrow, nerve
ACTIONS: Emmenagogue, diaphoretic, choleretic, diuretic, stomachic, orexigenic, vermifuge, bitter digestive, antibacterial, antifungal, antiviral
USES: Amenorrhea, anorexia, dyspepsia, threadworm, roundworm, nausea and vomiting
CAUTIONS: Pregnancy; may be toxic in large doses or with chronic use
PREPARATION AND DOSE: Infusion --1 tsp/cup water; 1:1 fresh tincture—1 to 20 gtt per day-4 times per day

Artemisias are found all over the world and is popular in Chinese medicine.

It is a specific herb for menorrhagia, when this excessive bleeding is caused by coldness.

It is useful in all cold, congealed conditions of the lower abdomen-dysmenorrhea, endometriosis and fibroids. It can also be used as douche for vaginal yeast and kapha symptoms.

It is antispasmodic in the intestines for vata cramps. Its affinity for the lower abdomen benefits all vata or nerve symptoms in this area.

The fresh leaf poultice is applied to remove warts. As a skin cream, or as a wash, it is used for itchy skin.

Musta

SCIENTIFIC NAME: *Cyperus rotundus*
COMMON NAME: Nutgrass
AYURVEDIC NAME(S): Musta
ENGLISH NAME: Nutgrass
FAMILY: Cyperaceae
PART USED: Rhizome
TEMPERATURE: Cooling
TASTES: Pungent, bitter, astringent
DOSHA EFFECTS: PK- V+ (in excess)
TISSUES: Plasma, blood, nerve, marrow, muscle
ACTIONS: Energizer, astringent, alterative, carminative, emmenagogue, antispasmodic, anthelmintic
USES: Menstrual disorders, menopause, dysmenorrhea, diarrhea, malabsorption, indigestion, sluggish liver
CAUTIONS: Constipation, high vata
PREPARATION AND DOSE: Decoction-low simmer; powder- 250 to 1 gram

Nutgrass is a common perennial weed with medicinal underground tubers. It is used across a wide swath of the globe, from southern Europe, across the Arabian peninsula to China. Today, it grows all over India.

The tubers are primarily anti-inflammatory and diuretic. With an astringent quality, musta is called for in ulcers and sores. Dioscorides notes it as a diuretic for ulcer and for use in warm plasters for sores. Since it lowers blood pressure, it is found in cardiovascular formulas.

Musta is a general tonic for women's issues, and is rich in minerals. It appears in many female hormone regulating and balancing formulas. It is a diaphoretic emmenagogue.

Musta's aromatic qualities make it suitable as a perfume ingredient.

Mustard

SCIENTIFIC NAME: *Sinapsis alba*
COMMON NAME: Mustard
AYURVEDIC NAME(S): Mustard
ENGLISH NAME: Mustard seeds
FAMILY: Brassicaceae
PART USED: Seed
TEMPERATURE: Hot
TASTES: Spicy, pungent
DOSHA EFFECTS: VK- P+
TISSUES: Lung, stomach, blood, muscle
ACTIONS: Expectorant, carminative, energizer, analgesic

USES: Coughs, body/joint pain, chronic sores/boils, improves digestion, dispels phlegm

CAUTIONS: Contraindicated in heating conditions

PREPARATION AND DOSE: Decoction, poultice, medicated oil, plaster, powder- 3 to 9 grams

Mustard is a very commonly used warming carminative, along the lines of cumin and clove.

Mustard oil is the main massage medium to treat kapha.

Baba Hari Dass recommends treating malaria by mixing chimney soot with ground mustard seed to form a paste. Apply this hot over the top of the big toe. Leave it on for two or three days. It cures in 2 to 3 days.[411] For bacterial blood infection (blood poisoning), he recommends heating a cotton ball in mustard or sesame oil, and applying this hot to the palm of the hand.

Myrrh

SCIENTIFIC NAME: *Commiphora myrrha* syn *C. molmol*

COMMON NAME: Myrrh

AYURVEDIC NAME(S): Bola

ENGLISH NAME: Myrrh

FAMILY: Burseraceae

PART USED: Resin

TEMPERATURE: Hot

TASTES: Bitter, astringent, pungent

DOSHA EFFECTS: KV- P+

TISSUES: Works on all tissues

ACTIONS: Antimicrobial, astringent, anti-inflammatory, expectorant, anticancer, anti-spasmodic, carminative, energizer

USES: Gingivitis, digestive problems, Athlete's foot, mouth ulcers, cold sores, common cold/sore throat, ulcerative colitis, amenorrhea

CAUTIONS: Pregnancy

PREPARATION AND DOSE: Tincture-orally- 1 to 2 ml 3 times per day, also taken as gargle and topical; capsules- up to 10 g (Khalsa)

Myrrh gum is first and foremost a detoxifier. It has strong antimicrobial properties. It increases circulation throughout the body.

Recent research has revealed its anti-inflammatory and analgesic qualities.[412]

As an oral care herb, myrrh can be used as a tooth powder or a wash. It is astringent and antimicrobial.

Myrrh gum rids us of suppressed emotions. It is closely related to guggul and salai guggul, and is essentially interchangeable with those resins.

Neem

SCIENTIFIC NAME: *Azadiracta indica*
COMMON NAME: Neem
AYURVEDIC NAME(S): Nimba
ENGLISH NAME: Neem
FAMILY: Meliaceae
PART USED: Bark, leaves
TEMPERATURE: Cooling
TASTES: Pungent, bitter, astringent
DOSHA EFFECTS: PK- V+
TISSUES: Plasma, blood, fat
ACTIONS: Bitter, digestive, alterative, antipyretic, antiseptic, antiemetic, antthelmintic
USES: Parasites, skin disease (eczema, ringworm, urticaria), malaria, fever, cough, vomiting, nausea, thirst, diabetes, tumors, jaundice, rheumatism, arthritis, obesity
CAUTIONS: Disease of tissue deficiency and cold temperature
PREPARATION AND DOSE: Infusion-hot or cold; paste; medicated ghee; medicated oil; powder- 250 to 500 mg

Neem is one of the most useful plants grown in Asia, and one of the most widely used. It is sometimes called "the village pharmacy," as people will plant a tree for the neighbors to share from the leaves, bark and seeds. Ayurvedic texts describe it as *sarva roga nivarini* (that which keeps all diseases at bay), or *arishtha* (reliever of disease). Neem offers the bitter and astringent tastes, so it is especially useful for balancing pitta and kapha doshas.

Neem leaves display a purifying effect on the blood, so cleanse the liver and skin of ama. A tea of neem leaf with honey can soothe an irritated throat.

Neem bark is cooling and astringent, and is taken internally for pitta issues. It is well suited for pitta eye conditions. In Asia, twigs of neem are widely used as primitive toothbrushes.

Neem is a *twacha rasayana*- a skin remedy. It draws out excess oil and smoothes blemishes, so it's wonderful for kapha skin. Due to its cooling nature, neem is also helpful for Pitta-related skin inflammation when applied externally.[413] Yogi Bhajan: "If you have got pimple which are not curable by any person or any reason, get those neem leaves. Put them in water and make a tea type situation or soup out of them. It is bitter, but it can purify you like an innocent, beautiful child. Very fantastic, it can kill any kind of germ or bacteria in the bloodstream. It is beautiful."[414]

Ayurvedic herb neem leaf is a broad spectrum antimicrobial that is popular in Asia for a wide variety of infections. It has shown results with Coxsackie virus in scientific experiments. Neem is a potent support for the immune system.

It stimulates insulin secretion in the pancreas, as well as possessing actions which support the immune system, which is often damaged as a complication of diabetes. Bitter neem has a general affinity for, and balancing effect on, the heart.

The antimicrobial properties lend neem to use in soap and shampoo, which are very popular in Asia. In addition to maintaining the color and strength of hair, it treats dry, flaky scalp.

All in all, neem is a classic folk herb. It does a plethora of things, yet it is mild and safe.

Nigella

SCIENTIFIC NAME: *Nigella sativa*
COMMON NAME: Black seed
AYURVEDIC NAME(S): Kalonjii, Mugrela
ENGLISH NAME: Small fennel, Black Cumin (incorrect), Fitch (Biblical), Love in the Mist
FAMILY: Ranunculaceae
PART USED: Seeds
TEMPERATURE: Heating
TASTES: Bitter, acrid
DOSHA EFFECTS: PV- K+
TISSUES: Blood, plasma, muscle, nerves
ACTIONS: Thermogenic, aromatic, carminative, diuretic, emmenagogue, anodyne, antibacterial, anti-inflammatory, deodorant, appetizing, digestive, anthelmintic, constipating, sudorific, febrifuge, energizer, galactagogue, expectorant.
USES: Skin diseases, hemorrhoids, cephalalgia, jaundice, inflammation, fever, paralysis, ophthamia, halitosis, anorexia, dyspepsia, flatulence, diarrhea, dysentery, cough, amenorrhea, dysmenorrhea, helminthiasis, especially tapeworm, stangury, intermittent fevers, agalactia
CAUTIONS: Not during pregnancy (history as abortifacient)
PREPARATION AND DOSE: Essential oil for insect repellent, used in cooking

This medicine is very popular in the Islamic world, and it is extensively used in the medicine of the Middle East. Jim Duke describes it as a Muslim Miracle Herb. An Arab Proverb says that, 'in the black seed is the medicine for every disease except death.'

It is a carminative and immune enhancer. As a culinary ingredient, it tastes a bit like fennel. The seeds are used as a condiment in bake goods and like pepper, or combined with cayenne in sauces.

It treats upper respiratory conditions, including ocommon colds, asthma and emphysema. At least a few of its constituents have shown an antihistamine-like action. Duke confirms its folk use for a wide variety of conditions, including bilious ailments, cancer, colic, headache, jaundice, stomachache, swellings, tumors of the abdomen and eyes, and warts. In Algeria, the roasted seeds are combined with butter for cough and honey for colic. The oils of the seed increase milk flow. In India, Nigella seeds are combined with various purgatives to dispel colic and also help kill and expel parasites.

Grind the seeds to a paste and mix with melted honey to make a type of halva (a Middle Eastern confection usually made with toasted sesame seeds and honey).

Externally, mix the powder with a little flour as a binder, and apply directly to abscesses, headache, nasal ulcers and rheumatic joints.

Nutmeg

SCIENTIFIC NAME: *Myristica fragrans*
COMMON NAME: Nutmeg, Jatiphala
AYURVEDIC NAME(S): Jatphalam (Sanskrit), Jaiphal (Hindi), Rou Dou Kou (Chinese)
ENGLISH NAME: Nutmeg
FAMILY: Myristicaceae
PART USED: Dried seed (commonly called nut) (oval, 2 to 3 x 2 cm), the kernel of a peach-like fruit[415]
TEMPERATURE: Hot
TASTES: Pungent
DOSHA EFFECTS: VK-P+
TISSUES: Plasma, muscle, marrow, reproductive, nerve
CHINESE CHANNELS ENTERED: Spleen, large intestine
ACTIONS: Aromatic, astringent,[416] carminative, circulatory enhancer (Ayurveda-"stimulant")[417], aphrodisiac (possible), rubefacient (oil externally)[418]
CHINESE ACTIONS: Warms middle burner, moves qi, eliminates pain
USES: Anxiety, insomnia, hypertension, indigestion, intestinal gas, suppressed appetite, vomiting, premature ejaculation,[419] diarrhea, cough, dyspnea, abdominal cramps[420]
CHINESE INDICATIONS: Diarrhea, especially from cold deficient spleen and kidneys[421]
CAUTIONS: Pregnancy, high pitta, diarrhea with heat, excessive tissue dryness, high heat, can cause mental dullness
TOXICITY: Myristicin strengthens the effect of tryptamine and moderately inhibits monoamine oxidases,[422] both in vitro and in vivo.[423] Even when high doses of 20-80 g of powder were consumed, a life-threatening situation never occurred.[424] [425] The acute toxicity of myristicin seems to be low, with no indications that it causes carcinogenic activity in short-term animal assays.[426] One study found, in vivo, that myristicin may be an effective cancer chemopreventive agent.[427]
Signs of overdose- vomiting, headache, tachycardia, dry mouth[428]
LD50 in rodents- 2600-6000 mg/kg
PREPARATION AND DOSE: Powder in capsules- 1 to 6 grams per day, decoction (Chinese) - 1.5 g to 6g (usually toasted before decocting), reports indicate

that in the human, 7.5 grams can lead to dizziness or stupor. However, for insomnia, this dose is routinely exceeded.

Nutmeg is cultivated in Southern India. [429] [430] Most nutmeg in the United States comes from the Caribbean, where it has become naturalized, especially on the island of Grenada. The outer covering of the seed, called mace, is also used as a cooking spice and herbal medicine.

Nutmeg contains a volatile oil and a fixed oil fraction. The essential oil contains a large proportion of monoterpene hydrocarbons (88%) and contains myristicine and related compounds. Pinene, eugenol, camphene, sabinene (major constituent in volatile oil).[431] Phenylpropanoids (myristicin, elemicin, safrole).[432] The fixed oil, or "butter of nutmeg" contains myristicin (methoxysafrole), myristic acid (tetradecanoic acid, the 14-carbon, straight-chain unsaturated fatty acid) and a portion of the essential oil.

The vast majority of nutmeg in the world is cultivated and harvested for culinary use. This is inferior medicine. The clinician should seek medicinal quality nutmeg that has been cultivated, harvested and prepared for medicine. Whole seeds preserve the active ingredients well, but the active ingredients degrade rapidly upon drying. If culinary quality is all that is available, freshly ground whole seeds will suffice. The seeds rapidly lose potency upon grinding. Bulk powdered seed must be freshly ground. However, nutmeg has a very strong taste and compliance is limited with powder. The author uses capsules prepared from seeds that are freshly ground and immediately encapsulated. Encapsulation retains the medicinal effects.

The psychotropic effects, and most other pharmacological properties, have been attributed to the compounds found in the essential oil, so it makes sense that the medicine needs to be protected so that the oil does not volatilize.[433]

Compared to other common herbal relaxants, nutmeg is powerful. If used in an excessively high dose while awake, the user will feel stupor and disorientation from the sedative effect, as with any other powerful relaxant.[434]

The strong psychoactive effects at high doses (feelings of unreality, euphoria, etc.) are believed to be due to myristicin, but there is little research to support this. Myristicin alone does not have the same effect as the whole seed. A 400 mg dose of myristicin, almost twice the amount present in 20 g of nutmeg (a 20 g dose produces psychotropic effects) produces only mild effects.[435] [436] [437] The MAO-inhibiting effects may be the cause for the sedation.[438]

Nutmeg is appropriate for sleep sustain insomnia. Extracts potentiated pentobarbitone-induced sleeping time in animals.[439] Whole oil of nutmeg increased the duration of sleep induced by ethanol in chickens.[440]

The sedating action of nutmeg begins after a predictable delay of 3 and one half to 5 hours, depending on the patient, and results in a prolonged somnolence of a predictable 8 hours. For insomnia, begin with a dose of one capsule at 6:00 p.m. The next night, increase the dose to two capsules. Continue increasing incrementally. Adjust the time of administration slightly to promote proper time of initiation of effects. The patient should feel profoundly drowsy at bedtime. Adjust the dose for the desired depth of sleep. Insomniac patients tend to under dose, as they often have not experienced truly deep sleep, and they tend to be satisfied with a less restful sleep. When the dose is increased incrementally to a higher amount, they often experience a profoundly rejuvenating sleep and awaken refreshed. Allow adequate time for the sleep effects, as patients will still be sedated if awakened before the full duration of action (8 hours). A typical dose for insomnia, given as one unit in the evening, is 3 grams.

Many sources[441] recommend taking small doses of nutmeg upon retiring, but this is problematic. The medicine will not take effect for 4 hours, so it is not appropriate for sleep onset insomnia when taken at bedtime. Since the duration is a solid eight hours, the patient will be sedated upon arising if taken at bedtime.

Administering nutmeg at bedtime with poppy seeds will produce 12 hour of sound sleep. Poppy takes effect immediately, so the patient is already asleep four hours later when the nutmeg becomes active. This can be of great value in convalescence.

Nutmeg has a delayed action, so it can be taken in divided doses throughout the day. A larger dose at night will produce a latent morning anxiolytic effect. A typical protocol would be 500- 1,000 mg at breakfast, lunch and bedtime. As the metabolism of nutmeg is gradual, patients often experience a sustained feeling of relaxed ease throughout the day, even if the dosing is irregular.

Nutmeg is a potent sedative and hypotensive.[442] The mechanism has not been well elucidated, but presumably it is through vasodilation. Nutmeg also retards pulse rate at appropriate doses. The author has observed clinically that nutmeg will reduce blood pressure, regardless of the severity, in virtually every case. It is an extremely effective short-term measure. The side effect is extreme fatigue. The patient will gradually adapt to the sedating effect over a few days if the dose is titrated. Higher doses of nutmeg extracts caused a precipitous fall in blood pressure not blocked by atropine in animals.[443]

This herb excels in treating premature ejaculation. The mechanism is obscure, but presumably is from the hypotensive effects.[444] Nutmeg is also mildly astringent. The most effective protocol is a modest daily dose that does not cause undue sedation, say 1 gram, longterm. The effect typically manifests in about 30 days, and continues.

Many sources describe nutmeg as aphrodisiac. It is one of the Ayurvedic "five aromatics" supposedly taken by kings to allow them to satisfy many women.[445] Considering its use in treating premature ejaculation, this is suspect. Some sources report that the action on the urinary tract is irritation. This might be responsible for purported action. (On the other hand, different sources report that the oil is used for urinary inflammation.)[446, 447] The authors do not consider it to be a clinically viable aphrodisiac. However, since nutmeg is a strong sedative, the relaxed mood it imparts may facilitate sexual interaction and performance. The hypotensive effects argue against an increase in erectile function.[448]

Usually it is a relatively minor ingredient in aphrodisiac formulas. One contemporary product, while touting the aphrodisiac effect, combines it with 22 other multipurpose herbs, many of which actually are herbs with targeted aphrodisiac effects, including saffron, shankpushpi, jyotishmati, jatamansi, ashwaganda and gokshura.[449]

Nutmeg is a moderately drying, astringent herb. It is constipating and diuretic, so it is used to treat diarrhea, for which it can be administered in milk or buttermilk.[450 451] Nutmeg is combined with opium for diarrhea and as a soporific. In North America, poppy seeds can be substituted. Nutmeg is particularly suited for diarrhea in children.[452 453]

A home medicine for diarrhea includes ghee, ginger powder, raw sugar and nutmeg.[454] The addition of the ginger increases agni, the digestive fire, to treat the underlying poor digestion, the cause of the diarrhea.[455]

As a carminative, Ayurveda considers nutmeg to be similar in action to cinnamon and clove. If necessary, any can be substituted for the other.[456] It reduces high vata. Baba Hari Dass says it opens up the nadis, purifies the blood and stops burping.[457] A typical combination for suppressed digestive function includes dry ginger, caraway and nutmeg, taken before meals.[458] A classical formula, *Jatiphala churna* ("Nutmeg powder"), combines nutmeg with cardamom seed, sandalwood wood, sesame seed, amla, pipali and miscellaneous other herbs. It is used for a variety of digestive complaints, including diarrhea.[459] Nutmeg is also used in formulas for hemorrhoids,[460] and applied externally as a paste with a solid fat.[461]

Nutmeg butter is an ingredient in ointments for joint symptoms (arthritis).[462] The nut is hepatoprotective.[463]

Ayurveda suggests nutmeg for runny nose in children. Jatiphala churna is also used for respiratory complaints involving excess mucus (cough, rhinitis, sinus congestion).

It is used as a minor medicine in diabetes.[464] In the Banda Islands, the oil is rubbed on the abdomen and forehead for headache and stomachache, respectively.[465] The pulp of nutmeg fruit is tough, woody and very sour. In Indonesia, it is used to make a delicious jam with pleasant nutmeg aroma. A nutmeg balm is produced in Malaysia that is used for headache, stuffy nose, minor skin itch and insect bites.[466] Dr. Lobsang Rapgay teaches that in the Tibetan tradition nutmeg essential oil can be mixed with coconut oil and applied for muscular stiffness.[467] It is used in infant teething (apply to gums), and as a vermifuge.[468]

Nutmeg is combined with saussurea root for digestive actions and with codonopsis and ginger for diarrhea. It is combined with pinellia root and ginger for vomiting, gas and decreased appetite and with pinellia, ginger, "massa fermentata" (nonstandard mixture of fermented wheat flour, various herbs, typically artemisia), grains of paradise seed (*Ammomum villosum*- relative of cardamom) for children with vomiting, gas and decreased appetite.

Ayurveda often combines nutmeg with banana and honey or other sweeteners, including sweet fruit.[469]

Peppermint

SCIENTIFIC NAME: *Mentha piperita*
COMMON NAME: Peppermint
AYURVEDIC NAME(S): Phudina
ENGLISH NAME: Peppermint
FAMILY: Lamiaceae
PART USED: Leaf
TEMPERATURE: Cold
TASTES: Pungent, sweet
DOSHA EFFECTS: PK- V=
TISSUES: Plasma, blood, marrow, nerves
ACTIONS: Anispasmodic, cholagogue, choleretic, carminative, antiseptic, analgesic (externally), diaphoretic, antiemetic
USES: Colic, flatulence, irritable bowel syndrome, indigestion, nausea, vomiting, gallbladder disease (Khalsa), common cold and flu, gallstones
CAUTIONS: Pregnancy, acute gallstones, hiatal hernia, GERD
PREPARATION AND DOSE: Infusion- 1 Tbsp/cup water; 1:1 tincture: 10-30 gtt per day-4 times per day, capsules- 3 grams per day (Khalsa)

Ever think there might be something more to peppermint that that after dinner candy and a sip of mint julep? Turns out that peppermint, as safe and mild as it is, is also powerful medicine.

Besides being a tasty tea and candy herb, peppermint is a widely used digestive aid that reduces gas. It has a long history of being employed in herbal medicine as an antispasmodic and carminative.

As an antispasmodic, it reduces gut cramping and excess movement. Peppermint is often used with other antispasmodics, including chamomile and thyme. Valerian root is another classic antispasmodic for digestive disorders. Since peppermint cools the digestive tract, and valerian has a warming energy, the combination is often effective and well tolerated across a broad range of people with tummy troubles.

This mint has a cooling temperature and a pungent taste. It decreases pitta and kapha doshas and is balancing for vata in typical doses. Spearmint is even more cooling, and might be a better choice for a fiery hot stomach.

The active ingredients in peppermint are mainly menthol and related terpenes (menthone, pinene, bornoel, cineole, and camphene). Historically, peppermint oil, containing menthol, has been employed for a wide variety of health conditions, including common cold symptoms, cramps, headache, indigestion, joint pain, and nausea.

Peppermint has shown promise for gallstone treatment. This safe preparation can be used for extended periods, up to several years. These terpenes reduce bile cholesterol levels, while also increasing bile acid and lecithin levels in the biliary system. Peppermint gives very good clinical success in reversing gallstone symptoms in cases diagnosed by ultrasound using peppermint powder in capsules, oral peppermint oil, and encapsulated camphor. In particular, the peppermint is very effective for the aggravating chronic burping that often accompanies this syndrome.

Peppermint oil works well to relieve the symptoms of irritable bowel syndrome (IBS).[470 471 472] Many people do just about as well with simple peppermint tea or capsules.

Traditional herbal systems value diaphoretics, including peppermint, for treating colds. Consumed hot, these perspiration-promoting medicines release waste materials and relieve congestion. Cooling diaphoretics are used to reduce fever and inflammation.

Topically, menthol is a good substitute for ice. Use a salve with menthol as a main ingredient.[473 474 475 476 477] Applied topically, menthol is a strong anodyne, local antiseptic, anesthetic and antipruritic (relieves itch). Peppermint oil is approved by German Commission E for myalgia and neuralgia. Menthol is effective for acute inflammation as well. It provides a deeply cooling sensation in therapy, even for the disease fibromyalgia, which is notoriously hard to treat. Even though fibromyalgia does not involve inflammation, many patients find great relief with menthol preparations.

At least two scientific studies have shown the value of herbal essential oils applied topically for headache.[478 479]

Peppermint has one drawback, compared to other mints. Its energetics are debated, but generally it's pungent in taste, with a cooling energy. Even the English name gives you a clue. Since it is hot, at least to an extent, the digestive effects can be contradictory. Pitta conditions can be aggravated by peppermint. You don't want that gastritis to be made worse. Other mints, including spearmint (*Mentha spicata*) and horsemint (or corn mint) (podina, *Mentha arvensis*) have a more overtly cooling energy.

Pipali

Scientific Name: *Piper longum*
Common Name: Pipali
Ayurvedic Name(s): Pipali
English Name: Long Pepper
Family: Piperacae
Part Used: Fruit (peppercorn)
Temperature: Hot
Tastes: Pungent
Dosha Effects: VK-P+
Tissues: Plasma, blood, fat, marrow, nerve, reproductive
Actions: Energizer, expectorant, aphrodisiac, carminative, anthelmintic,

analgesic

USES: Colds, coughs, asthma, bronchitis, laryngitis, arthritis, abdominal tumor, lumbago, sciatica, epilepsy, paralysis, worms, rheumatism, gout, dyspepsia, flatulence

CAUTIONS: High pitta inflammatory conditions

PREPARATION AND DOSE: Infusion, milk decoction, medicated oil, powder- 100 to 500 mg

Pipali is a pepper approximately one to two inches in length. It is used in Ayurvedic and Chinese herbalism.

Ayurveda considers pipali to be a powerful blood cleanser. It is also renowned as a beneficial herb for both the digestive and respiratory systems. Unlike black pepper, to which it is related, it is a rejuvenative.

Long pepper enhances turmeric bioavailability. Turmeric mixed with 10% long pepper has the equivalent bioavailability of 95% curcumin standardized extract and has the full range of constituents available in the whole root vs. the refined standardized extract (and is much cheaper). Moreover, curcumin in high doses may cause gastric damage, whereas whole turmeric does not show such activity in high doses. To the contrary, it appears to be protective for the gastric mucosa.[480]

Pipali is moistening, whereas black pepper is drying. The two are often combined to offset the energetics.

Pomegranate

SCIENTIFIC NAME: *Punica granatum*

COMMON NAME: Pomegranate

AYURVEDIC NAME(S): Dadima

ENGLISH NAME: Pomegranate

FAMILY: Lythraceae

PART USED: Fruit rind, root bark, fruit

TEMPERATURE: Cooling

TASTES: Astringent, bitter (fruit rind and root bark), sweet or sour (dependent on fruit variety)

DOSHA EFFECTS: Sweet variety -VKP= (may increase Ama)

Sour variety - may aggravate Pitta

TISSUES: Plasma, blood, marrow, nerve, muscle

ACTIONS: Astringent tonic, alterative, homeostatic, anthelmintic, refrigerant, stomachic

USES: Worms, sore throat, ulcers, conjunctivitis, anemia, chronic bronchitis, tuberculosis, colitis, diarrhea, dysentery, prolapse of vagina or rectum, leucorrhea

CAUTIONS: Constipation

PREPARATION AND DOSE: Decoction, fresh juice, paste, powder- 250 to 500 mg

Pomegranate is an astringent fruit that is mainly used as tea or food for sore throat.

This purple fruit has very high amounts of colored pigment flavonoids that are potent antioxidants, which reduce free radicals.[481] Pomegranate juice shows three times greater antioxidant activity than other well known sources, such as red wine or green tea.[482]

Numerous recent studies have shown it to reduce cholesterol and have an anticancer effect.[483]

Poppy

SCIENTIFIC NAME: *Papaver somniferum and spp.*
COMMON NAME: Post dana
AYURVEDIC NAME(S): Ahiphena
ENGLISH NAME: Poppy seeds
FAMILY: Papaveraceae
PART USED: Seeds (non-narcotic)
TEMPERATURE: Heating
TASTES: Pungent, astringent, sweet
DOSHA EFFECTS: VK-P+
TISSUES: Plasma, blood, muscle, bone, marrow, nerves
ACTIONS: Astringent, carminative, antispasmodic, sedative, analgesic
USES: Diarrhea (especially in children), dysentery, abdominal pain, poor absorption, insomnia, nerve pain, cough
CAUTIONS: Gastritis, colitis, high pitta
PREPARATION AND DOSE: Infusion, powder – 250 mg to 1 gram

The poppy plant contains small quantities of opioids, including morphine and codeine, so it is mild.

Poppy seed is a warming sleep remedy that acts immediately. Brew 4 Tbs as a decoction. Drink the tea one half hour before bed. The effect typically lasts for about 4 hours. Use this same decoction to rapidly relieve cough, similar to codeine (another opiate) cough syrup.[484]

The presence of another alkaloid, papaverine, in the seeds, explains why the plant parts relax muscles and reduce stomach and respiratory spasms. The seed is safe and effective for pediatric diarrhea.

For pain relief, drink the tea throughout the day.

The flowers have a similar effect. Long term use can be constipating. Sometimes the seeds are ground and mixed with raw sugar and cardamom for diarrhea, asthma and cough.

Extracts of poppies have been used to treat fevers, tuberculosis, liver and kidney problems and diseases of the urinary tract.

Cold pressed poppy seed oil is used in food, mainly on salads. Ground poppy seeds are common thickening agent in Northern Indian food. They give a sweet, mild, nutty flavor and aroma.

Poppy seed chutney is a tasty way to ingest the somnolent benefit of the seeds.

1 tsp poppy seeds
1 tsp grated coconut
1 tsp ghee
One eighth tsp cumin powder
One eighth tsp turmeric powder

Mix poppy seeds with the coconut. Add water to form a paste. Heat ghee in a skillet. Add cumin and turmeric. Remove from heat. Stir. Add spiced ghee to the poppy seed mixture, stirring. Let it cool.

Punarnava

SCIENTIFIC NAME: *Boerhaavia diffusa*
COMMON NAME: Punarnava
AYURVEDIC NAME(S): Punarnava – what renews us
ENGLISH NAME: Punarnava, Spreading Hogweed
FAMILY: Nycyaginaceae
PART USED: Whole plant, root
TEMPERATURE: Heating
TASTES: Bitter, sweet, pungent
DOSHA EFFECTS: KV- P+
TISSUES: Plasma, blood
ACTIONS: Alterative, blood tonic, rejuvenative, diuretic
USES: Edema, anemia, difficult/burning urination, kidney stones, heart disease, alcoholism, hepatitis, hemorrhoids
CAUTIONS: Dehydration
PREPARATION AND DOSE: Decoction; powder- 250 to 500 mg

The plant is found throughout India, especially during the rainy season.

All the parts of the plant are used, although each part has a different therapeutic value and must be prepared in its own way for maximum benefits.

Punarnava is a unique herb that helps maintain efficient kidney and urinary functions. It protects the kidneys, especially the nephrons, which are damaged by long-term diabetes. Punarnava is a well known diuretic, anti-spasmodic and anti-inflammatory agent in urinary tract infections.

The antiedema action is beneficial for congestive heart failure, when it is often administered with arjuna bark.

A mild and well tolerated medicine, it is anti-inflammatory, stomachic laxative, myocardial stimulant, antibacterial and antiviral. It is useful in asthma, anemia, jaundice, ascites, anasarca, scanty urine, internal inflammation and as an antidote for snake venom.

The root of this plant is a powerful rasayana. It pacifies vata and kapha. The roots have anti-convulsant, analgesic, laxative and expectorant properties. They also have hepatoprotective actions.

Punarnava supports the quality of 6 of the 7 categories of bodily tissues, including nutrient plasma (Rasa Dhatu), blood (Rakta Dhatu), muscle (Mamsa Dhatu), fat (Meda Dhatu), bone marrow and nerves (Majja Dhatu) and reproductive fluids (Shukra Dhatu).

Psyllium

SCIENTIFIC NAME: *Plantago psyllium*
COMMON NAME: Psyllium
AYURVEDIC NAME(S): Snigdhajira
ENGLISH NAME: Psyllium
FAMILY: Plantaginaceae
PART USED: Seeds, seed husks
TEMPERATURE: Cooling
TASTES: Sweet, astringent
DOSHA EFFECTS: PV- K and Ama+
TISSUES: Plasma, blood
ACTIONS: Laxative, demulcent, emollient, astringent, expectorant
USES: Chronic constipation, chronic diarrhea/dysentery, catarrh, colitis, urethritis, cystitis, gastritis, ulcers
CAUTIONS: May create food stagnation and congestion in gastrointestinal tract
PREPARATION AND DOSE: Infusion, paste, powder- 500 mg to 2 grams

Psyllium seed, a common bulk fiber laxative, relieves constipation.

It balances bowel function and relieves pain in Irritable Bowel Syndrom (IBS).[485] Psyllium's capacity to absorb fluids means that it is useful for treating diarrhea, a common IBS symptom. As it travels through the gut, the mucilage in psyllium creates a soothing benefit, which may relieve cramping. An English study revealed that constipation significantly improved in patients taking psyllium. Eighty-two percent of the subjects had IBS symptom relief.[486] A study to determine the optimum dose recommended 20 grams per day.[487]

Bulk fiber promotes a sensation of fullness and helps with weight loss.

Psyllium seed looks especially promising. A triple-blind experiment done last year in London with non-dieting subjects revealed that the participants felt much fuller than normal one hour after the meal, and ended up eating 15 grams less fat per day than usual. A whole grain breakfast cereal with added psyllium is a tasty way to get soluble fiber into the diet.

The typical dose of fiber used in such studies is 5 to 7 g per day. Aside from the occasional feeling of fullness, fiber rarely has any side effects.

Rauwolfia

SCIENTIFIC NAME: *Rauwolfia serpentina*
COMMON NAME: Indian snakeroot
AYURVEDIC NAME(S): Sarpagandha
ENGLISH NAME: Indian snakeroot
FAMILY: Apocynaceae
PART USED: Root
TEMPERATURE:
TASTES: Bitter
DOSHA EFFECTS:
TISSUES: Nerve, blood, plasma
ACTIONS: Hypotensive, febrifuge, sedative
USES: Lower blood pressure, mental illness, insomnia, anxiety, psychosis, historically used as antidote to poisonous snakebites, dysentery, abdominal pain, fever, colic
CAUTIONS: Contraindicated in pregnancy (teratogen and abortifacient), depression, peptic ulcers, hyperprolactinemia.
PREPARATION AND DOSE: Powder- 50 to 300 mg daily, or more, if supervised

This herb is the source of the valued hypertension drug, reserpine. It is superb herb for reducing blood pressure at low doses.[488] It is so effective for lowering blood pressure it will actually create low blood pressure if not monitored carefully.

Historically, it was used to treat snakebite.

Sarpagandha is indicated in mental disorders.[489] It is said to remove evil spirits.

Khalsa has been very successful in using it for autism, especially in autistic children with a profile of anxiety and insomnia, which is common.

It can act as a strong aphrodisiac, including producing erectile difficulties from lowered blood pressure.

This is a very potent herb, and must be used with caution. It is difficult to find in America.

Rhubarb

SCIENTIFIC NAME: *Rheum spp.*
COMMON NAME: Rhubarb
AYURVEDIC NAME(S): Amla-vetasa
ENGLISH NAME: Rhubarb
FAMILY: Polygonaceae
PART USED: Root
TEMPERATURE: Cooling
TASTES: Bitter, pungent
DOSHA EFFECTS: PK-V+
TISSUES: Plasma, blood, fat
ACTIONS: Purgative, alterative, hemostatic, antipyretic, anthelmintic

USES: Jaundice, liver problems, skin inflammation, pitta type diarrhea/ dysentery, constipation with accompanying fevers, ulcers, or infections
CAUTIONS: Pregnancy, chronic diarrhea, chills, hemorrhoids, vata -type
PREPARATION AND DOSE: Infusion, powder – laxative 1 gram, purgative 3 grams

Rhubarb root is a cold, bitter, anthraquinone containing laxative.

Rhubarb promotes bile, which "drains damp heat." We see that these qualities make it suitable for jaundice.

It is suited to geriatric constipation. Use it with warming carminatives to avoid cramping.

This herb is milder than senna or cascara and two to four capsules a day would be appropriate. Widely well tolerated, rhubarb root can be used for a broad range of patients and conditions.

Rose

SCIENTIFIC NAME: *Rosa spp.*
COMMON NAME: Rose, Gulab
AYURVEDIC NAME(S): Shatapatri
ENGLISH NAME: Rose
FAMILY: Rosaceae
PART USED: Flower petals, hips (fruit)
TEMPERATURE: Cold
TASTES: Bitter, astringent, pungent, sweet,
DOSHA EFFECTS: VPK=
TISSUES: Plasma, blood, marrow, nerve, reproductive
ACTIONS: Flower- antibacterial, antidepressant, anti-inflammatory, antiseptic, antispasmodic, antiviral, aphrodisiac, aromatic, astringent, blood tonic, carminative, expectorant, kidney tonic, and sedative
Hips- astringent, blood tonic, diuretic (mild), kidney tonic, laxative, nutritive, tonic, astringent, carminative, diuretic, digestive, anti-inflammatory (topical), laxative
USES: Anger, anxiety, catarrh, depression, diarrhea, dysmenorrhea, frequent urination, hypercholesterolemia, tonsillitis, vertigo, kidney and bladder infections, exhaustion, gout, rheumatism, amenorrhea, colic, external inflammations
CAUTIONS: Ingestion of seeds (theoretical)
PREPARATION AND DOSE: Infusion- 1 to 2 tsp hips (without seeds)/cup boiling water, decoction- ½ to 1 tsp powder achenes/1 cup water, boil until 1/2 cup of liquid remains

Rose flowers, seldom used here, are popular medicine in the Middle East and India. They are especially good for reducing pitta, and are a good laxative for people of pitta constitution.

They soothe inflamed surfaces and regulate menstruation.

Commonly, rose petals are mixed with honey or raw sugar and allowed to marinate for a year. The jam is a tasty confection with a cooling laxative effect.

Safed Musali

SCIENTIFIC NAME: *Asparagus adscendens* (*Chlorophytum borivilianum*)
COMMON NAME: Safed musali
AYURVEDIC NAME(S): Shreta musli
ENGLISH NAME: Asparagus (Indian, not the common vegetable)
FAMILY: Liliaceae
PART USED: Root
TEMPERATURE: Cooling
TASTES: Sweet
DOSHA EFFECTS: VP-K+
TISSUES: Reproductive
ACTIONS: Tonic, demulcent, aphrodisiac
USES: Premature ejaculation, low libido, bladder infection, diarrhea
CAUTIONS: Very high doses may lead to gastric upset
PREPARATION AND DOSE: Powder-1-10 grams per day, often as milk decoction

Safed (white) musali tuber, a relative of shatavari, is a potent Ayurvedic aphrodisiac plant that has been used since the 11th century A.D. Like shatavari, it is a general tonic.[490]

It contains various stigmasterol derivatives and various steroidal glycosides.[491] It has a very high 12-17% total saponin content.

It is nutritive and demulcent, as asparagus roots tend to be, so it suits urinary disorders. It is also been shown significant effect in increasing semen volume and total sperm count. Clinical trails also showed it to enhance working capacity.[492] Similar to ashwaganda, it imparts strength and aids immune function. Safed Musali in traditionally used for lack of libido and impotence in males and is well known for treating premature ejaculation. As a general health promoting, anti-aging tonic, it has an affinity for the pelvis and rectum. It is a common, safe ingredient in sexual tonic formulas. It is an ingredient in Chyvanprash.

Safed musali is now seeing use for diabetes and arthritis.[493] It is a minor remedy for diarrhea.

The tuberous roots are used as pickles.

For general sexual weakness and impotence, cook safed musali in milk. It is often used at a dose of 1-2 grams per day as a maintenance food.[494] For acute low libido, use 15 or more grams per day. This variety of asparagus is a food so high doses are safe.

Saffron

SCIENTIFIC NAME: *Crocus sativus*
COMMON NAME: Saffron
AYURVEDIC NAME(S): Nagakeshara, kesar
ENGLISH NAME: Saffron
FAMILY: Iridaceae
PART USED: Flower -stigma
TEMPERATURE: Cold
TASTES: Pungent, bitter, sweet
DOSHA EFFECTS: VK=P-
TISSUES: Works on all tissues but especially the blood
ACTIONS: Alterative, emmenagogue, aphrodisiac, rejuvenative, energizer, antispasmodic, carminative
USES: Menstrual pain/irregularity, menopause, impotence, infertility, anemia, enlarged liver, hysteria, depression, neuralgia, lumbago, cough, asthma, chronic diarrhea, rheumatism
CAUTIONS: Pregnancy, because it can cause a miscarriage. It is a narcotic in large doses.
PREPARATION AND DOSE: Infusion, milk decoction, medicated oil, medicated ghee, powder- 100 to 250 mg; use in small dosages as a pinch with other herbs

Saffron has been used as a versatile medicine more than 3,600 years. Historical evidence suggests that it was used in Greece for skin ulcers, wounds, thrush, cardiac arrhythmias, smallpox, measles, jaundice, constipation, eye diseases, liver diseases, joint pain, earaches, diarrhea, vomiting, and headaches.[495] It has historically been used in treating gynecological conditions- to regulate menstruation and fertility. Studies have identified steroidal estrogens and other substances in saffron that mimic female sex hormones. Saffron and its constituents (crocin and crocetin) have antitumor activity against different malignancies in humans and animals.

Ayurveda considers it to be one of the finest blood revitalizers. Saffron is a very potent herb, which enhances circulation throughout the body, but particularly in the female reproductive tract. Even though it has pungent taste, the overall energy is cold, making it a favored herb for combating pitta.

Salai Guggul

SCIENTIFIC NAME: *Boswellia serrata*
COMMON NAME: Boswellia, Sallaki
AYURVEDIC NAME(S): Salai guggul
ENGLISH NAME: Boswellia
FAMILY: Burseraceae
PART USED: Resin
TEMPERATURE: Cooling
TASTES: Bitter, sweet, astringent
DOSHA EFFECTS: VPK=
TISSUES: Blood, muscle, fat, reproductive
ACTIONS: Alterative, antispasmodic, analgesic
USES: Arthritis, rheumatism, gout, nerve pain, muscle spasms
CAUTIONS: None known
PREPARATION AND DOSE: Purified powder- 250 mg to 1 gram

Salai guggul has become well known in North America over the last decade for its pronounced effects on joint disorders. The medicine is a gum resin that exudes from the bark of a large branching tree that grows in semi-arid areas of South Asia. Extracts of this gummy exudate have been traditionally used in the Ayurvedic system of medicine as an anti-arthritic. In Ayurvedic herbalism, medicinal preparations of gum are known as "gugguls."

This gum contains constituents, boswellic acids, which inhibit inflammation producing substances, leukotrienes, in the body. In fact, boswellia gum inhibits inflammation through several mechanisms in the body. Scientific experiments showed that the herb "was found to exhibit marked sedative and analgesic effects."

Boswellia gum treats pain, another reason it should be used for advanced osteoporosis. While Ayurveda recommends this herb for arthritis, studies using humans for this disease are lacking. Boswellia has been shown to reduce inflammatory processes in humans with colitis, however, which is a step in the right direction.

These days in America, Boswellia is usually administered as a purified extract. For the initial treatment dose, 400 mg three times per day is suggested.

Sandalwood

SCIENTIFIC NAME: *Santalum album*
COMMON NAME: Sandalwood
AYURVEDIC NAME(S): Chandana
ENGLISH NAME: Sandalwood
FAMILY: Santalaceae
PART USED: Wood, volatile oil
TEMPERATURE: Cooling

TASTES: Bitter, sweet, astringent
DOSHA EFFECTS: PV- K or Ama+ (in excess)
TISSUES: Plasma, blood, nerve, reproductive, muscle, marrow
ACTIONS: Alterative, hemostatic, sedative, refrigerant, antiseptic, antibacterial, carminative
USES: Eye disease, cystitis, urethritis, vaginitis, herpes zoster, acute dermatitis, bronchitis, palpitations, gonorrhea, sunstroke
CAUTIONS: Severe lung congestion, high kapha
PREPARATION AND DOSE: Infusion- hot or cold, decoction, medicated oil, powder- 5 grams to 15 grams per day

Many of us are familiar with the wonderful aroma of great quality sandalwood oil.

This medicine is one of the best cooling remedies for pitta. As such, it is used to treat a spectrum of hot diseases, internally and externally, from jaundice and fever to herpes and skin rash. Mix 10% sandalwood oil with zinc oxide ointment and apply it to herpes blisters.

The essential oil is a very popular remedy for disorders of the urinary tract, including cystitis and gonorrhea. It is also used for irritating coughs and bronchitis.

An emulsion of the wood mixed with sugar, honey and rice treats an upset stomach.[496]

Sandalwood is the main external treatment for acne and similar inflammatory skin diseases. Khalsa created, and has used, with great success, a water based gel containing sandalwood oil, aloe gel, menthol, borax and a few other minor ingredients, for very serious cases of adolescent and adult acne.

Chandana means "gladdening." It has a prabhava for giving happiness. It is a medhya remedy.

Sandalwood is a vajikarana medicine.

Chandana is hemostatic and is used to staunch bleeding from simple wounds. Khalsa leaned to use sandalwood oil as a treatment for nosebleeds (a type of rakta pitta) from Yogi Bhajan. It is still the most effective treatment he has seen to instantly stop a bleeding nose. Tip the head back and insert 2-3 drops of the oil into the afflicted nostril. The bleeding stops immediately. The only objection people mention is the strong lingering scent of the sandalwood, which smells nice when dabbed on as a perfume, but can be a bit overpowering when up the nose!

To take the essential oil internally, put 20 to 50 drops per day in empty capsules and swallow.

Sarsaparilla

SCIENTIFIC NAME: *Smilax officinalis*
COMMON NAME: Sarsaparilla
AYURVEDIC NAME(S): Dwipautra, Copchini
ENGLISH NAME: Sarsaparilla
FAMILY: Liliaceae
PART USED: Rhizome
TEMPERATURE: Cold
TASTES: Bitter, sweet
DOSHA EFFECTS: PV- K=
TISSUES: Plasma, blood, nerve, reproductive, marrow
ACTIONS: Alterative, diuretic, diaphoretic, antispasmodic, antisyphilitic, antirheumatic
USES: Venereal disease, herpes, skin disease, arthritis, rheumatism, abdominal distention, intestinal gas, debility, impotence, turbid urine, gout, epilepsy, insanity, chronic nervous disease
CAUTIONS: None known
PREPARATION AND DOSE: Powder or decoction, 3-12 grams per day

Sarsaparilla kindles agni and reduces intestinal vata, so it finds use in nervous system conditions.

Sarsaparilla, though native to tropical America, has a history of use in Europe as a blood purifier dating back to the 16th century. Sarsaparilla is a well-known herb in many areas of the world, and used extensively in global herbalism.[497] Smilax species also grow in Asia and have similar properties.

Primarily, sarsaparilla root is a tissue detoxifier, especially for the urinary tract. It is an active diaphoretic. As is typical with alteratives, it has wide applications for the skin, and has a long history of use for inflammatory skin disorders including psoriasis. Sarsaparilla is a famous liver herb.[498] Its alterative functions also lend it to use in joint diseases, for which it is widely respected. For hot conditions, use it with gentian.

Several saponin ingredients in sarsaparilla have been shown to be effective in treating psoriasis.[499 500] In a controlled study, one of these constituents, sarsaponin, greatly improved psoriasis in 62% of the patients and completely cleared the disease in 18%.[501]

Sarsaparilla binds endotoxins, cell wall constituents of bacteria that are absorbed from the digestive tract. If these endotoxins are allowed to bypass the liver and circulate in the blood, they contribute to gout, arthritis, psoriasis, and fever - just the conditions sarsaparilla has historically treated. The saponins in sarsaparilla act as phytohormones in the body, and may aid in enhancing male functions.

Take 3-12 grams of sarsaparilla root per day as a tasty tea, or the equivalent in capsules.

A different herb is also called sarsaparilla in Asia. This is Indian sarsaparilla root (*Hemidesmus indicus*), called Sariva, or Anantamool, in the family Asclepiadaceae. It is sometimes substituted for Smilax, and has similar properties (tonic, antibacterial, diuretic, demulcent, diaphoretic and blood purifier). It is employed in syphilis, chronic rheumatoid arthritis, urinary stones and skin inflammation.

The roots yield essential oil containing p-methoxy salicylic aldehyde as the major constituent. It contains coumarins and triterpenoid saponins, which, as a whole, tend to promote circulation, reduce inflammation and promote stamina.

Senna

Scientific Name: *Cassia angustifolia*
Common Name: Senna
Ayurvedic Name(s): Rajavriksha- king of the trees
English Name: Senna
Family: Fabaceae
Part Used: Leaves, pods (milder)
Temperature: Cold
Tastes: Bitter
Dosha Effects: PK-V+
Tissues: Plasma, blood, fat
Actions: Purgative, anthelmintic, antipyretic, alterative
Uses: Constipation, inflammatory skin conditions, hypertension, obesity
Cautions: Hemorrhoids, inflammation of the gastrointestinal tract, diarrhea, pregnancy
Preparation and dose: Infusion- hot or cold; powder- 1 to 2 grams as purgative

Senna leaf is a strong purgative that is used only in acute constipation. It may also be used to detoxify the body, lower fever, expel worms or act as a diuretic. Ayurveda adds inflammatory skin conditions, hypertension and obesity.

Senna is a 2 foot high shrub with grayish to yellowish green leaves. "Cassia senna" or "Alexandrian senna" (Cassia acutifolia) is native to tropical Africa and cultivated in Somalia, Egypt, Sudan and elsewhere. "Tinnevelly senna" (Cassia angustifolia) is native to India and cultivated mainly in India and Pakistan.[502]

Strangely, senna is a member of the bean family, Leguminosae, so senna bushes produce pods, which also have purgative action. The pods are flat and kidney shaped, with the imprint of the seed showing through the pod. They are milder than the leaves.

Senna leaf has a bitter taste and cold energy. Ayurveda says that it will reduce kapha and is employed for clearing pitta from the small intestine. Though senna is a laxative, which theoretically should be good for vata, it is a peristalsis enhancer that will provoke vata in the long run through its bitter taste and cold energy.

Peristalsis is the wave-like motion that propels feces out of the large intestine.

When the bowel is functioning properly, muscles squeeze briefly every few seconds and then relax, propelling stool towards the rectum (*transit*). So called "stimulant" laxatives promote this wave. Among the best are senna leaf, cascara bark and aloe leaf, all of which contain closely related ingredients. They should be used only short term for brief episodes of acute constipation.

The active ingredients in senna are anthraquinone compounds. The principal active constituents are called sennosides A, B, C, and D. All the four glycosides are responsible for the activity. They are composed of various configurations of *aloe-emodin* and *rhein*, and occur as glycosides in the plant. The sennosides are water soluble, so the herb works well as tea. The anthraquinone glycosides pass unchanged into the colon where bacteria hydrolyze the glycoside bond yielding the free anthraquinones (aglycones). These free anthraquinones are absorbed into the blood, and then re-secreted into the large intestine, where they stimulate smooth muscle contraction and defecation.[503]

Because of its substantial squeezing action, senna is usually used along with warming carminative herbs, such as ginger and fennel, which reduce potential cramping.

If the herb is soaked in cold water, these resins are not extracted, so a cold infusion does have less of a laxative action. A hot senna tea is a stronger laxative.

Use caution with senna where there are hemorrhoids, inflammatory conditions of the gastro intestinal tract, diarrhea or pregnancy. Repeated use of senna or similar strong purgatives may and weaken the tone of the colon. In some people, moistening therapy and by laxative oil might be a better way to deal with chronic constipation.

Use senna tea. Brew 1-2 grams of dried leaf per day, in a combination with warming carminative herbs, such as anise, cardamom and ginger.

Sesame

Scientific Name: *Sesamum indicum*
Common Name: Sesame seeds
Ayurvedic Name(s): Tila
English Name: Sesame seeds
Family: Pedaliaceae
Part Used: Seeds
Temperature: Heating
Tastes: Sweet
Dosha Effects: V- PK or Ama + (in excess)
Tissues: Works on all tissues, especially bone
Actions: Nutritive tonic, rejuvenative, demulcent, emollient, laxative
Uses: Chronic cough, weak lungs, chronic constipation, hemorrhoids, tooth decay, receding gums, hair loss, weak bones, osteoporosis, emaciation, convalescence, dysentery, amenorrhea, dysmenorrhea
Cautions: Obesity, high pitta

PREPARATION AND DOSE: Decoction; paste; medicated oil; powder- 500 mg to 2 grams

Sesame seed is the source of most Ayurvedic massage oil.

Sesame seeds are rich in calcium. Ayurveda considers the Asian black variety to be superior.

For juvenile bed wetting, sesame seed is a miracle. The child should take 1-2 tbs of ground seeds at bedtime.

Shankpushpi

SCIENTIFIC NAME: *Evolvulus alsinoides*
COMMON NAME: Shankpushpi
AYURVEDIC NAME(S): Shankpushpi
ENGLISH NAME: Shankpushpi
FAMILY: Convolvulaceae
PART USED: Plant, juice
TEMPERATURE: Hot
TASTES: Astringent
DOSHA EFFECTS: VPK=
PRABHAVA: Improving mental clarity
TISSUES: Nerve
ACTIONS: Nervine, sedative, brain tonic
USES: Nervous debility, mental or emotional exhaustion, epilepsy, insomnia, insanity
CAUTIONS: None known
PREPARATION AND DOSE: Decoction; powder- 250mg to 1 gram

When we need mental piece and sleep, we may call upon shankhapushi to help restore clear quality of the mind and relaxation. Its flowers resemble the shankha or conch shell, thus the name. It usually is a foot tall plant, with dome of flowers, in open fields in North India.

This herb is an outstanding rejuvenative tonic for the mind and nerve tissue. The plant is said to have profound mystical properties, with an affinity for the heart, throat, third eye and crown chakras.

The herb is especially effective for mental disorders of anxiety and fear. Often taken with or prepared in ghee, it promotes tranquility without dulling the mind. In depression, it uplifts. In mania it is calming. Students may use it for exam phobia. For attention deficit disorders, it combines well with brahmi, jatamamsi, calamus and licorice.

Dr. Dever calls this herb "A Godsend for the stressed out people of the twenty first century."

For sleep, use shankpushpi at a dose of about 6 grams at bedtime.

According to the *Astanga Hridyam*, ghee, cooked three times with shankpushpi juice and milk, makes even the dullest mind sharp.[504]

Shatavari

SCIENTIFIC NAME: *Asparagus racemosus*
COMMON NAME: Shatavari
AYURVEDIC NAME(S): Shatavari ("hundred husbands")
ENGLISH NAME: Indian Asparagus
FAMILY: Liliaceae
PART USED: Root
TEMPERATURE: Cooling
TASTES: Sweet, bitter
DOSHA EFFECTS: PV- K or Ama+ (in excess)
TISSUES: Works on all tissues
ACTIONS: Tonic (general, reproductive, nervine), nutritive, rejuvenative, antacid, demulcent
USES: Debility of female organs, infertility, sexual debility, impotence, menopause, ulcers, hyperacidity, dehydration, lung abscess, cough, cancer, herpes, leucorrhea, chronic fevers
CAUTIONS: High ama, excessive mucus
PREPARATION AND DOSE: Lifetime as a tonic- 1 gram per day, acute conditions, use up to 8 grams per day as necessary.

Shatavari is the main building tonic for women in. Shatavari means "hundred husbands." I think you get the idea.

This relative of the vegetable asparagus is particularly rejuvenative to the female reproductive tract and the blood, and to build the body.

Shatavari is taken for a wide variety of acute female hormone complaints, including dysmenorrhea. This herb increases fertility, and balances female hormones, making it valuable in treating menopausal complaints, such as vaginal atrophy. It does contain phytoestrogens triterpene saponins, including shatavarin.

Shatavari is used to strengthen the immune system, increase milk and sexual secretions, and as an aphrodisiac. It increases intellect, digestion, and physical strength. A recent study found that a medicine containing shatavari reduced stress effects substantially.[505]

This herb is used as an effective moisturizer for the membranes of the lungs, digestive tract, and, like other asparagus species, the kidneys and urinary tract. The fresh root juice is used with honey for dyspepsia.[506] The tubers are candied and used as snacks.

A 1990 study revealed that shatavari is at least as effective as metoclopramide, a commonly used drug, for dyspepsia.[507] We like it as a milk decoction combined with ghee, raw sugar, and honey.

Shatavari infused oil or ghee is used for massage for nerve, joint and urinary disorders.

Shatavari is related to the Western asparagus root, which has similar properties Women in Asia start shatavari at puberty, and often take 1-2 grams per day for long periods. In many ethnic groups in Asia, menopausal complaints are almost unknown. To treat a wide variety of female hormonal symptoms (PMS, menstrual cramps, mood changes, menopausal hot flushes, etc.), higher doses can be used. Work up gradually to the dose that is effective, about 7 grams per day.

Shigru

SCIENTIFIC NAME: *Moringa oleifera*
COMMON NAME: Malunggay
AYURVEDIC NAME(S): Shigru
ENGLISH NAME: Drumstick tree
FAMILY: Moringaceae
PART USED: Leaf, seed
TEMPERATURE: Cooling
TASTES: Sweet
DOSHA EFFECTS: VPK=
TISSUES: Plasma
ACTIONS: Nutritive
USES: Food, infectious diseases, diabetes
CAUTIONS: None
PREPARATION AND DOSE: Food and beverage

The shigru tree is truly remarkable. Yet it has gone virtually unknown, except to botanists and Ayurvedic herbalists.

Moringa is a common tree, native to northern India, and cultivated throughout sub-tropical areas from West Africa to Fiji. Also known by its common names of malunggay, drumstick plant (the four foot seed pods look like drumsticks),[508] ben tree, benzolive, kelor tree and horseradish tree, it is a food and medicine source like almost no other. Probably the fastest growing tree known, it commonly reaches three meters in height just 10 months after planting. The hardy tree can grow well in the humid tropics or hot drylands, in blistering heat, desiccating dryness and impoverished soils. It campares to corn and soy in terms of food and medicine value.[509]

The Moringa tree has an impressive range of dietary benefits. According to Trees for Life, the dry leaves have four times the calcium of milk, triple the potassium of bananas, more than twice spinach's hefty iron quotient, and seven times the vitamin C of oranges.[510] They contain 17 percent protein (double that of milk) and very high amino acid content, [511] including good amounts of the sulfur-containing amino acids, methionine and cysteine, are a good source of B vitamins, are low in fat and carbohydrates and contain two to four times the beta carotene found in carrots.[512] [513] A study measuring the calcium metabolism in young mammals found that drumstick plant had close to the absorption of a milk diet.[514]

People cook and eat young tender shoots, whole young leaves and leaflets of older leaves like spinach.[515] Leaf powder can be added to sauces, soups or chowders. The seeds can be prepared as peas or roasted and eaten like peanuts.[516] The young pods are a vegetable reminiscent of asparagus. In India, Moringa fruits are added to curries.[517]

It has been estimated that a glassful of fresh leaves contains the daily requirement of vitamin A for ten people. Charities are using Moringa to prevent vitamin A deficiency childhood blindness in developing areas.

Moringa has a long history in medicine. Ayurveda has used shigru as a source of vitamin C, and for colds, boils, fever, joint pain and gout.[518] [519] Ayurveda says Moringa leaves prevent 300 diseases.

It contains compounds, including beta-sitosterol, that show hypotensive activity. Indeed, it is used in India to treat high blood pressure.[520]

The seeds and roots contain an antibiotic that treats skin infections.[521] The seeds are anti-inflammatory, antispasmodic and diuretic.[522] Moringa flowers taste like radish. They are a nectar source for honey, and can be steeped to make a tea for treating colds. The roots are a source of a spice resembling horseradish. Moringa is now available in powder, capsules, and processed for tea.

Spearmint

SCIENTIFIC NAME: *Mentha spicata*
COMMON NAME: Spearmint
AYURVEDIC NAME(S): Phudina
ENGLISH NAME: Spearmint
FAMILY: Lamiaceae
PART USED: Leaves
TEMPERATURE: Cold
TASTES: Pungent
DOSHA EFFECTS: KP-V=
TISSUES: Plasma, blood, marrow, nerves
ACTIONS: Diuretic, relaxant, carminative
USES: Urinary inflammation, digestive upset, nervousness, headache
CAUTIONS: Severe chills
PREPARATION AND DOSE: Powder -½ to 6 grams

Spearmint is mildly soothing when applied to digestive disorders, and slightly relaxing overall.

Ayurveda says that this herb clears the mind and senses, and that it is superior to peppermint as a relaxant and as a diuretic. Whereas peppermint is hot and cold, which can cause problems, spearmint is completely cooling. For an even cooler mint, see horse mint.

Use spearmint as a culinary ingredient in chutney or raita.

As are all mints, spearmint is a mild diaphoretic that is employed in cold and flu. For a diuretic effect, use spearmint as a hot tea.

As a general digestive remedy, shred a handful of washed spearmint leaves. Mix in one half teaspoon of salt, 2 teaspoons of lemon juice, one teaspoon of coriander seed powder and one teaspoon of cumin seed powder. Consume one teaspoon of the paste with each meal for a few days.

Tulsi

SCIENTIFIC NAME: *Ocimum sanctum*
COMMON NAME: Tulsi, Vishnupriya ("the beloved one of Vishnu")
AYURVEDIC NAME(S): Tulsi ("The Incomparable One"), Surasa
ENGLISH NAME: Holy basil
FAMILY: Lamiaceae
PART USED: Herb
TEMPERATURE: Hot
TASTES: Pungent, bitter
DOSHA EFFECTS: VK- P+
TISSUES: Plasma, blood, marrow, nerves, reproductive
ACTIONS: Diaphoretic, febrifuge, nervine, antispasmodic, antibacterial, antiseptic
USES: Colds, cough, sinus congestion, headaches, rheumatism, arthritis, fevers
CAUTIONS: High pitta
PREPARATION AND DOSE: Infusion, medicated ghee, powder-250 mg to 1 gram

This unassuming little garden plant plays a central role in the folk medicine of South Asia. According to de Jager, it is one of the three most sacred herbs of India, along with soma and lotus.[523] This mild medicinal herb and vegetable is cultivated near temples and private homes, where it is believed to purify the air and to sanctify the environs. The name comes from the reverence with which it is regarded in Indian culture. Tulsi is a considered to be a Goddess herself, and to serve humanity daily bey her presence here. Tulsi is considered to expand and sharpen awareness, aid meditation, and promote compassion when taken as a medicine.

Although a member of the basil genus (*Ocimum*), this particular type of basil hardly resembles the culinary variety we are used to seeing in pesto here. Much more pungent, the plant has a bitter taste, and larger leaves. Though the seeds and root are used in medicine, the leaves are the main therapeutic part of the plant.

In India, three main varieties of tulsi are available.

Rama tulsi ("Svet", or "Shukla"- white) is actually deep green, and used more for digestion. It is 3 feet high, with stems about 1/2 inch thick.

Krishna tulsi ("Shyama"- black) is deep magenta, close to purple, is used more for its detoxifying action and is hotter. It can be over 6 feet tall and 5 feet across with stems over 2 inches thick- essentially a small tree.

For the most part, though, these two varieties can be used interchangeably. The chemotypes of the two types can vary substantially, depending on where they grow.

Vana ("grove") tulsi is *Ocimum gratissimum*. It has many of the same properties as Rama and Krishna tulsi. For regular use, de Jager recommends a a blend of Rama, Krishna and Vana, 2:2:1.[524]

In Ayurvedic herbalism, sattvic tulsi is used as an expectorant and anti-mucus herb, for respiratory diseases like cold and flu.[525] It is quite warming to the body, so it will make you sweat (a diaphoretic), a characteristic that also lends itself to fever [526] and flu treatment. Diaphoretics are commonly taken internally for skin disease and itch in all systems of herbal medicine, and tulsi is no exception. A hot infusion of dried leaves is an excellent anupan for other treatments.[527] For kaphaja kasa (kapha coughs), use fresh Krishna tulsi (or substitute regular basil) juice with honey. (Juice tulsi in a wheat grass juicer.)

Tulsi's ability to bring down fever is a prabhava, or special action. Tulsi's febrifuge property works through a process that impacts more the core dynamics of the body, and so can affect deep, old, mysterious and periodic fevers, for which it is sometimes used with black pepper. A folk fever remedy includes cooking onion and tulsi in coconut oil and applying the infused oil to the head.

As a warming digestive aid, it is given for indigestion from overeating.[528] For this use, the gentle tridoshic nature is so mild that most everyone tolerates it. Tulsi strengthens all the agnis at every level.

Holy basil is a muscle relaxant, and kills intestinal parasites. Rice pudding is prepared with the soaked seeds to treat serious diarrhea.

Quite recently, tulsi is getting serious attention in the scientific literature for its exciting potential uses in several important conditions. Most important, tulsi treats diabetes, normalizing blood sugar and blood fats,[529] including cholesterol and triglycerides, factors that are integral to diabetes, as well as to other cardiovascular diseases. A recent animal study led the researchers to conclude that "The results indicated a significant reduction in fasting blood sugar, uronic acid, total amino acids, total cholesterol, triglyceride, phospholipids and total lipids. In the liver, total cholesterol, triglycerides and total lipids were significantly lowered. Total lipids were significantly reduced in the kidney. In the heart, a significant fall in total cholesterol and phospholipids was observed."[530] A paper (double blind, placebo controlled) published on stress related arterial hypertension found that, in two weeks, tulsi powder dropped the blood pressure in 25 patients an average of 26 mm Hg.[531]

For an excellent general heart tonic, combine it with the cooler arjuna.

Tulsi works for diabetes in humans. A significant, placebo controlled, crossover study showed a 17.6% reduction in blood sugar, and led the scientists to conclude that tulsi was of value in mild to moderate diabetes.[532]

The herb seems to prevent cancer and to protect against radiation damage, at least in laboratory animals. A study published in 1999, from Madras, demonstrated that hamsters were protected from developing cancer of the mouth by taking holy basil.[533] Mice survived radiation exposure when they had been administered the herb.[534] [535]

Tulsi helps shortness of breath and bronchiospasm in asthma. Holy basil kills microbes, including bacteria and fungi.[536] It has now been shown to stimulate the immune system, confirming the historical use.[537]

This versatile herb also benefits ulcers. It has been shown to reduce acid production in the stomach and increase protective mucus secretion.[538]

Tulsi is anti-inflammatory[539] and it is now presumed to have adaptogenic benefits. Traditionally, tulsi was thought to protect against damage from stress. Modern research now confirms it.[540] As a tonic, de Jager compares it to ginseng and maca.[541]

Finally, research reveals that tulsi is an antioxidant- not surprising, considering its high flavonoid content, and its clinical effects.[542]

Tulsi treats gray hair (palita), a pitta condition. The same special property that allows warming tulsi to reduce fever is at play here. Oils with tulsi are available for scalp application, or nasya, or drink tulsi tea.

Traditionally, tulsi is given as a tea, in a dose of 3 tsp. of dry herb, brewed into water, per day. Tulsi is a very mild and safe herb, however, and some people have more success with higher doses. Gradually increase the amount of tea until you get the results you are looking for, or until you have any digestive distress, which is very unlikely. You may also drink the fresh juice, taking about one-half ounce three times a day. It has been historically combined with ginger and black pepper for asthma, or combined with honey for bronchitis for cough.

The essential oil is inserted in the ear for ear infection. Make an infused tulsi ear oil by cooking tulsi leaf in mustard oil and adding fresh garlic juice.

Tulsi opens the heart and mind, and encourages devotion. Using tulsi herbally supports the energy of attachment, the energy that draws prosperity near, and keeps it in our lives. Energetically, tulsi also clears the aura and stimulates the immune system.

Turmeric

SCIENTIFIC NAME: *Curcuma longa*
COMMON NAME: Turmeric
AYURVEDIC NAME(S): Haldi, Haridra
ENGLISH NAME: Turmeric
FAMILY: Zingiberae
PART USED: Root (rhizome)
TEMPERATURE: Hot
TASTES: Bitter, astringent, pungent (mildly)
DOSHA EFFECTS: K- PV+ (in excess)
TISSUES: Works on all tissues
ACTIONS: Antihepatotoxic, anti-inflammatory, antiarthritic, cholagogue, choleretic, carminative, cyclooxygenase inhibiting, antifertility, topical antibacterial and antifungal, hypotensive, anti-atherosclerotic, anticancer

USES: Jaundice, gallstones, hemorrhage, bruises, colic, arthritis, sprains, wounds, toothache, flatulence, prevents cataracts

CAUTIONS: Pregnancy, bile duct obstruction

PREPARATION AND DOSE: Infusion- 1 tsp/cup water; 1:0.85 tincture- 10 to 40 gtt per day-4 times per day; raw powder- up to 30 grams per day (Khalsa)

Sally Manday had eczema. Her skin was so damaged that blood soaked through the bandages in which she was forced to wrap her arms. Already 40 years old, Sally has endured chronic eczema since childhood. Over the decades it had worsened until it covered every inch of her body below the neck. She was miserable and depressed about her future.

Ironically, Sally was very conscious about her health. She ate an excellent diet, used herbs and vitamins, and had a generally healthy lifestyle, but she had never been able to get control of her skin, despite numerous programs from various practitioners. The dose of steroids necessary to control the eczema produced intolerable side effects.

When a friend asked Sally if she'd finally had enough, she replied that she was willing to try anything Yogi Bhajan recommended a rigorous program of herbs and diet, centered on turmeric, in the startling (to Sally, at least) dose of one ounce per day. She was desperate though, and began the treatment. The results were dramatic.

Within days, Sally's skin began to respond. She faithfully continued to take her turmeric. By the end of the six weeks, she had a patch the size of a dime on one hand, which was shrinking rapidly. The entire rest of her body was covered with fresh new skin!

All this happened fifteen years ago. Sally has not had a speck of eczema since then. She now manages her skin only with diet, and one or two capsules of turmeric per day, or perhaps a pinch in her food. For such a mild mannered kitchen herb, turmeric sure packs a punch.

This valuable medicine, said by many in India to be the most important, is my (Khalsa's) favorite herb. After learning about it over thirty years ago from Yogi Bhajan, I've gotten to know it as an old and trusted friend. In fact, I'm known in the herb world as "Mr. Turmeric." The more I use this yellow wonder, the more uses it seems to have. I call it "the medicine cabinet in a jar."

Turmeric is a perennial herb of the ginger family. The yellow rhizome is the medicinal portion. Grown in South Asia, turmeric, sometimes called Indian saffron, is the ingredient that gives the yellow color to curry powder and Yellow Thai dishes. It is extensively used for flavor and color in many foods around the world. India, which produces nearly the whole world's crop, uses 80% of it. The United States is the largest importer of turmeric in the world, where it is used almost exclusively to color prepared mustard.

Turmeric has wide application and is used to treat, among other conditions, arthritis, ulcer, flatulence, bloody urine, bruises, colic, chest pain, jaundice, menstrual difficulties, hemorrhage, and toothache. Yoga practitioners take it to benefit the musculoskeletal system.

Fresh turmeric has an aromatic and spicy fragrance, which gives way to a more medicinal aroma when dried. Over time, the smell becomes earthier. It has a warm, bitter taste. In India, it is used in almost every dish- especially with lentils and potatoes. Use it sparingly in vegetable or bean dishes, along with other warming spices like garlic and cinnamon, and to offset sweet tasting condiments such as dried fruits or onions.

In herbal terms, turmeric is described as aromatic, stimulant, tonic, carminative, anthelmintic, vulnerary and antibacterial.

Turmeric has adaptogen-like properties. Although adaptogens typically act on the endocrine system, turmeric's effects do not seem to be by this route. Perhaps its benefits are better termed "protective."

The active principles, "curcuminoids," are recognized for broad range of activity and safety. In addition to strong antioxidant properties, these compounds are strongly anti-inflammatory, as well as broadly immune enhancing and detoxifying. Turmeric contains powerful free radical scavengers.[543]

Turmeric is very safe, and is widely used in food, so modest doses are fine to use. Amounts of as little as 1 gram per day have been shown to have clinical effects.

Curcumin is the compound that makes turmeric yellow. It is the most researched constituent of the herb, and is mainly responsible for turmeric's anti-inflammatory properties. It is unlikely, however, that curcumin accounts for the totality of the broad spectrum action of the herb. Subjectively, herbalists say that for many conditions, they have seen better results with the whole herb than with curcumin alone.

Curcumin is one of the diaryl heptanoids known collectively as curcuminoids that comprise about 5 % of turmeric. A polyphenol, curcumin (chemically termed "diferuloyl methane"), has actions similar to other polyphenols.

Curcumin has no known toxicity. Extremely high doses of turmeric, its alcohol extract, and pure curcumin do not produce undesired effects in any animal studied.

The mechanism of action is not well understood in curcumin's case. Some evidence suggests that it acts to promote steroid secretion in the adrenal glands, while other evidence contradicts this theory. We do know that two primary actions are inhibition of lipoxygenase, and antioxidant effects, similar to other polyphenols.

One study demonstrated that curcumin has a novel mechanism of action, distinct from the main categories of anti-inflammatory drugs, such as salicylates (like aspirin) and glucocorticoids (like prednisone). Finding an anti-inflammatory different from these typical categories is truly a breakthrough.

First and foremost, turmeric curbs inflammation. One of the active ingredients, curcumin, the pigment that give turmeric its distinctive yellow color, has anti-inflammatory effects comparable to cortisone and phenylbutazone, the standard in drugs for inflammation.[544] Curcumin is nonsteroidal, so it has none of the ravaging side effects of steroid anti-inflammatories.[545] One of the most famous uses for turmeric is the treatment of inflammatory skin disease. These anti-inflammatory qualities make turmeric suitable for the treatment of conditions as diverse as gum disease and carpal tunnel syndrome.

Curcumin also treats pain directly. Like another medicinal spice, cayenne, it depletes nerve endings of substance P, the pain receptor neurotransmitter.[546] Research shows that curcumin and related compounds suppress pain through a mechanism similar to many drugs (COX-I and COX-II enzymes).[547] Recently, turmeric has been shown to enhance wound healing. Recently, a study looked at a combination of exceptional herbs, including turmeric. Forty-two patients with osteoarthritis were randomly assigned to receive an Ayurvedic preparation, containing (per capsule) 450 mg of ashwaganda, 100 mg of Boswellia, 50 mg of turmeric, and 50 mg of a zinc complex, or a placebo, for three months. The dosage was two capsules three times per day, after meals. The treatments were then crossed over. Compared with placebo, the herb combination significantly reduced the severity of pain and the disability score. No side effects required discontinuation of treatment.

An animal study from England, published in 2003, found that turmeric improved osteoarthritis.

Turmeric has historically been used as an external poultice for sprains and sore joints.

Turmeric has a wealth of benefits for the digestive system. Historically, this medicine has been used to reduce gas (a *carminative*),[548] a function that is now getting increasing scientific support. Another compound in this herb, *p-tolymethylcarbinol*, increases the production of several important secretions in the digestive tract.

Turmeric is widely use for indigestion, and there is some scientific evidence that curcumin treats dyspepsia. A double-blind placebo-controlled study with 106 patients measured the effects of 500 mg curcumin 4 times daily against placebo. Seven days into the study, 87% percent of the curcumin group experienced full or partial dyspepsia symptom relief, compared to 53% of the placebo group.[549]

With its ability to suppress inflammation, increase mucin content of the stomach, and stop bleeding, turmeric prevents and treats ulcerations of all types, including gastritis, peptic ulcer, and irritable bowel syndrome/ colitis.[550] Turmeric is a wonder for colitis, with its pain, inflammation, mucous membrane damage, and diarrhea. Use two heaping Tablespoons of turmeric powder, and two heaping tablespoons of slippery elm bark powder, mixed into a paste with water or maple syrup, per day.

Hemorrhoids respond particularly well to turmeric, which, in addition to oral use, can be applied topically as a paste. Apply a paste of turmeric, mustard oil and onion juice. Turmeric based hemorrhoids creams are widely available in Asia. This paste is bright yellow, however, so remember, you may end up being yellow where you won't want to be yellow! (Only temporarily, though.)

One of the most famous uses for turmeric is the treatment of inflammatory skin disease, for which it is used internally. Use up to 15 grams per day.

In fact, turmeric is a good general treatment for all connective tissue. Being a polyphenol, curcumin has the property of stabilizing collagen. It is used to enhance healing after surgery, reducing adhesions and scarring.

Turmeric is particularly appropriate in treating inflammatory skin diseases, such as psoriasis and eczema, as it reduces heat and cleanses the liver. These qualities make it perfect to consider for all herpes diseases (oral, genital, shingles). It is also touted for urticaria.

Externally, haldi is the supreme skin medicine. In Asia, a myriad of turmeric ointments is available for acne, dermatitis, and psoriasis. Of course, they turn your skin yellow for a while...

Or use it as an ubtan. Mix turmeric with garbanzo flour, sesame or almond oil, a little fresh cream and honey.[551] Herbalist de Jager, who is known in India as "Haldi Baba" (Sir Turmeric), suggests treating a bleeding cut by pressing the cut into a small cup of turmeric powder. When it happened to him, he said, "After a few seconds I took my finger out and the bleeding stopped. The wound never bled again and healed quickly. I am still amazed every time I use this trick for cuts and lacerations."[552]

Since turmeric both kills insects, and heals skin lesions, it's not surprising that a combination of turmeric and neem, another Ayurvedic insecticidal herb, applied topically, eradicated scabies in 97 % of the people treated, within 3 to 15 days. This formula is also traditional for ringworm.

Turmeric is a significant antioxidant. Again, curcumin is the main recognized constituent, but other ingredients are also active. This herb works about as well as vitamin C or E.[553]

Turmeric has been shown, at least in rats, to prevent cataract formation.[554] This remedy is a classic Ayurvedic treatment for all "leaky" conditions. An astringent, it helps curb bleeding or other fluid excesses, and pulls in tissue that's prolapsed, so it's appropriate for "wet" macular degeneration. It's also a very effective anti-inflammatory, and works well for inflammatory conditions in the eye. A typical dose of turmeric to control active inflammation would be about ½ ounce of the powder per day, and for prevention, a teaspoon, or 2 capsules, would do. Applied as a wash, it can used for inflamed eye conditions (conjunctivitis, opthalmia).

Since macular degeneration is strongly associated with atherosclerosis, any treatment that remediates that condition could be beneficial.

Modern research suggests that turmeric has broad anticancer effects. It affects cancer during initiation, promotion, and progression of the tumors.[555] Several studies suggest that turmeric can also cause cancer to regress.

Turmeric and curcumin have action against several potent carcinogens, including cigarette smoke.[556] In smokers, turmeric given at 1.5 grams per day for 30 days substantially reduced the formation of mutagenic (cancer causing) chemicals. It is estimated that 500mg (less than 1/2 a teaspoon) of turmeric per day in the diet could eliminate DNA damage characteristic of the development of cancer.

Another recent study reported a 68% reduction of cancer in animals following treatment with curcurnin.

Turmeric is also used in the treatment of benign tumors. Ayurveda recommends it specifically in the treatment of breast or uterine cysts and tumors.

Bitter herbs are generally known to promote bile flow. Curcumin has been shown to increase bile acid output by over 100%, and to increase the solubility of the bile, all qualities that lend turmeric to the treatment of gallstones. Classically, it is used mixed with barberry.

Antioxidant curcumin protects the liver about as well as licorice root and milk thistle, well known herbs for that use, which supports the historical high regard in Asia for turmeric as a liver herb. It also reduces liver enzymes, clinical signs of inflammatory liver disease.[557] [558] These same qualities indicate the use of turmeric for the treatment of alcohol abuse.

As a liver cleanse, Yogi Bhajan recommended a 72 hour monodiet of a milk decoction of turmeric, cinnamon, clove, black pepper, ginger and cardamom, as much as desired.[559] Break the monodiet with kicharee or light fruit.

Turmeric is called a blood purifier, and has been compared to the herb chaparral in its action. It should be noted that the molecular structure of curcumin is very similar to that of NDGA, the active constituent of chaparral.

Turmeric normalizes cholesterol. One constituent, dimethylbenzyl alcohol, reduces serum cholesterol (in the blood), while curcumin removes accumulation of cholesterol in the liver. The anticholesterol action includes reducing intestinal cholesterol uptake, increasing the conversion of cholesterol into bile acids, and increasing the excretion of bile acids.

As a hemostatic, turmeric is effective at reducing bleeding. One herbalist reports seeing an emergency oral dose of two heaping Tablespoons of turmeric powder control the crisis in a case of bright red blood pumping from the rectum.

Turmeric reduces arterial plaque. Since it inhibits platelet aggregation, it can benefit circulation in many ways, including reducing the accumulation of deposits on arterial walls. A recent study showed that it reduced smooth muscle damage in the artery, the beginning step in atherosclerosis (hardening of the arteries). Turmeric would wisely be used in artery disease or in recovery from bypass surgery or angioplasty.

Anemia benefits from turmeric, as it facilitates the production of new blood cells. Its unique combination of characteristics makes it suitable in the treatment of varicose veins.

Long used as a respiratory herb, turmeric excels in reducing cough, for which it is often mixed as a household remedy with coriander and cumin. Gargle with warm turmeric tea, or drink turmeric boiled in milk to relieve coughs and sinus congestion.

As an astringent and anti-inflammatory herb, turmeric is effective as a gargle for sore throat. Bitter herbs, generally, are known to be cooling. Turmeric can be used for severe sore throat with fever. It is often administered in combination with ghee (clarified butter) for this condition.

Clearly, its anti-inflammatory and anti-bacterial properties make turmeric ideal for treating bronchitis. Asian herbalists use it for asthma.

Turmeric has a long history as an antimicrobial, which is now being supported by modern research. The herb inhibits a wide variety of microbes, including staph, strep, amoebas, and several disease-causing fungi. Curcumin evens inhibits HIV.[560] Ayurveda recommends it as an antibacterial for those chronically weak or ill.[561] Turmeric is used, internally and externally, for the treatment of boils. It is also antifungal and anthelmintic, acting especially against Entamoeba histolytica.

This herb is antidiabetic in its action, and will help normalize blood sugar. Its action on the liver, cholesterol levels, and lipids generally assist in diabetes. It treats diabetic ulcer, whether used orally or applied to the wound.

Turmeric is an emmenagogue and a mild menstrual regulator. As such, it is the best general spice for women to move stagnant blood.

Conditions which are treated with nervine and anti-spasmodic herbs can respond to turmeric, for which it is often used with bayberry.

Body weight and appetite will respond to turmeric. It is used in Asia to reduce obesity and in the treatment of anorexia.

Being anti-inflammatory and astringent, it is a superb medicine for oral care. Many Asian tooth and gum preparations are made with turmeric. As well, it can be used for toothache.

Though supported by scant scientific literature, turmeric is widely used in Ayurvedic asthma regimes, with the same use being clinically supported by several American herbalists.

With its noted anti-inflammatory and skin healing properties, turmeric is applied as a cream or pack for connective tissue conditions. In Asia, it is mixed with honey and rubbed on the body for strains, sprains, bruises, and itching.

As a paste it is a first aid treatment for wounds. When prepared as an eye wash, it shows effectiveness in conjunctivitis and opthalmia.

Remember that turmeric is bright yellow, and stains the skin (and everything else it touches, like your toothbrush and your pajamas)! American patients may have difficulty with compliance, as bright yellow skin has not yet become fashionable here.

Turmeric is a mild herb. For acute inflammation, like a sore knee from a long bike ride, the dose might be as high as one ounce (4 Tbs.) per day. Stir the powder into water and swallow, or make it into a paste with honey or a bite of oatmeal. For smaller doses, less serious conditions or ongoing health benefit, use 1 gram per day in capsules. If using standardized extract, containing a high proportion of curcumin, the dose is 1500 mg of total curcumin content per day.

Getting the Turmeric Down

1) Golden Milk: increase turmeric proportion if desired. Prepare in two parts:

a)Prepare a golden yellow turmeric paste by mixing a 1/4 cup of turmeric powder to 1/2 cup of pure water and boiling in a saucepan until a thick paste is formed. This paste may be stored in the refrigerator.

b)After the paste is made, for each cup of golden milk, blend together 1 cup of milk, 1 teaspoon almond oil or any vegetable oil, 1/4 teaspoon of turmeric paste prepared above (or more if necessary), and honey to taste. While stiffing on a low heat, bring the milk just to the boiling point. The mixture may then be blended in an electric blender to make a beautiful foamy drink. Fruit may be added before blending. Serve with a little cinnamon sprinkled on top.

2) Stir in water/milk/juice/tea. Swallow quickly.

3) Stir into sweetener (honey, maple syrup) to make a paste, swallow from spoon.

4) Mix with thick, strong tasting food (i.e. peanut butter), swallow.

5) Mix with water to form *soft* paste. Spoon to the back of throat. Swallow. Follow with water/juice/tea.

Mix: 1/2 pint sesame tahini
2 Tbs. sesame oil (or other)
1/4 cup honey
1/4 cup lemon juice
1/4 to 1/2 cup turmeric powder

6) Sandwich: Make turmeric paste as in golden milk recipe. Spread paste ¼ inch thick on both slices of broad. Add condiments: lettuce, parsley, etc. Include cucumber slices. Close and eat.

Valerian

SCIENTIFIC NAME: *Valeriana officinalis*
COMMON NAME: Valerian
AYURVEDIC NAME(S): Tagara
ENGLISH NAME: Valerian
FAMILY: Valerianaceae
PART USED: Root
TEMPERATURE: Hot
TASTES: Pungent
DOSHA EFFECTS: VK- P+
TISSUES: Plasma, muscle, marrow, nerve
ACTIONS: Sedative, hypnotic, nervine, hypotensive, antispasmodic, anticonvulsant
USES: Insomnia, exhaustion, restlessness, hysteria, pain, anxiety, cardiovascular arrhythmias, Attention deficit hyperactivity disorder (ADHD), gastrointestinal and menstrual cramping, shingles, backaches
CAUTIONS: Potentiates sleeping time induced by barbituates
PREPARATION AND DOSE: Infusion- 1 to 2 tsp/cup water; 1:1 tincture: 10-60 gtt

per day-4 times per day; capsules: 2-10 grams (Khalsa)

Valerian is a relaxant herb that has a calming effect on the autonomic nervous system. It is a good short-term sedative that works quickly, offering a healthy, nontoxic alternative to strong prescription drugs. [562 563]

For insomnia, valerian is taken right at bedtime to help induce sleep quickly.[564] Valerian is best for insomniacs who have trouble falling asleep, because it decreases the amount of time it takes to fall asleep, but doesn't necessarily work on the length of sleep.

Because this is a mild herb, you may need five to ten capsules to get the desired result; valerian cannot be thought of like a "sleeping pill" which is generally much stronger and just requires just one or two tablets. One or two valerian capsules or tablets may work simply for calming nerves, but more may be required as a sleep aid. Start with a lower number and work up till you get the desired result.

Valerian is used widely in Europe and many of the studies showing its effectiveness have been conducted there. In the past 35 years, more than 200 scientific studies have been done on valerian. In much of Europe, physicians are more likely to recommend valerian instead of pharmaceuticals. Valerian is an active ingredient in about 150 over-the-counter medicines in Germany, including some preparations for children. (In fact, some studies have shown positive effects on hyperactive children.)

It has antispasmodic action, so it is used for cramps of all types, including menstrual cramps. Antispasmodics reduce gut cramping and movement. Valerian root is a classic antispasmodic for digestive disorders.

Ayurveda considers valerian to be one of the best all around remedies for vata disorders, including intestinal gas and pain. As a warming herb, relaxing valerian is an excellent balancing remedy for the coldness of vata.

In the U.S. its recommended that valerian not be used by children, pregnant women or nursing women, except on the advice of a health practitioner.

A typical dose of valerian root, powdered in capsules, would be 1,000- 3,000 mg, as necessary, several times per day, for anxiety, or 5,000 mg or more, as necessary, as a one-time dose, before bed, to relax for sleep.

Jatamansi root (*Nardostachys jatamansi* syn *Valeriana jatamansi*) is a close relative of valerian, and is used in essentially the same way. They are, for all intents and purposes, interchangeable. Jatamansi is more tridoshic than valerian, with a cooler energy. Either might be used under the name Tagara. Use them as alternates. It never hurts to have alternative remedies for anxiety and insomnia. Some folks may resond to one more than the other.

Jatamansi is antispasmodic and carmintive, so it is used for colitis. It is sedative, and widely used in relaxant formulas.

Vamsha Rochana

SCIENTIFIC NAME: *Bambusa arundinaceae*
COMMON NAME: Tabasheer
AYURVEDIC NAME(S): Vamsha-rochana
ENGLISH NAME: Bamboo Manna
FAMILY: Graminaceae
PART USED: Milky bark of the plant, or sap can be used as substitute
TEMPERATURE: Cooling
TASTES: Sweet, astringent
DOSHA EFFECTS: PV- K+
TISSUES: Plasma, blood, marrow, nerve
ACTIONS: Demulcent, expectorant, tonic, rejuvenative, hemostatic, antispasmodic,
USES: Colds, coughs, fever, asthma, bleeding disorders, emaciation, debility, dehydration, palpitations, vomiting
CAUTIONS: Can increase congestion (to avoid- balance out with pungent herbs like pippali and ginger)
PREPARATION AND DOSE: Decoction; milk decoction; powder 250mg to 1 gram

Bamboo manna (milky bark) is mainly used in cold and flu preparations as an expectorant and cough remedy. It is a main ingredient in Sitopladi Churna, a cold and flu remedy. It is demulcent, and could increase congestion, so it is combined with warming herbs, especially ginger.

It is also demulcent and tonic, so it lowers vata, and all vata related disorders. It nurtures the heart and liver and soothes vata in the nervous system. Vata disorders of anxiety and tissue depletion respond to vamsha-rochana.

It is a mild, food-like medicine that is often given in milk decoction.

· NINE ·

NON-HERBAL AND MINERAL MEDICINES

According to Ayurveda, any substance can be used as a food, a drug, or a poison. Ayurveda also says that the best medicines make the best poisons, and the best poisons make the best medicines. All this is just another way of saying that "the dose makes the poison."

While most Ayurvedic medicine is herbal, there are some notable exceptions. Ayurveda uses a wide array of substances from the earth as medicine. In particular, Ayurveda has developed a system of preparing and administering mineral medicines that is quite extraordinary. Things as various as mineral pitch scraped from a warm cliff face in the summer to ground diamonds have their place. We will discuss a selection of these famous Asian medicines and compare them to the herbal medicines that make up the backbone of Ayurvedic therapeutics.

Bhasma

Bhasmas are preparations in which metals, after purifications, are reduced to their oxide or sulfide form, while pishti is a preparation in which they are treated with rose water washes, called *Bhawnas*, and dried.

Rasa Shastra (rasa, mercury, shastra, literature) is the science of metals, minerals, gemstones and their processing.[565] Metallic medicines have several advantages over herbs. The doses are smaller, and there is no bad taste, so compliance is good. They assimilate very rapidly. They penetrate deeply into all the tissues. They last a long time, as they never spoil. They become more potent as they age, and have no date of expiration date. They have no seasonal harvest issues.

Here's an explanation from Yogi Bhajan. "Herbs are very slow, snail type of remedies. They are not extract, they don't go right in and push in, they change the metabolism slowly and work on the root cause of what the disease is about. Allopathic medicine goes in, turns the disease upside down, and goes out, so you get it again every six months or once a year, you know."

"Ayurveda can be so potent, and they know how to make it potent- so potent that some of the medicine they give you on the tip of the match stick. They just put on the match stick and they put it on your tongue and give you a little water, and say that's it- you are cured- and you get cured. It takes about ten, twenty days for you to get cured."

"I saw this happening. I took my friend from London. He has a tumor in the brain, and they said if they will operate the chances of life is sixty/forty- sixty percent he will die, forty percent he will live. It was not sixty/forty that way."

"So I took him to this vaidya of mine and he asked me privately, "Does he have money?" I said, "Sure he has a lot of money." He said, "Well, then we can make the medicine."

"You know, we made a medicine in India. It cost us lot. I mean, doctor, you know how much money it cost. It costs tons of money because they use gold, they use diamond, they use lot of stuff. They make ash out of the whole thing."

"What was that? Twelve carats of diamond, of one carat each, without a black spot. So we found it. We brought it and gave it to him- something like that- gold and sliver leaves and this and that. So he burned it to ash- the whole thing, the whole thing- and he gave it to him. He just put it on that stick and put it in his mouth- that's all. It was a lot- it was almost a cup. And he said, "You are cured. The rest I'll keep, because lot of poor people will come who can't afford it, and I'll give it to them free, but at your expense. Now you are cured."

"He came in he said, "My God, thousands of pounds," (He is an Englishman.) "Thousand of pounds have been spent and, God, he just put it on and I didn't even feel it on my tongue. It was kind of a sand."

"I said, "Whatever it is, just see."

"So after ten day we were returning. I said, "Go and get your that brain thing done."

"They couldn't find a thing. They said, "You are all right."

"And he was telling the doctor, "I still feel pressure."

"He said, "For what? There is nothing" He said, "Look at your own picture. It's gone. The whole tumor in the brain got dissolved."

He was okay.

"So that is Ayurvedic medicine. If they can't diagnose you, they can pinpoint. They can really take care of you." [566]

The most important bhasma, rasa, is made from incinerated mercury. It is the only remedy to contain all six tastes. It is a long acting energizer and general tonic that nourishes all tissues, starting with rasa. Substitute mercury with magnetic iron if desired. Ghandak bhasma (purified sulfur oxide) is a remedy for mercury poisoning. Tillotson says, "They say that the sulfur bhasma removes the mercury from the system, and they have lots of experience as they work with mercury in their medicine making."[567]

Makaradhwaj is a well known bhasma made from mercury. It is a sublimed material made from mercury, sulphur and gold. Eight parts of mercury and one part of gold leaf are mixed together to form an amalgam. To this mixture, 16 parts of sublimed sulphur are added, and the mixture is pulverized very thoroughly in a stone mortar for 24 hrs, or longer, until the whole is converted to a dull powder of uniform consistency. This powder is placed in a narrow mouthed bottle and gradually heated on a sand bath. The bottle becomes filled with red fumes. On cooling, the red Makaradwaj has sublimed on the inner surface of the neck of the bottle.

It is seldom used alone, but usually given with honey or other anupans. It is used for adults and children, the dose adjusted according to age. Makaradwaj is thought to be a wonderful tonic and is said to increase longevity. It is used in debilitating conditions and after acute illness, in failing circulation and cardiac asthenia. It increases the red blood cells and improves general nutrition. It is said to be of great value in gas and indigestion. It is used widely as an aphrodisiac.

Cinnabar (shingraf, hingula) is a fine grained, dark red, very heavy mineral ore of mercury. It has the same chemical composition as Makaradwaj, but does not have the same properties, as it has not been incinerated and prepared as a bhasma. Purified cinnabar (Shuddha hingula) is made by grinding the raw ore with goat's milk for 6 hours, after which it is ground with lime juice for another hour. This cycle is repeated 7 times!

Purified mercury (often called parad) is thought to be tonic, detoxifying, purgative, cholagogue, antibacterial and sialagogue. It incrcases red blood cell count. In large doses, it is toxic. It has all six tastes, and nourishes all the dhatus. It is the ultimate yogavahi, and will carry many medicines to any tissue.

Hingula is used in liver disorders, such as the early stages of cirrhosis, dyspepsia and chronic diarrhea. It also finds uses in diabetes.

Of course, contemporary medicine does not agree with using mercury in any form.

Medhya therapy promotes intellect, or wisdom. For medhya, anything that promotes the sattva guna can be considered. Ayurvedic alchemical bhasma preparations, including panna (emerald), swarn (gold) and heera (diamonds) can be effective.

MINERAL BHASMA PREPARATIONS

Medicine	Active Ingredients	Therapeutic use	Dose
Abhrak Bhasma	Mica & juices of several indigenous drugs	Tonic & hematinic, used in chronic asthma, phthisis, old age debility, gives strength, whooping cough, asthma, semenuria, diabetes, carbuncle, puerperal disease, diability, dry cough, chronic diarrhea, colic, abdominal tumor, loss of appetite, anorexia, hyperacidity, hemorrhagic jaundice and bleedings piles, heart disease, epilepsy, dysuria	250 mg

DIAMOND BHASMA	Diamond ash	Strength, tissue firmness, aphrodisiac, eyesight, chronic debilitating diseases (cancer, diabetes)	50 mg
GANDHAK RASAYANA	Sulfur bhasma prepared with cow's milk, cardamom, cinnamon, guduchi. Triphala, dry ginger, Bringraj, fresh ginger	Blood purifier. Gout, skin disease, dental abscess, arthritis, diabetes, hemorrhoids, used to treat mercury poisoning	500 mg
KANTLAUH BHASMA	Magnetic iron	Antirheumatic & hematinic. Used in anemia.	125 mg with honey
LAUH BHASMA	Iron	Restorative, hematinic & astringent. Indicated in anemic conditions, disorders of liver & spleen, jaundice, edema and general debility. Increase hemoglobin content of blood. Anaemia, seminal weakness, leucorrhoea, obesity, leprosy, abdominal and vata diseases	125 mg with honey
MAKARADHWAJ	Red mercuric sulfide with gold	Strong heart tonic, aphrodisiac, rejuvenator. Respiratory disease. (Seldom used alone. Usually with anupan.)	50 mg
MANDOOR BHASMA	Reduced iron	Alterative, hematinic & diuretic. Used in anemia, edema, rickets & jaundice. Liver problems caused due to anemia, dyspepsia and jaundice.	250 to 750 mg with honey
MANIKYA BHASMA	Ruby	Nervine & heart tonic. Used in nervous & general debility	65 to 130 mg with honey
MAYUR CHANDRIKA BHASMA	Mayur pankha (peacock feather)	Antispasmodic & antiemetic. Useful in urinary disorders, female disorders and general debility.	250 mg with honey
MOTI BHASMA	Pearl and ghritkumari rasa	Antacid, nervine, sedative & alterative. Used in hyperacidity, asthma, cough & nervous excitement, growing children & pregnant women.	65 to 130 mg with honey
PRAWAL BHASMA	Coral	Antacid, used in cough, scrofulous affections, spermatorrhea, pulmonary hemorrhage & calcium deficiency	125 to 750 mg with honey

Raupya Bhasma	Purified silver	Cool, sour. Cools mind and emotions. Nervine sedative & aphrodisiac. Used in mental diseases, general debility, uterine diseases & irritability of uterus.	65 to 130 mgs with honey
Shankh Bhasma	Conch shell	Carminative & analgesic. Used in colic and flatulence.	250 to 750 mgs with honey
Swarna Bhasma	Pure gold	Sweet, bitter, hot, oily, heavy, nervine tonic, aphrodisiac, emmenagogue & increase sexual power, stimulates activity of stomach, skin and kidney causing diaphoresis. Intelligence and memory. Is a very potent medicine. Can revive a dying patient. Indicated in tuberculosis, chronic fever, general weakness and impotence.	32 to 125 mgs with honey
Tamra Bhasma	Copper	Bitter, hot. Strongly detoxifying for kapha and vata. Astringent, sedative, antispasmodic, antiseptic. Used in cough, asthma and liver disorders.	65 to 130 mgs with honey
Vanga Bhasma	Tin	Inflammation of stomach and other mucous membranes. Mix with shilajit and mica bhasma. Diuretic & urinary antiseptic. Used in urinary disorders and general debility. Impotence, diabetes, peptic ulcer, skin diseases.	125 to 250 mgs
Yasad Bhasma	Zinc	Alterative, diuretic and hypoglycemic & astringent. Internal hemorrhage, diabetes, urinary disorders and night sweats in tuberculosis. It is the remedy of leucorrhoea, cough, gonorrhea, diarrhea, semenuria, chronic fever, anemia, dyspnea, scrofula, goiter, tuberculosis and edema.	125 to 250 mgs with honey
Akik Bhasma	Akik & Ghrit Kumari rasa	Haemostatic & antacid, used in hemorrhage, epilepsy, weak heart or eye, asthma, bronchitis & restores strength & vigor.	375 mg with honey

Baikrant Bhasma	Baikrant (Tournabin) & juices & indigenous drugs.	Used in old age, in TB, general debility and as a substitute for Diamond Bhasma.	130 mg with honey
Godanti (Harital) Bhasma	Godanti & Ghritkumari rasa	Emmenagogue, anti-spasmodic, tonic, antacid. Used in influenza, cough, headache, malarial fever. Cephalgia, vomiting, leucorrhoea, constipation, dyspepsia and malarial fever.	375 mg with honey
Hazrulyahud Bhasma	Hazrulyahud	Antacid, bladder stone, suppression of urinary secretion & burning urination.	375 to 750 mg with milk
Kansya Bhasma	Kansya	Used in asthma, cough, diabetes, debility.	125 to 375 mg with honey
Kapardak Bhasma	Yellow Kapardaka & lemon Juice	Antacid, carminative & antispasmodic. Used in abdominal colic, dyspepsia, diarrhea, anorexia & calcium deficiency.	250 to 500 mg with honey
Kasheesh Bhasma	Kasheesh & amla juice	Hematinic & alterative. Used in anemia, enlargement of liver and spleen, abdominal diseases, cough & general weakness, low blood pressure, emaciation, leprosy, vata disease.	125 to 250 mg with milk
Kukutandtvak Bhasma	Kukukutandatwak	Tonic & alterative. Used in rickets, leucorrhoea, seminal defects & night discharge.	250 to 375 mg with honey

Figure 24 Bhasma Preparations

Shilajit

This famous medicine is a tarry black or brown substance that exudes from rock cliffs, primarily in the Himalayas. It is thought to be an aged form of a prehistoric herb which is seeping to the earth's surface, but its origin still remains obscure. The tar is purified, dried, and encapsulated.[568]

While not an herb per se, shilajit is a very popular remedy.

Shilajit has a great reputation as a prime drug in a variety of diseases. Shilajit is strongly rasayana, and yogavahi. It helps in revitalization of tissues and improves assimilation and metabolism. It strengthens the nervous system and increase sexual stamina. It is unusual for one medicine to be strongly detoxifying and simultaneously building, so shilajit is a treasure. It will increase strength and stamina, even for a healthy person.

Shilajit is a general detoxifier and rejuvenator, and is particularly useful in diabetes.

It is the best medicine for tonifying the kidneys and urinary system. It dissolves kidney stones.

Stir shilajit into warm milk for a rasayana effect, or obtain it encapsulated. The tar consistency makes it messy and difficult to deal with.

The dose of shilajit is quite small, so compliance is good. That is a big advantage. A typical dose is only 1 to 2 grams per day.

Here is one program for a deep cleanse with shilajit:[569]

- Prepare the body with oleation.
- Purify the body with appropriate therapies (cleansing the stomach, small intestine and large intestine)
- Consume ghee prepared with drugs of bitter taste for three days
- Take shilajit with the decoction of triphala for three days

Sulfur Preparations

Sulfur is an essential nutrient in the human body. We actually use a considerable amount of sulfur for our daily lives. In fact, about 0.25% of our body weight is sulfur. Generally, sulfur performs a detoxifying function. In plant medicines and foods, sulfur is the active ingredient in onions, garlic and cabbage, and the chemical that gives them their characteristic smell. Ayurveda uses many forms of sulfur as medicine.

Sulfur is part of the chemical structure of numerous necessary nutrients in the diet, and we all eat a small amount in food every day. It is abundant in keratin, a protein that strengthens hair, nails, and skin.

Sulfur plays a role in the production of collagen, a skin protein that helps keep connective tissue elastic and healthy.

Yogi Bhajan taught about the combination of sulfur, cloves and honey as a blood cleanser. Khalsa has used this formula in scores of cases to treat inflammatory skin conditions, such as acne, whether in a teenager or an adult. The regime includes powdered mineral sulfur (flowers of sulfur) in a capsule (it tastes terrible). Taken internally, mineral sulfur loosens stool and creates strong smelling intestinal gas. Carminative herbs (Khalsa uses cumin, ginger and turmeric) can be taken concurrently to reduce the gas.

Kajjali is a specially prepared substance made using a unique Ayurvedic method. It is formed from mercury and sulfur. Ayurveda teaches that this form of mercury is safe, though opinions differ on that subject these days.

Gandhak Vati is a famous rasayana remedy containing sulfur. It contains kajjali, ginger, black pepper, cloves, rock salt, sauchar lavan, chanak kshar, mulak kshar and nimbuk drava. This formula acts as an appetizer and digestive. The sulfur is deeply detoxifying. The cloves are aromatic, energizing and carminative. The ginger root is included to relieve nausea and vomiting, to correct gas and to promote digestion. Salt increases hydrochloric acid in the stomach. Use Gandhak vati for lack of appetite, anorexia, abdominal pain, acidity and indigestion. The dose is 2-4 g twice daily with water.

Medicated Ghee preparations

India is a tropical country, and in the hotter areas, it's difficult to dry herbs in the sun in the conventional way. They mold from the humidity. So Ayurveda has concocted numerous low technology methods to preserve the active ingredients from plants. Medicated ghee is just such a method.

Herbs are simmered in ghee and water until the water evaporates. The spent herb (the marc) is removed. That way, the fat soluble and the water soluble herb constituents are extracted and remain in the ghee. Every trace of water must be removed, or spoilage must occur. Medicine so produced is called ghrita.

Ghee is self preserving, so medicated ghee lasts forever, if well cared for. Medicated ghee can be used internally or externally. Ghee is the ultimate remedy for pitta, so most medicated ghee preparations are pitta remedies. Brahmi ghee is an example.

Shata Dhaut Ghrita (100 times washed ghee) is a traditional preparation made from ghee. Hundred times washed ghee is prepared from organic cow milk ghee by washing it in water, repeatedly, 100 times, using a specific prescribed method.

This procedure transforms the ghee into a soft, cooling, nourishing, silky cream. It is used as a traditional Ayurvedic skin cream. It produces radiant and glowing skin, especially for people with a pitta skin type.

It is an astringent, moisturizer and anti wrinkle cream. It can be used as a daily face and body moisturizer or for facial massage. Apply it for the pitta issues of sunburn, eczema and rosacea.

· TEN ·

AYURVEDIC FORMULAS

People have been using Asian herbs for a very long time. Just about every possible combination of these herbs has been tried. Ayurvedic herbalists found that formulas were preferable to single herbs. The herbs in a formula act synergistically or perhaps offset side effects from one or more of the ingredients. In fact, it would be exceedingly rare for a single herb to be employed, absent the arena of teas made at home by Grandma.

The best formulas were used repeatedly, and became widely used classics. They developed names and were written down in the scriptures.

These formulas are more along the lines of a concept than a recipe. The classical formula appears in some sutra somewhere, but the ingredients and instructions might be a bit vague. Like Grandma's apple pie, everyone makes them a little differently. Each version of a classical formula is intended to be used for the same conditions. Slightly varying recipes might be made by the pharmacist or the many commercial manufacturers.

For example, triphala, the most widely used formula, is made by some with equal parts of the three fruits. Others make it with varying proportions, and some even add small amounts of other herbs, such as pipali.

There are hundreds of these formulas. We will discuss several of the most popular and effective classical combinations.

Agnitundi Vati

Agnitundi Vati is indicated for a range of common gastric problems including lack of appetite, indigestion, gas, stomach acidity and stomachache. It contains powerful digestion stimulants that increase the flow of digestive juices. Bowel movements become regular and constipation is eliminated.

Uses: Lack of appetite, gas, indigestion and fullness
Ingredients: Cumin, Vidanga, Triphala, Hordeum vulgarae, Psyllium, Ajwain
Dose: 2 grams twice or thrice daily, with meals, with water

Ajmodali Churna

Ajmodali Churna has ingredients known for their effectiveness in alleviating aggravated vata. It is used in rheumatoid disorders with body and joint pain. The herbs detoxify the accumulated ama in the body channels and enable circulation, creating better tissues nourishment. The rejuvenating properties of the churna are legendary.

Uses: Edema, rheumatoid arthritis, gout, backache

Ingredients: Vacha, Musta, Gercinia pedunculata, Black pepper, Saussurea lappa, Haritaki, Ginger

Dose: 2-4 grams per day

Arjunarisht

This medicated wine is a major heart tonic. It is a convenient way to get in arjuna bark, and is used for a wide variety of cardiac and respiratory conditions, including tachycardia and congestive heart failure.

The liquid format allows it to work rapidly, and makes it a good choice for acute conditions like arrythmias.

Uses: Arrhythmia, Angina

Ingredients: Arjuna, Munakka, Modhuka puspha, Dhataki, Jaggery

Dose: 1 ounce, with equal quantity of water, 3 times daily

Avipattikar Churna

Avipattikar Churna is designed to strengthen digestion without aggravating pitta. Excess pitta aggravates and inflames the digestive fire, creating acidic conditions. The herbs cool and sooth the internal membranes, neutralize acid and remove excess heat from the digestive system. This is the "Tums" of Ayurveda. Amla is anti-inflammatory, while toning the intestine. Haritaki pacifies vata and promotes stool movement. The mild carminatives gently increase agni.

Uses: Gastritis, hyperacidity, dyspepsia, gas, constipation and lack of appetite.

Ingredients: Ginger, pipali, triphala, musta, vid namak, vidanga, cardamom, cinnamon, operculina turpethum, rock sugar.

Dose: Take 3-5 g twice daily with milk or lukewarm water.[570]

Chyavanprash

This ancient tonic is used by all ages to improve mental and physical well being. As a mild all around health tonic, Chyavanprash can be used by people of all ages. It is named for its inventor, Chyavan, a forest monk, who developed it for his own sexual potency before a late-in-life marriage. "Prash" means jelly.

Amla is the basis for Chyavanprash, the most famous Ayurvedic rejuvenating jelly. Chyavanprash is the multiple vitamin of Ayurveda, and the most consumed Ayurvedic formula. Fifty percent of all Ayurvedic sales is for this jelly![571]

As a mild all around health tonic, Chyavanprash can be used by people of all ages. Yogi Bhajan said that it is the healthiest thing in the world ever got produced by a human being.[572]

It is good for almost any weakness or as a general energy supplement.[573] It's also used for cough, lung diseases, wasting, loss of voice, cardiac disorders, thirst, gout, impotence and to promote growth of children.[574]

Chyavanprash is about 80% amla fruit. According to the *Charaka Samhita*, this classic remedy is comprised of 42 other herbal ingredients.[575] Into a base of fresh amla fruit, the herbal ingredients are added for their synergistic effects, including ghee, sesame oil, sugar cane juice, raw honey, clove, and cinnamon.

As a long term, slow acting remedy for chronic inflammation, use 1-2 grams per day.

Modern scientists say that chyavanprash protects the liver from damage[576] and reduces blood sugar and cholesterol significantly.[577]

For sexual rejuvenation, stir chyavanprash into warm milk or spread on toast, and consume 1-2 tbs. every day. Yogi Bhajan told Khalsa that one ounce, in sliver leaf, with a glass of milk, would make an excellent everyday breakfast.

Chyavanprash Geneal Formula

500 parts	*Amla fruit, fresh*
50 parts	*Vetasa (raw cane sugar)*
6 parts	*Sesame seed oil*
6 parts	*Ghee*
6 parts	*Honey*
5 parts	*Vamsalochana (Bamboo manna)*
2 parts	*Pipali*

1 part each of around 38 other herbs (recipes vary slightly), including cinnamon bark, cardamom seed, bala root, gokshura, grape fruit, lettuce, hatritaki, guduchi, musta, punarnava and sandalwood.

Dashmula

Dashmula is the famous "ten roots" formula. These ten warming roots are used in cold conditions, and to treat vata generally. The warming nature also pacifies kapha.

As kvath, it is prescribed to patients suffering from cough, cold and fever, especially when accompanied by a headache. The kvath is also the most commonly used solution for Ayurvedic enemas.

Dashmula oil is a wonderful warming massage oil for vata conditions.

As is common with Ayurvedic formulas, this formula may contain ingredient variations from different sources.

Uses: Fever, anorexia, anemia, body ache, edema, coughing and breathing problems, pharyngitis, vertigo

Ingredients: Gokshura, Bilwa, Desmodium gangeticum, Vraria picta, Solanum surratense, Solanum indicum,

Premna mucronata, Oroxylum indicum, Umelina arborea and Stereospermum suaveolens

Dose: 10 g, dry herb weight, brewed as tea, per day

Hingvastak

This is a very well known digestion formula for vata. It is pungent, salty and warming. It balances vata and kapha, but may be too hot for pitta. It prompts appetite, stimulates normal preristalsis and props up apana.

Hingvastak is a general remedy for all types of indigestion of fullness, and for disorders of reversed energy in the GI tract, such as hiccups. Due to enhancing apana, it is not suitable in substantial doses during pregnancy.

Tierra recommends 10 to 20 grains of the powder is taken with the first morsel of rice and ghee at breakfast.[578]

Uses: Indigestion, constipation and hiccups.

Ingredients: Cumin seed, ajwain seed, Nigella seed, ginger root, black pepper fruit, pipali fruit, mineral salt and asafoetida.

Dose: 1-2 grams after a meal. The powder can also be made into pills with lemon juice, or commercial tablets are available.

Guggul Formulas

Gugguls are remedies made by mixing resinous guggul with dry powdered herbs. Generally, they are detoxifying and anti-inflammatory.

Triphala guggulu

This formulation of herbs acts as a rejuvenator and removes aggravated vata disorders. It is used in constipation conditions resulting in hemorrhoids, fistula and edema. It also works as a laxative, an appetizer and blood purifier.

Uses: Constipation, hemorrhoids, detoxification, obesity

Ingredients: Guggul, triphala, pipali

Dose: 1-3 g per day

Amritadi Guggulu

This guggul treats joint conditions caused by vata.

Uses: Rheumatism, gout, arthritis, leprosy, edema

Ingredients: Guggul, vidanga, black pepper, pipali, triphala, ginger

Dose: 1-3 g per day with water

Punarnavadi guggulu

Punarnavadi Guggulu works a broad-spectrum remedy for patients suffering from gout, sciatica, arthritis, edema and pain in the lower abdomen and bladder areas. This is a powerful, deep acting detoxifier and diuretic. Punarnava is a major diuretic remedy. The downward energy of this herb, and the detoxifying effect of the guggul recommend the combination for prostatic hypertrophy.[579]

Uses: Rheumatism, gout, arthritis, edema, prostatic hypertrophy

Ingredients: Punarnava, castor oil, ginger, guggul, Operculina turpethum, Baliospermum montanum, guduchi, black pepper, pipali, triphala, psyllium, rock salt, Semicarpus anacardium, vidanga, Swarna makshik

Dose: 1-3 g per day with water or punarnava tea

Yograj guggulu

Yograj Guggulu is a version of guggul that is more well balanced, tridoshic and suitable for long term use. It is a classic formula for chronic arthritis. There are many variations of this classic formula. It includes triphala and trikatu, which serve to make it tridoshic and contribute to mild detoxification.

Uses: Chronic arthritis, deep detoxification (long term use), facial paralysis, edema, anemia, inflammatory skin disease, genitourinary disorders, obesity

Ingredients: Guggul, Pipali, Ajwain, Caraway, Vidanga, Celery seed, Cumin, Cedrus deodara, Piper chaba, Cardomom, Rock Salt, Costus speciosus, Vanda roxburghii, Gokshura, Coiander seed, Triphala, Musta, Trikatu, Cinnamon, Lemongrass, Hordeum vulgare, Abies webbiana, Cinnamomum iners

Dose: 2 grams per day or as needed

Kumariasava

This asava is based on its main ingredient, kumari (aloe). It is alterative, tonic and hematinic. Use kumariasava for anemia, liver inflammation, fatigue, cough, asthma and constipation. Based on cooling aloe, is is mainly an anti-pitta medicine.

Uses: Hepatitis, gallbladder symptoms, cough

Ingredients: Ghrit kumari (aloe vera gel), Iron, Triphala, Trikatu, Chaturjat, Dhaniya, Chitrakmool, Deodar, Punarnava, Rasna, Danti, Motha, Aparajita, Chavya, Pipali, Dhataki, Jaggery

Dose: 1 ounce, with an equal quantity of water, 3 times per day

Mahasudarshan

Mahasudarshan (literally "the great formula for good vision"- *maha*, great, *darshan*, vision) contains bitter herbs that cool and cleanse the eyes.[580] The formula contains chiretta, guduchi, barberry, black pepper, long pepper, ginger root and the triphala combination. The combination is bitter, pungent and astringent.

Chiretta herb is a variety of gentian, and is probably the bitterest herb in the Ayurvedic pharmacopoeia. As gentians are, it is strongly cooling and detoxifying. A major anti-pitta remedy, it detoxifies kapha and ama toxins very well. However, it is very cold, so may aggravate kapha overall. For this general formula, it needs to be balanced by the other warmer herbs in the formula.

Guduchi is another anti-pitta herb, also used for fever and infection, sometimes called "Ayurvedic quinine." Barberry root is a cooling, detoxifying liver remedy. Black pepper is the most respected alterative, it is quite drying. Its warming nature balances the cold herbs in the formula. It is ideal for kapha conditions, such as glaucoma. Long pepper is a powerful, rejuvenating, warming alterative, which moistens the tissues and offsets the drying action of the other herbs. It is especially complementary to the drying nature of black pepper. Ginger root, the Ayurvedic universal medicine, is a detoxifier. The triphala combination is included as a general eye nutrient, liver cleanser, and detoxifier with tridoshic effects.

Mahasudarshan may also be used in immune support, detoxification, upping agni and supporting the liver.

Uses: Poor eyesight, eye inflammation, detoxification, bitter digestive aid, antipyretic, diaphoretic, diuretic,

Ingredients: Chiretta (or other bitters), trikatu, triphala (often includes many other minor, mostly cooling, herbs, including guduchi, musta, neem, pushkarmula, ajwain, tagara and licorice).

Dose: 1-3 g with each meal

Narayan Oil

Narayan oil is the main abhyanga oil for arthritis. It feels simultaneously hot and cold, due largely to its natural camphor content. Narayan oil stimulates circulation when used in massage. As is common, this formula is a concept, rather than a specific recipe. The older formulas contain a dozen or so herbs infused into a base of sesame oil. Modern formulas may be simpler, and based on mint, clove and eucalyptus oils.

Maha Narayan oil is a more complex formula ("maha" means great), containing 42 herbs. Its actions are comparable to Narayan oil, adding more alterative and pain relieving properties.

Uses: Massage in arthritis

Ingredients: Sesame oil, bala, ashwagandha, salai guggul, guggul, wintergreen, calamus, licorice, triphala, angelica, shilajit, fenugreek, turmeric, horsetail nutmeg, clove, camphor, myrrh, jivan

Dose: Apply liberally as a massage lubricant.

Sanjeevani Vati

Sanjeevani vati is a diaphoretic formula that increases sweating. It is a detoxifying formula that reduces ama. As a digestive formula, it reduces gas. Triphala detoxifies the digestive tract and loosens stool. Ginger is a universal digestive aid. Calamus warms the digestion effective for indigestion. The vidanga fruit is an anthelmintic, diuretic and carminative. It is a typical people's remedy for common cold with fever.[581]

Uses: Indigestion, fever, cholera, detoxification

Ingredients: Vidanga, ginger, black pepper, triphala, vacha, guduchi, Semicarpus anacardium, Aconitum ferox

Dose: 100- 300 mg twice daily with ginger juice or honey

Saptamrita Lauha

In one of the most important modern formularies of *Ayurveda*, the *Bhaishajyaratnavali* suggests a formula called *Saptamrita Lauha* ("sevenfold nectar") in the treatment of *timira* (blindness).[582] The efficacy of *Saptamrita Lauha* was assessed in a clinical trial of 48 retinopathic eyes. The formula was found to be highly effective, with the rapid clearing of retinal hemorrhaging, observed in both diabetic and hypertensive subjects. In three eyes the hemorrhage was cleared completely. The recurrence of a hemorrhagic episode was found to be statistically lower in eyes treated with *Saptamrita Lauha*.[583]

Uses: Eye disorders (of diabetes and others)

Ingredients: Licorice root, triphala, iron bhasma, ghee, honey

Dose: 100- 300 mg twice daily with water

Saraswat Churna

Saraswat Churna is a brain building combination. Vacha is one of the main brain herbs, with warming temperature. Shankpushpi is a standout as a brain and nerve rejuvenative, with a cooling temperature.

Uses: Anxiety, panic, epilepsy, cognitive debility, memory loss

Ingredients: Ashwaganda, vacha, shankpushpi, ajwain, cumin, trikatu, rock salt

Dose: 1 to 3 g twice a day with honey and ghee

Sitopladi Churna

Sitopladi Churna is used in a wide variety of breathing problems, coughing, fever and tuberculosis. It is a mucus thinning formula with cooling properties. It is a widely popular cough and sore throat remedy in folk use.

Uses: Cough, flu, fever, tuberculosis, anorexia, tongue numbness
Ingredients: rock sugar, bamboo manna, long pepper, cardamom, cinnamon
Dose: 1 tsp 3-4 times per day, or more, if necessary

Talisadi Churna

Talisadi Churna is a variation on the popular Sitopladi, to which are added Abies webbiana, black pepper and ginger. It is hotter and stronger than Sitopladi. It is used in a wide variety of breathing problems, common colds, coughing, asthma and to liguify plegm for expectoration. It can also be a warming digestive aid.

Uses: Cough, flu
Ingredients: Rock sugar, bamboo manna, long pepper, black pepper
Dose: 1 tsp 3-4 times per day, or more, if necessary

Trikatu

Another widely used tonic goes by the name "trikatu" ("three pungents"). Composed of ginger root, black pepper, and long pepper ("pipali"), it is used as a mildly warming tonic for enhancing digestion and circulation. This three part mix is often listed as an ingredient in formulas.

Baba Hari Dass' version was powdered ginger, black pepper and anise seed. For mucus and springtime allergies, he liked to mix equal parts with honey to form a paste, and take a teaspoon two or three times daily. It is described as "Medicine that is like a mother to a child."[584]

Uses: Alterative, warming digestive
Ingredients: Black pepper, pipali, dry ginger
Dose: 2-6 grams per day

Triphala

The name means "three fruits," referring to the fruits of amla, bibitaki, and haritaki that comprise the combination. These special fruits have many common names in different dialects. The fruits are dried, powdered, mixed together, and encapsulated.

This blend is about the most compatible medicine there is, and will benefit literally anyone who takes it. Since it contains all six tastes in proper proportion, it is suitable for all people from childhood to elderhood. It is used by itself, or as an ingredient in numerous formulas. It serves as a tridoshic anupan for just about any medicine. It is so safe and highly esteemed that a common aphorism among many practitioners is "when in doubt, use triphala."

The uses for triphala fill volumes in the Ayurvedic literature. Besides being a general tonic, it is a light laxative, skin, eye, and liver nourisher, and a general detoxifier. It is used in applications as diverse as a cleansing throat gargle, to a dry massage powder.

Ancient authors noted that it contains every taste except salty, and it is the ultimate tridoshic remedy.

In the *Sharngadhara Samhita,* a 14th century (CE) text on pharmacy, triphala is described as one part haritaki, two parts bibitaki, and four parts amla.[585] In contrast, *The Ayurvedic Formulary of India* notes that it is prepared by mixing equal parts of the three fruits.[586] *Sharngadhara* states that, consumed with honey and ghee, it is an effective stimulant to digestion, acting to reduce the vitiation of kapha and pitta.[587] *The Ayurvedic Formulary of India* adds gas, constipation, diabetes and eye diseases, all classic uses much in evidence today.[588]

Amla is the best single remedy for pitta, and is a tonic for the blood, bones, liver, and heart. It enhances production of red blood cells and strengthens the teeth, hair, and nails, as well as improving eyesight and regulating blood sugar. It is one of the strongest rejuvenatives, and an extraordinarily rich source of vitamin C and bioflavonoids. Recent scientific evidence shows that amla prevents lipid peroxidation in cell membranes.

It is the most frequently used cataract medicine. Amla generally benefits the eyes, and is known to improve eyesight.[589]

In his excellent book, *Ayurvedic Ophthalmology*, esteemed herbal eye expert Alan Tillotson confirms that amla is generally good for all types of ametropia (focus disorders like nearsightedness).[590]

Khalsa counseled an otherwise healthy 30-year old female with poor acuity, impaired night vision, and myopia. The treatment protocol was centered upon the usage of amla at a dose of 7 g daily for 15 months. At the end of the treatment period the patient's vision was normalized, corrective lenses were eliminated, and full night vision was restored as measured by the state driving vision test.

Bibitaki is the best single herb for generally controlling kapha and excess fat toxins. This herb nourishes the lungs, throat, voice, eyes, and hair. It excels at removing stones and accumulations of toxins (mucus, cholesterol, mineral deposits) in the digestive, urinary, and respiratory tracts. It is unique in being both laxative and astringent, so it purges the intestines, while simultaneously toning the tissues.

Haritaki is the best single herb for vata and for generally controlling dryness and constipation, and is thought by many to be the single most important Ayurvedic herb. Widely used in Tibetan medicine, it is called the "king of herbs" there. Sacred paintings depict haritaki in the hand of the Medicine Buddha. The gentle laxative qualities of haritaki are perfect for easy detoxification. It nourishes the brain and nerves. It is strongly astringent, contracting tissues, and is therefore used for various ulcers, prolapses, and fluid discharges. Haritaki is called "the mother," and is thought to increase mental/spiritual awareness. It is given to children upon the premature loss of a parent.

Triphala is included as an essential part of variety of classical *Ayurvedic* formulations. One simple recipe told by *Charaka* is to prepare a paste of triphala powder with water and smear it within an iron vessel, where it is kept for 24 hours. The paste is used with honey and water, followed with ghee. *Charaka* says that "by using this recipe continuously for one year, one can live for a hundred years, free from aging and diseases."[591]

As a simple rasayana, the *Charaka Samhita* suggests triphala with bamboo manna, pipali, ghee, honey and raw sugar.[592] The *Ashtanga Hrdaya* lists a combination of madhuka flower *(Madhuka indica)*, tvakshiri sap *(Bambusa arundinaceae)*, Pipali, rock salt, Suvarna (gold bhasma), vacha rhizome and iron bhasma, mixed with equal quantities of triphala. This may be taken with honey, ghee, or sugar, and when taken repeatedly, "acts as a rasayana, cures all diseases, bestows intelligence, longevity and good memory."[593]

To increase stamina, take a small dose of triphala and honey at night, followed by molasses and fresh ginger in the morning, before breakfast.[594] And triphala is mixed with shilajit for stubborn kidney conditions, including nephritis and diabetes.[595]

Mixed with such herbs as guduchi, kutki and vacha, it can be used as a decoction (warning- very bad taste ahead) for treatment of fever with cough and mucus.[596] Mixed with neem, kutki and senna, with honey, can be given as a decoction (ahem) to alleviate pain and/or fever with a burning sensation.[597]

Applied topically, the three fruits powder is a strong agent for wound healing. K.M. Nadkarni's modern classic *Indian Materia Medica* recounts how a surgeon named Dr. A. Lakshmapathi applied triphala powder to a cut he sustained from a dirty razor, and covered it with a bandage. The cut completely healed within 72 hours with no evidence of a scar. Subsequent to this, Dr. Lakshmapathi routinely applied a dusting of triphala powder for healing fresh surgical wounds with great success.[598] We, and our close colleague Alan Tillotson, have also had occasion to use triphala, in many forms, and in many cases, as a dressing for wounds, with similar, excellent results.[599]

Triphala churna can also be used as a medium for dry massage, particularly suitable in the treatment of Kapha conditions. Mixed with water it can be employed as a shampoo, a gargle *(kabalagraha)*, or for nasal administration (*nasya*). As a decoction it can be employed for enema *(basti)*. Use triphala as a rapid-acting expectorant, say, during hay fever season, infusing 5 g of the churna in 8 ounces of water overnight. Consumed first thing in the morning upon arising, a dramatic expectoration follows within minutes. Khalsa learned this remedy from Yogi Bhajan.[600]

For inflammatory skin eruptions (erysipelas) with pus, and severe fevers, *Chakrapani's* famous *Ayurvedic* recipe book *Chakradatta* suggests triphala can be mixed in equal parts with guggul. This combination can also be used topically to heal wounds that are large and painful with weeping and discharge.[601] Ulcers and herpes sores can be washed with triphala decoction, and a purgative dose of triphala and guggul can be taken internally.[602]

Triphala nourishes the eyeball, and strengthens the nerves and other tissues involved in the eye.[603]

Eye washes are popular in Ayurvedic ophthalmology. Triphala may also be administered as an eyewash. You may use triphala water. Add 1 tablespoon triphala powder to 10 oz. water. Cover and let sit for 12 hours. Filter and apply with an eyedropper or eye cup.[604] A cold infusion of *amla* only may be substituted.[605]

Modern science revealed a definite weight loss benefit, when used with guggul.[606]

The three fruits that were shown, in a scientific investigation, to lower cholesterol significantly, although bibitaki proved slightly stronger than amla. [607]

Triphala is commonly found as a *churna*, a finely sieved powder, which can be mixed with water, ghee or honey, but it can also be encapsulated for the discerning palate.

And there are many other ways of preparing triphala- medicated oil, decoction, confection, asava and arishta among them. The finely filtered decoction can be used as a morning eyewash. Triphala is a rasayana, for which purpose it is traditionally prescribed for a year or more in doses of up to 2 grams, taken twice daily, and may even be taken throughout one's life on a semi-regular basis to cleanse the tissues, strengthen digestion, and sharpen the senses.

Most practitioners will agree that in small doses (1–2 g) is an unusual combination of rejuvenating tonic and alterative, and safe for long-term use, whereas in large doses (10–5 g) it is a purgative, used for shorter periods of time. As a purgative, it is safe and effective, even for geriatric and pediatric use.

We both use, recommend and teach about triphala extensively. As a long term basic tonic herb, there is fundamentally no better choice to add to your routine than triphala.

As a general lifelong tonic, take 1 gram of triphala per day. For a light laxative effect, increase the dose gradually to up to 5 grams per day as necessary. Triphala's laxative quality is fast acting, but its tonic properties are long term. Although it is common to have every patient take a daily maintenance dose of triphala, right from the start of treatment, this uses up a valuable part of the individual's compliance potential. Perhaps some folks need to experience fast acting herbs initially, to stay emotionally committed to the process of healing, with the less dramatic maintenance herbs coming later, after symptoms have subsided.

To keep the bowels open during a gentle cleanse, start triphala at 3 grams per day, and increase by one gram per day until the bowels are comfortably regular.

The laxative action of this formula promotes the downward moving apana. According to Yogi Bhajan, if this gets excessive, add yogurt to the diet to offset the extreme downward moving nature of the triphala.[608]

Let's admit it- triphala tastes bad. Khalsa was siting with Yogi Bhajan one day when another student mentioned that she had tried triphala, "You said that you could take triphala with butter and honey. I tried it and it tastes awful." Yogi Bhajan replied, "It should be mixed with ghee and honey just to digest it properly and to give it time so that it does not leave without those stomach juices which are required.

Indian medicines always need to be taken with ghee because they are so powerful that they must not leave the stomach fast. It is very difficult to digest oil, but ghee is timed according to body temperature. It is very digestible, but assimilates a lot of stomach juices. Triphala is also very bitter, by the way."

"Can you put it in a capsule?"

"No. Because it is bitter, it should touch the tongue. The bitterness is what straightens out the head the moment it touches the tongue. People are supposed to chew triphala. Did you taste? It's terrible. It really straightens out the entire head."[609]

· ELEVEN ·

AYURVEDIC HOME REMEDIES

Food has been the medicine of humanity since the dawn of time. Many herbs that we associate only with seasoning our food are, in fact, potent herbal medicines. Take ginger and black pepper as examples.

The complex cuisine of India began, thousands of years ago, as recipes to get healing herbs and foods into people. Gradually, as the process evolved, complicated mixtures of food ingredients, herbal medicines, and flavorings coalesced into a tasty amalgam that warms the soul, heals the body, and pleases the palate.

Although the list of herbal medicine foods is huge, here is a selection of remedies that are easy to find, and particularly effective.

Acne

Green vegetables are an important tool in the treatment of inflamed skin. Considered the most anti-inflammatory of foods, they are even more cooling when used raw. Any green vegetables will work - spinach, celery, cucumber - even green beans.

High amounts of green vegetables will bring acute acne, psoriasis, and dermatitis under control quickly, say natural healing experts. Because it is easy to fill up quickly on fibrous raw green vegetables, juicing is a good choice for getting in large amounts of the active ingredients. Try a couple of tall glasses of cucumber or celery juice per day.

Backache

Turmeric curbs inflammation and lowers pain. Like cayenne, it depletes nerve endings of substance P, the pain receptor neurotransmitter. Ginger combines well with turmeric for back pain. Turmeric is used as an external poultice for sprains and sore joints.

Willow bark tea is effective for low back pain.

Bad breath

Ever eat in an Indian restaurant? Did you notice the dish of fennel seeds by the exit? You just ate a meal of beans, onion and garlic- time to produce some intestinal gas. Grab those fennel seeds, pop 'em in your mouth, and chew them slowly, to evade the gas and sweeten the breath. Same for chewing fresh basil leaves.

Cold and flu

Chrysanthemum flower is the flower you see at the florist, but get it from your herbalist, please. This cooling, immune enhancing herb treats fever and red, dry, swollen eyes and strengthens the lungs. It kills many pathogenic bacteria, including strep. Chrysanthemum is often combined with honeysuckle flower for a delicious, effective drink, especially for inflammation.

Cough

Marshmallow root excels in cough treatment. The modern campfire food is a descendant of an old-fashioned medicinal candy made from marshmallow herb. But marshmallow has been used medicinally since ancient Greece, and Roman physicians suggested marshmallow for irritated tissues.

The root contains very high levels of mucilage, which is made of large sugar molecules, which have a soothing effect on mucous membranes, so modern herbalists recommend marshmallow primarily for relieving respiratory problems, such as coughs. It quells irritation and associated dry cough.[610]

Gargling with sesame oil, bibitaki or turmeric will suppress the urge to cough.

Earache

Khalsa has raised three children. With these Ayurvedic methods, none of them have ever had an ear infection. Herbal ear oils are the pillar of a natural treatment program for acute earache. First on the list is garlic. The classic herbal ear treatment, it is rapidly effective. Khalsa keeps a bottle of liquid aged garlic at home to treat childhood ear infection. Try it by squirting the ear full of the liquid. Insert a cotton ball and tape in place. Send the child to bed. In the morning, the aged garlic will have penetrated, and the earache will be gone.

An Israeli study done in 2001 looked at one hundred three children aged 6 to 18 years who were diagnosed with earache. An herbal ear oil (garlic, mullein, Calendula, St. John's wort) was compared to an anesthetic drug ear drop. The herbal ear oil was as effective as the drug.[611]

Headache

Willow bark is nature's aspirin for headache. It contains salicylates, which are the herbal forerunners of aspirin.[612]

Aspirin thins the blood, but willow bark does not,[613] so it won't cause the bleeding problems common with aspirin. You won't experience the typical digestive disturbances of aspirin when using willow.

Use a tea brewed from up to 1 oz., dry weight, of the raw herb, per day, or an extract containing 240 mg total salicin per day. Willow can be used for as long as necessary.

Hemorrhoids

Beet root is a superb treatment for hemorrhoids. It causes the liver to manufacture bile, and promotes liver blood circulation, lowering blood pressure in the portal vein, the site of the hemorrhoid (actually a varicose vein in the rectum). Milder carrot will work, a bit more slowly. Eat several servings of beet root or beet greens per day, or a monodiet of these foods, until the problem diminishes. Continue until you get complete relief.

Treat hemorrhoids with turmeric. Swallow up to 4 Tbs. per day of the bulk powder per day until the pain is gone. As an astringent, apply it topically as a paste to shrink the hemorrhoids.

Menstrual Cramps

Treat menstrual cramps, caused by vata, with cinnamon bark. Many women have found it to be a striking remedy, often giving relief on the first try, after years of monthly pain.

Cinnamon warms the torso. This quality makes it a very good choice to promote menstruation. Since cinnamon enhances circulation to the uterus, the warm relaxing blood can relieve the cramps.

Two weeks before the period, take one gram of cinnamon in a capsule or an appropriate anupan. Increase by one gram per day until the period. If no cramps develop, that's your dose. If cramps were there, increase the dose slightly next time. Most women get good results with about 10 grams per day, starting about 2 days before the period, and continuing through the cramp days.

Nausea

Ginger's effect on motion sickness and nausea has been thoroughly proven, so it's not surprising that Europeans practitioners use ginger in tea for indigestion. It reduces spasm, absorbs and neutralizes toxins in the gastrointestinal tract and increases the secretion of digestive juices, including bile and saliva.[614] Ginger contains ingredients that soothe the gut and aid digestion by increasing peristalsis that moves food through the intestine.

Baba Hari Dass recommended putting a piece of copper in the mouth for seasickness.[615]

The Flu

Yogi Bhajan taught a recipe for persistent cold and flu, based on ajwain.

He said, "So you can take millet, and boil it with a black jira, and ajwain. To their taste, I mean, they all know what to do. And please cook it hard, and if you want to add little taste to it, you can put corn in it. That's admissible. And once you do all that, make it really good. And then that will become your thing, and you can make pancakes out of that. And you can use mustard oil, or you can use virgin olive oil. The rest, you can add anything you want. And you can put little black pepper or cayenne if you want to make it hot or not, that's your choice. And once it's very well cooked, it will become kind of a thing, like a dough with which we have to make pancakes. The mustard oil, when taken cold crushed into the body, it kills everything which kills the body. Straightforward, right on. I mean to say, in our villages, nobody cares for anybody. If the cow is sick, they take a bamboo stick and fill it with the oil, and pour it in with the milk. Three days later there's no problem. So they do to the man, too. Amazing. But this thing works.

"Something again happened before, in Los Angeles. We were all very sick and nobody knew what to do. We made those pancakes, remember? And we got out of the trouble. You will have bad sore throats, you will be having sneezing. You know this feeling? Exact. I'm not kidding. This exactly will happen, many of you."

"It takes about two, three hours to go into the body to start giving you some sort of relief. As simple as that."[616]

· TWELVE ·

SPECIFIC DISEASES AND TREATMENTS

When We Need Some Help

Some of us, the fortunate few, are natural peak performers, with strong prakruti, excellent lung capacity and strong digestive systems. Some may have hardy skeletons with large reserves of minerals. They seem to thrive on stress, eat the standard American diet with less ill effects, require hard endurance exercise and rarely get ill. And they age more slowly, to boot. Their natural edge on the rest of us shows up in extraordinary health and stamina.

But even if you didn't start with a naturally robust constitution, you can regain the balance in your body. Would you like to regain your physical stamina, your optimism, and ability to be sociable? To say nothing about thriving on the stresses of career and family. When you're in balance, you can again think clearly. You resist disease. Even if illness and injury should strike, you recover rapidly.

It just takes some study and determination to change the way you always do things. Ayurveda gives you a plan to follow.

The Elder Years

As we age, many factors conspire to pull us out of balance.

Roberta Lee, M.D., who practices complementary medicine with a specialty in herbal therapeutics, is the medical director of the Center for Health and Healing at Beth Israel Medical Center in New York City. Dr. Lee sees a lot of osteoporosis at her clinic. She reminds us that hypochlorhydria (low agni in the digestive tract) is common in aging people.[617]

The aging stomach begins to produce less acid, further retarding mineral absorption and protein digestion. To add to this problem, many seniors do not consume enough protein. This is a catabolic situation- it causes accelerated tissue destruction and loss, weakening a body that is perhaps already frail- a drastic slip toward exaggerated vata. Assess the pitta of the digestive tract, make the proper adjustments and compensate by upping protein sources. Elders may require 1-2 extra servings of protein each day to maintain bone and protein reserves.

Ayurveda and Women

Ayurveda aims to nourish, restore and balance the body functions that have been taxed by the wear and tear of daily life. Signs of aging are all marks of lack of "juice," from arthritis with lack of joint fluids, to fatigue with lack of endocrine hormones, to menopause difficulties with vaginal dryness.

Generally, compared to men, women tend to drift in the direction of being colder (think those cold feet under the covers), drier (who hasn't seen all those bottles of moisturizers?) and lighter- all vata characteristics. Over a lifetime, the goal for a woman is to stay warm, juicy and grounded.

Diet is the first and most basic building block of good health, and can be an effective treatment for disease, even when used alone. Women generally do better with a diet of mainly cooked, easy to digest, moist food.

Sweet taste (not white sugar), contained in whole carbohydrates and good quality fats, is the most rejuvenating, so sweet food, including milk, ghee (clarified butter), and especially honey, is recommended to rebuild body tissues and restore sexual juices.

Honey rejuvenates your body.[618] With sweet taste, and is predigested, so it nurtures all parts of the body. Use it in your herbal tea to allow the honey to act as a vehicle for the active principles of the herbs. Ghee also is a prime revitalizing food. It enhances tissue lubrication, increasing digestion and liver health.[619] Add ghee to the diet for the brain and intellect, bone marrow, and reproductive tissue.

Onion and garlic increase sexual energy, libido, and sexual secretions.

Shatavari root is the main Ayurvedic sexual rejuvenating tonic for women. A builder and balancer for the reproductive organs, it increases milk and sexual juices, increases fertility, balance hormones and improves menopausal complaints, such as vaginal atrophy.

Shatavari detoxifies the blood, enhances the immune system, promotes the intellect, and enhances digestion and physical strength. One study determined that a medicine containing shatavari markedly reduced stress effects.[620]

Through moderate and consistent lifestyle and health building practices, it is clear that women can enjoy life at a level that is far beyond what most people have learned to tolerate. Happiness, in all areas of your life, including the bedroom, is your birthright.

Treatment of individual diseases

Ayurveda is, first and foremost, a system of preventive care and maintenance. However, things do happen. Sometimes, even with the best intentions, the doshas can get unruly and end up causing problems.

For the convenience of discussion, Ayurveda does name diseases, but the focus is much different than conventional medicine. Regardless of what we call a disease, the Ayurvedic treatment is always individualized. The balance of the energies is always the focus. And bringing things back to balance is the paramount goal.

Ayurveda does have some outstanding treatments for acute illnesses. Let's investigate some of them.

Acne and Dermatitis

You spend a lifetime living in your skin, and a good chunk of your paycheck indulging it. It is the barrier between you and the hostile world outside you. Clearly, it's very important to keep your skin strong and healthy.

In Ayurvedic physiology, the skin has six layers, and these layers are located not only superficially but extend to the deeper levels of the body. A "skin" disease is not just 'skin-deep'. It is generally rooted in the various *dhatus*, like fat, muscles and blood. In fact, this disorder is called "that which comes out from the inner part to the outer part." Acne is the classic hot, inflamed, toxic, pitta condition.

Incorrect diet and lifestyle are the main causes of this disease. Pursuing a diet or lifestyle that is against one's prakruti creates an imbalance in the bodily energies, which leads to contamination of the body tissues, leading inevitably to skin diseases. In Ayurvedic terms, the prime dosha involved is pitta. Hot, spicy, fried, oily and greasy foods, overexposure to heat and sunlight, drinking too much tea or coffee, alcohol consumption and smoking can aggravate pitta and bring on dermatitis.

Herbal medicine focuses on reducing inflammation in the skin, healing the tissue of the skin if necessary and eliminating the source of the irritating toxins through the liver, kidneys, and large intestine.

After you begin to apply Ayurvedic balancing principles, and the skin begins to settle down, it's time to heal the underlying structure of the tissue. Gotu kola is the most spectacular herb for treating damage, not only to skin, but to all types of connective tissue. Gotu kola has the ability to heal and regrow new skin, repairing even long-standing, painful lesions, skin ulcers and scars.

Another excellent herb that reduces inflammation in the skin is licorice root, which contains steroid-like substances, which, consumed internally, or even applied topically, provide relief.

Ayurvedic barberry and other herbs that contain berberine are good for reducing inflammation of the skin, whether taken internally or applied as a cream.[621]

When it comes to detoxifying the liver, few herbs are better known than burdock root, which is used across Eurasia for skin inflammation. It is rich in anti-inflammatory flavonoids, lignins, and bitter constituents.

In keeping with Baba Hari Dass' ideas, for liver diseases, peel a green papaya, slice and cover with blackberry vinegar for 10 days. Each day eat one slice of the papaya and/or drink some of the blackberry vinegar.[622]

Green vegetables treat inflamed skin with their cooling energy, which is even cooler when they are used raw. Use any green vegetable, including pea pods, celery, lettuce and sprouts.

It may be the high magnesium content in the chlorophyll, which is known to cool inflammation, or some yet to be identified constituent, possibly bioflavonoids, but high amounts of green vegetables will bring acute acne, psoriasis, and dermatitis under control quickly. Because it is easy to fill up quickly on fibrous raw green vegetables, juicing is a good choice for getting in large amounts of the active ingredients. Try a couple of tall glasses of cucumber or celery juice per day.

Aloe leaf is a popular Ayurvedic remedy for skin healing. This remarkable plant is applied directly to the damaged skin in the form of a cream or gel. It heals the skin quite effectively, due to its actions as anti-inflammatory, antimicrobial and analgesic. A scientific experiment, mice with damaged skin were treated with aloe gel, aloe cream or a placebo cream. After two weeks, the aloe had significantly delayed inflammation in the skin, and had noticeably reduced healing time, compared to the controls. New skin growth was also enhanced in the aloe treated mice.[623] Aloe can also be taken internally. Use the dried aloe leaf in capsules or drink the gel. Aloe is laxative, so adjust the dose accordingly.

Triphala is a detoxifying laxative. Use enough to maintain two or more easy bowel movements per day. Or, prepare a powder of equal quantities of turmeric, amla, and neem leaves. One teaspoonful of this powder can be taken twice a day with water. One or 2 grams of mineral sulfur powder per day will detoxify the skin.

On the whole, topical treatments offer, at best, temporary relief for dermatitis. For the short run, though, they can offer some relief. Boil neem leaves in water and wash the affected area everyday. Make a paste of fresh spearmint and leave it on pimples overnight.[624]

Mix 50 grams of powdered yellow sulfur in 8 ounces of mustard oil or coconut oil. Apply this mixture to the affected area every morning. Sit in the sun or in a warm place after applying this oil. Wash after one half hour.

Baba Hari Dass offers burning coconut fibers to ash. Mix this with sesame oil and apply to the skin.[625]

Ubtan therapy has a long history in acne and for facial skin healing. We discuss ubtan elsewhere in this book. These are a few suitable recipes.

Dermatitis is a condition that offers you the chance to see herbal medicine at its best. Be patient - the long-term approach really is the only way to have long-term success. With diligent effort and a consistent approach, you will be very satisfied with the long-term result. Apply these remedies. The fruits of your labors will make you glad you did.

Allergy

Allergies are the body's immune overreaction to specific substances that it misidentifies as harmful.

This happens when the immune system is weakened, and the ahamkara cannot separate the self from the non-self.

Allergies are a sign of depleted ojas, which is closely associated with the immune system. Each time one is exposed to an allergen, the doshas become imbalanced, and ama is created, according to the particular imbalanced doshas, leading to dosha related symptoms of allergy.

Pitta dosha may be imbalanced. Aggravated pitta releases heating ama. Pitta ama accumulates in deep tissues- rasa, rakta, mamsa and lasika (lymph). This ama in turn causes contamination of yet deeper tissues, leading to characteristic symptoms, such as allergic skin disturbances.

If kapha takes the hit, the aggravated kapha ama accumulates in the respiratory channels, leading to respiratory allergies.

Medicines to detoxify, strengthen agni, strengthen ojas and then address the individual symptoms treat allergy.

Rice and honey invigorate ojas. Tonic medicines, including ashwaganda, bala and shatavari, support the immune system. Saffron promotes synergy of tonic medicines. Anti-pitta remedies that restrain inflammation in acute episodes include bringaraj, chiretta and aloe. Anti-kapha medicines that lessen mucus include garlic, pipali and hing.

Anxiety

Anxiety is a prime example of a vata symptom. Warming, grounding, carminative remedies that sedate and promote digestion are used for anxiety.

Valerian is a relaxant herb that has a calming effect on the autonomic nervous system. It is a good short-term relaxant that works quickly, offering a healthy, nontoxic alternative to other measures.

In the past 35 years, more than 200 scientific studies have investigated valerian. In much of Europe, even physicians are likely to recommend this remedy. This herb is an active ingredient in about 150 over-the-counter medicines in Germany, including some preparations for children. (In fact, some studies have shown positive effects on hyperactive children.)

Chamomile flower is used as a mild relaxant for nervousness and anxiety. A cup of chamomile tea is a time-honored remedy for taking the edge off. Since it is mildly relaxing it finds a use in the treatment of headaches. As an antispasmodic, it is used for cramps. Chamomile has recently been shown to bind to the same brain receptors as the tranquilizer Valium.

Arthritis

Nothing could be more miserable than the prospect of facing the rest of your life with round the clock increasing pain, leading eventually to a slow slide into disability. Yet, for millions of osteoarthritis sufferers, that's what the future holds.

The term *arthritis* literally means "joint inflammation," but it also is used to refer to a diverse collection of more than 100 rheumatic diseases that cause pain, stiffness, and swelling in joints and may also affect other parts of the body, primarily other sites of connective tissue. One form or another of the disease afflicts nearly 43 million Americans.[626] Arthritis is the most prevalent cause of disability in people 65 and older.[627]

Osteoarthritis (OA), or *degenerative joint disease* (DJG) is the most common form of joint disease.

This 78 million-strong aging baby boomers are focused on remaining fit, fending off typical geriatric health concerns and assuring that their bodies are as healthy and active as their minds.[628] With OA looming, they are eager to try natural therapies to stay active and pain-free.

OA is typified by erosion of joint cartilage. As people age, the water portion of cartilage increases while the protein composition degenerates, causing the cartilage to form tiny crevasses. The result is that cartilage surfaces fray, wear, ulcerate and in extreme cases, wear away completely, leaving the joint to slide bone-on-bone, causing pain and limiting joint mobility. Bony spurs may form at joint edges.

The disease increases in prevalence with age.[629]

In the long run, OA causes joint pain, loss of function, reduced joint motion and deformity. OA most often affects the knees, hips, spine, and hands, and sometimes other joints. Ultimately, disability may result from disease in the spine, knees and hips. [630] It is now known, however, that of the disease can be arrested or reversed.[631]

The energy of osteoarthritis is cold and dry. Osteoarthritis usually occurs in vata prakruti people- those with low body temperature and slow metabolic rate. These bodies have difficulty retaining fluids in the tissues, so there is a general lack of lubrication, including the joint surfaces. The overall result is stiffness and pain.

Of course, pain is the first symptom that comes to mind when most people think about the misery of arthritis. But it turns out not to be the case for those who have the disorder. Lost sleep, another vata symptom, is among the main grievances of arthritis victims, according to University of North Carolina researchers. [632] [633] Sleep disruption overshadows problems such as reduced mobility, fewer visits to family and friends and missing work or favorite recreational activities. Not only does arthritis disrupt sleep, but sleep disruption also makes pain worse, all signs of increasingly disordered vata.

Amavata

Amavata is a presentation of chronic joint and body pain, with swelling at some or all of the synovial joints. As the condition progresses, the pain may migrate and develop into burning sensations. Amavata resembles rheumatoid arthritis (RA), but the Ayurvedic concept is broader, and may describe persons who have modern diagnoses of OA, ankylosing spondylitis, or other joint disorders.

Other associated symptoms include stiffness, indigestion, fatigue, emotional withdrawal, loss of taste, thirst and dryness, insomnia, constipation, dizziness and fever.

When digestive agni is weak, ama may accumulate and make its way to the joints, where it slowly damages the structures and may provoke inflammation and swelling. Amavata is treated by detoxifying the tissues of ama, promoting digestion, and repairing the joint tissues. This is a classic opportunity for panchakarma. Because vata is the main dosha involved, enema is especially indicated.

Herbal Medicine for OA

Because arthritis and related osteoporosis are among the leading ailments affecting aging baby boomers, the search for alternative methods of combating this looming duo is leading them to dietary supplements in droves.dcxxviii

Cyclooxygenase-2 (COX-2) is a key enzyme helps the body produce the inflammatory compounds prostaglandins and cytokines. When the body overproduces COX-2, though, the result is chronic inflammation and pain. Turmeric, holy basil, grape juice or stuffed grape leaves and green tea appreciably inhibit COX-2.[634 635]

Indian Salai Guggul (Boswellia) gum contains components, boswellic acids, which inhibit inflammation-producing substances, leukotrienes, and inhibits inflammation through several mechanisms in the body.[636 637 638]

Turmeric has profound anti-inflammatory properties, and is a staple in Ayurvedic arthritis treatment.[639 640 641 642 643 644 645 646 647]

Recently, a study looked at a combination of these exceptional herbs. Forty-two patients with OA were randomly assigned to receive an Ayurvedic preparation, containing (per capsule) 450 mg of ashwaganda, 100 mg of Boswellia, 50 mg of turmeric, and 50 mg of a zinc complex, or a placebo, for three months. The dosage was two capsules three times per day, after meals. The treatments were then crossed over. Compared with placebo, the herb combination significantly reduced the severity of pain and the disability score. No side effects required discontinuation of treatment.[648]

A traditional pain reliever, willow has an outstanding reputation. It contains salicin and other related compounds (salicylates), which are the herbal predecessors of aspirin.[649 650 651]

Ashwaganda builds and solidifies tissue growth- it is "anabolic". Since OA is a disease of "catabolism," or tissue destruction, ashwaganda seems like a good choice. Modern research is bearing this out.[652]

The demonstrated effectiveness of ashwaganda in a variety of rheumatologic conditions may be due in part to its anti-inflammatory properties, which have been established in several studies.[653 654]

Baba Hari Dass suggested a tea of star anise for lower back pain.[655]

Simple topical preparations are widely used. Baba Hari Dass recommended several. For backache, warm and liquefy the fresh sap of the pine tree, apply on a cloth and apply to the affected area. For knee pain, mix cow dung ash with water. Bring it to a boil to form a paste, and apply directly on the knee.[656]

Ayurvedic Massage for Osteoarthritis

Massage for vata arthritis should be done in a warm room, with warming oils.

The focus should be on gentle increase of joint range of motion. Since osteoarthritis patients have a lack of oily, lubricating "slime" in the tissues, abhyanga should be done liberally. Olive oil, warming mustard and Narayan oils are good choices. The patient should not feel any pain. Sand, since massage therapy is renowned for promoting sleep, it can have a dramatic benefit in sleep loss from osteoarthritis.

Asthma

Bronchial asthma, now properly called reactive airway disease, or RAD, is a disease of the airways of the lungs, characterized by tightening of these airways, coughing, wheezing and shortness of breath. It's a chronic condition. People with asthma live with it every day and for their whole lives.

Asthma involves three major features. First, there's airway obstruction. In people with asthma, allergens and environmental triggers make the bands of muscle surrounding the bronchials tighten, and air cannot move freely. The air moving through the tightened airways causes the whistling sound we know as wheezing.

Then there's inflammation, which causes red and swollen bronchial tubes. Inflammation contributes greatly to the long-term lung damage. In the long run, treating inflammation is key to managing asthma. Finally, there's airway irritability. Asthmatic airways are extremely sensitive. Even the slightest triggers, such as pollen or animal dander may cause the airways tend to overreact and narrow.

Respiratory diseases can certainly be miserable. And sometimes they are life threatening. They certainly are common, and prevalence is rising in epidemic proportions.[657 658 659 660]

Long-term resolution of asthma involves treatment of the adrenal glands to increase production of adrenal hormones, both stress hormones and anti-inflammatory hormones. Usually, that resolves asthma very rapidly. We want to treat the lungs as well with specific pulmonary herbs to tonify, soothe and strengthen lung tissue. Short-term asthma symptoms can be relieved with natural remedies, but the exciting part is that even lifelong asthma can eventually be resolved *permanently* with the use of long-term adrenal and lung tonics.

The natural medicine asthma strategy will include all these elements:

- For acute symptoms- herbs for immediate bronchodilation
- For chronic tightness- herbs to maintain daily bronchodilation
- For chronic inflammation- anti-inflammatory herbs
- For chronic lung tissue stress- herbs to support lung tissue and function
- For chronic mucus- herb to reduce mucus (herbal astringents, expectorants)

Start with herbs to open the airways for the short term. Bala root contains a mild constituent related to ephedrine. It will bring some airway opening effect.

Probably the preeminent herbs for asthma are the peppercorns (black pepper and pipali). Warming peppercorns are long-term lung tissue builders and detoxifiers. They do a good job of keeping the airways open over time. Take 10 capsules or 1/2 oz as tea per day.

Relaxing nervines can be useful for asthmatics. Calming herbs such as valerian may help in stressful situations when the asthmatic may be more vulnerable to an attack. Turmeric is widely used in Ayurvedic asthma regimes. It's anti-inflammatory (this in some way is most likely related to the mechanism for asthma), antioxidant, immune-supportive and broadly anti-microbial. Turmeric can reduce coughs, especially when mixed with coriander and cumin.

Licorice root is another good choice as a long-term builder, since it is a lung tonic and has adrenal effects (it contains compounds that are similar to the adrenal cortical hormones) and in the short-term it is expectorant. Licorice is a powerful and diverse tonic in its own right. Basil helps shortness of breath and bronchiopasm in asthma.[661] Garlic sometimes helps.

Bitter herbs reduce the long-term accumulation of mucus, and these include turmeric, dandelion, yarrow, yellow dock, barberry and goldenseal; pungent herbs thin mucus and aid expectoration and these include black pepper, garlic, cinnamon, cloves, ginger, rosemary, sage and thyme.

Foods and nutrients for asthma

Another element of long-term asthma treatment is to include anti-inflammatory herbs and foods in the diet, since asthma involves inflammation of the bronchi and an inappropriate inflammatory reaction by the body to certain substances.

Onions and garlic are excellent anti-allergy herbs, especially for asthma. Onions contain the bioflavonoid quercetin, but both of these lily bulbs also inhibit an enzyme, lipoxygenase, which generates an inflammatory chemical.[662]

Chilies are effective food for allergies, especially asthma, both to prevent or treat an attack. In addition to being immune-boosting long-term, the capsaicin in chilies desensitizes airway mucosa. The effect is long-lasting, so chilies can be used preventively; there is also clinical evidence that capsaicin can break an attack once it has started.

Athlete's Foot

Itching, burning, aching, smarting, flaky feet - is athlete's foot just for jocks? On the contrary, athlete's foot is, in fact, incredibly common, even among those whose heaviest workout is picking up the remote control. It occurs at all ages, from preadolescence to high school students, to aging weekend athletes.

Robert Landis, 43, of Vashon Island, Washington, knows all too well the itching and distress of athlete's foot. An avid outdoor athlete and long distance bicyclist, Robert picked up the dreaded fungus. Four years later, the pain and scaly skin was still bugging him almost constantly.

Robert describes his condition as "itch, especially between the toes and on the sole, with scaly, red skin that itched all the time. The toenails were discolored with white lines."

After several unsuccessful attempts with various external preparations, Robert sought Khalsa's help. After a careful analysis of his condition and metabolism, Khalsa suggested garlic as a remedy. Robert took nine capsules of garlic per day. Within six weeks, the itch was gone for the first time in four years. Gradually, the inflammation and redness subsided, the pain disappeared, and the skin returned to normal, with no scales.

Now, several months later, Robert's toenails are growing in normally, and the condition is completely reversed. Robert feels like his treatment was "easy, user friendly, and less expensive than drugs."

Internal remedies

Almost all herbs containing significant amounts of essential oils are antifungal, and many are used in treatment. Some of these herbs are for internal use, while others are applied topically.

Garlic is a widely recommended and well researched antifungal, proving to be more effective against many fungi than several antifungal drugs. A typical, but by no means absolute maximum, dose is three cloves per day (6-9 capsules).

Berberine containing herbs are generally antifungal. They certainly are effective for yeast, so many herbalists recommend them for internal treatment of athlete's foot fungus.

Turmeric root is beneficial for the redness, swelling, and pain of athlete's foot. Turmeric kills a wide variety of microbes, which could enhance your effort to kill the fungus. Use as many capsules of this mild herb per day as you can comfortably swallow, up to four tablespoons of powder stirred into water.

Khalsa has used cayenne with good results. A few others to consider would be thyme, aloe, and ginseng, all of which have worked well at one time or another in the past.

Most treatments for athlete's foot, of course, focus on external application. While this can be beneficial in the short run, or as part of a more complete program, success really depends on using internal remedies as well. Liquids can be applied to the feet with a swab or eyedropper, or, for milder herbal solutions, a foot bath works well. Foot baths or washes are made from, essentially, herb tea. Place the brewed tea in a pan and enjoy a healing soak.

In Khalsa's experience, the essential oils of clove and cinnamon are very reliable. Both these oils are *HOT*, though, so you need to be cautious in applying them. Dilute the essential oil with any vegetable oil, such as almond, or hand lotion, or even rubbing alcohol. Start with a 10% solution, and work up to a strength that is effective. Infected toenails will often tolerate applications of pure clove or cinnamon oil. The thin oil penetrates very well into the tissues under the nail. Apply the oils once or twice daily.

Vegetable oils in general have a mild healing effect on foot fungus. Oils with herb constituents, called "infused oils," are a good way to get the best of both. A common hair and body oil, used in India, contains amla, which has antifunga properties. Interestingly, there is very little tinea in India, even though it is a hot and humid climate.

Bad Breath

In the final analysis, at least 90% of all bad breath starts off in the mouth, and the crud that collects between your teeth isn't the main storehouse of smell. The stench comes from the ama on the back of your tongue. In fact, this is the location of the most concentrated ama in the body. The offenders are sulfur compounds, created when anaerobic bacteria break down food. These bugs thrive in a dry mouth, so it's important to keep the saliva flowing and the oral cavity moist.

Cleaning the tongue is a critical part of maintaining oral health. Ayurveda, in particular, emphasizes this daily practice. Brush your tongue while brushing your teeth, or use a tongue scraper. Tongue cleaning reduces bad breath, and helps prevent plaque.[663] Nasal washing with a neti pot will clean out any accumulated ama from the sinuses.

Mouthwashes made with essential oils are for canker sores, bad breath, and sore throats. Put 1-2 drops of essential oil in a cup of water. Use peppermint, eucalyptus, lavender, clove or rosemary.

Add some apple cider vinegar if you like. Salt may also be added. Gargle. Use this 2-3 times a day as needed. Or chew a few cardamom seeds for a quick breath cleaning.

Green and black tea polyphenols kill the bacteria that cause bad breath. In a "bad breath" study, scientists combined tea extracts with three species of bad breath bacteria for 48 hours. Tea polyphenols suppressed the growth of bacteria by 30% and reduced the production of compounds that cause bad breath.[664] It looks like rinsing with black tea keeps plaque from forming and also destroys tooth decay causing acids.

Benign Prostatic Hyperplasia

The pelvic area is seen as a particularly critical area in which it is necessary to keep energy balanced to retain homeostasis. (The other critical body areas are the heart and the head.) Prostate problems, which occur with aging, happen during the time of life when vata is dominant. It's not surprising that the aging prostate is connected to disordered vata. BPH is an *udavarta* disorder, one involving the reverse direction of vata. As previously mentioned, apana in the large intestine and genitals rises upwards, leaving prostate energy diminished.

Ayurvda has talked about BPH for a long time- it appears in the classic scriptures. Ancient works describe that below the *nabhi* (navel) there is a hard gland that can bulge. It is like a small stone. This gland, when affected by unbalanced vata, can cause disease *vataashteela* (that we now name BPH).[665]

Ayurveda maintains that overindulgence in sex will downgrade prostate health.[666] (This will vary with each person.) Ayurveda says that we should never suppress natural urges (yawning, belching, gas, etc.). Doing so will aggravate vata and contribute to *udavarta*.[667] Habitually ignoring the urge to urinate can irritate the prostate. Other contributing factors include excesses in physical labor, fasting, pungent, bitter and astringent foods, wine and meat. Clinical observations show that BPH is becoming more common in Japan. Those who consume more meat and milk appear to be at greater risk.[668] A Finnish study from 2000 found that meat consumption increased lower urinary tract symptoms (hesitancy, incomplete emptying, incontinence, nocturia and daytime frequency) and vegetable intake decreased these symptoms.[669] In fact, The **American Dietetic Association and Dietitians of Canada say that vegetarians have lower rates of prostate cancer.[670] Other studies confirm this.[671] (By definition, the cells in BPH are benign, not cancerous. BPH is not thought to be a risk factor for prostate cancer by some authorities in conventional medicine. Others reason that any unhealthy condition in the prostate is cause for future problems, and are convinced there is a link. Studies are equivocal.)**

Ayurveda sees BPH not so much as a problem in itself (of course it can make a man miserable), but a sign of a much more serious syndrome. Vata reversal is a big problem, and will eventually bring all bodily processes to a grinding halt. It is the antecedent to a cascade of problems that flow in a predictable way. It goes like this. The apana vata ascends into the liver, creating an imbalance in the pitta of the liver. This draws ama from the gut into the liver, and later into the blood. This pitta disordered blood accumulates in areas of weakened areas, which can be anywhere, but can include the disordered apana. As the ama accumulates in the urogenital tract, it has no way out, as the apana that would normally assist it to exit is now reversed. Inflammation ensues. Certain men are more susceptible to the collected effects of this problem than others, but the sum total of these disruptions of the doshas often settles in the prostate and blooms as BPH.

In general, udavarta conditions are treated with remedies to assist vata back into its proper directions of movement. Medicated enemas promote bowel function. Barley, oil and meat soup in the diet nourish and balance disordered vata. Herbs that generally balance this condition include haritaki, asafoetida and calamus.[672] A rectal suppository made from asafoetida, honey and rock salt, smeared with ghee for insertion, can be used.

So any given case of BPH can involve any of the doshas in any proportion. The boggy, wet, swollen prostate is a kapha excess. The inflamed tissue is a manifestation of pitta. The blockages and reversed energy flow comes from vata. The diet appropriate to the offending dosha is indicated.

A multipronged approach is likely to be successful. Maintaining the quality and quantity of the reproductive fluid (shukra) will stabilize the testosterone level and sexual desire. Ayurveda will also focus on promoting the unobstructed flow of urine, easing the pressure on the genitourinary tract upping immune function and purifying the urine to avoid infections and preserving the normal size of the prostate.[673] The prostate is sensitive to the accumulation of ama, so detoxifying programs are necessary to prevent problems. Turmeric, cumin and fennel can help purify the urine.

Punarnava, the above ground, herbaceous portion, is a diuretic, anti-spasmodic and anti-inflammatory agent, with analgesic qualities, in urinary tract infections. Unlike most diuretics, which are catabolic by definition, Punarnava is a rasayana. This herb is perfectly designed for prostate problems. Use 4 grams per day with hot water, or use Punarnava Guggulu at 1 gram per day, or as needed.[674]

Men can use shatavari root as a soothing general remedy for the genitourinary system. Considered a builder and balancer for reproductive organs, as a rasayana, it increases semen and sexual juices in general. This cooling herb acts as a blood cleanser and supports the immune system. Shatavari as a soothing treatment for dry or inflamed membranes of the sex organs. As a mild diuretic, with a tropism for the urinary tract, it can relieve the congestion of the prostate. It can be prepared as a milk decoction combined with ghee, raw sugar, and honey. Shatavari is related to the Western asparagus root, which has similar properties, but which is a stronger diuretic.

Zinc is critical for prostate function. Black pepper, cumin and coriander increase bioavailability of the zinc. Black pepper peppercorn is also a drying herb that will reduce the size of wet, boggy tissues in general.

Radish is diuretic and detoxifying. Maintaining proper bowel volume and movement regularity is necessary to prevent aggravation of apana vata, the force that governs elimination. Testosterone enhancing foods, such as asparagus, bananas and dates will delay prostate swelling. A few other foods have general benefit for the urinary tract. Most are diuretic. Included are beets greens (try as a monodiet for two weeks), coconut, grapefruit and melon.[675]

Banyan tree sap is a folk remedy for the prostate. Banyan trees, huge behemoths that dot north India, have spongy wood filled with milky sap. The sap is easily extracted. It is a sweet sticky liquid somewhat like honey. It is a general tonic remedy for the prostate. Use about a teaspoon per day, especially combined with yogurt. This is a favorite of my mentor.

One possible herbal combination for BPH is shilajit, purified zinc mineral ash, kachnar, guduchi, turmeric, punarnava, sandalwood and sarsaparilla. Another proprietary mixture contains Mimosa pudica, Argyreia speciosa, Orchis mascula, tulsi, black pepper, gokshurs, guggul and shilajit.

Amla, turmeric, shilajit and guggul are anti-inflammatory, if inflammation is a paramount symptom.

Another formula would be equal parts of ashwaganda, gokshura and shatavari. Use 6-10 grams per day of this mixture, in a vehicle appropriate to the condition.

Castor oil to bowel tolerance will reverse the vata of the large intestine.

Since BPH results in nighttime urinary dribbling, using diuretics during the day, and then abstaining from water in the evening can reduce nocturnal pilgrimages to the bathroom. Use a tea of holy basil leaf and coriander seed.

Try a healing recipe for the prostate. This is basically a taste way to ingest a large dose of diuretic, detoxifying, anti-inflammatory parsley.

Parsley Prostate Rasayana

1 cup Basmati rice
1 cup Parsley, dried, or fresh, chopped, to taste
2 cups Potato, chopped (skins on)
2 Onions, chopped
2 tsp. Ajwain seed
1 tsp. Red pepper, ground (or more to taste)
1 Tbs. Turmeric
1 tsp. Black pepper
2 Bay leaves, crushed
1/2 cup ghee

Sauté onions in ghee. Add spices. Cook until browned. Add rice, potato and parsley. Stir until mixed. Add water (to steam rice), cover, and cook for another 15 minutes. Can be eaten as a mono diet. Serves 4-6. Serve with yogurt for extra stamina.

Canker sores

Since mouth ulcers stem from a breakdown in tissue structure, the herb gotu kola can be quite effective. Gotu kola is widely known to heal wounds and promotes connective tissue growth. The dose is 1 oz. of dry weight of herb, brewed as tea, per day, or a smaller dose, to tolerance, in capsules. This tea can also serve as a rinse for connective tissue disorders in the mouth.

Consider high oral doses of acidophilus and an acidophilus mouth rinse.[676] Other rinses that can help include alum, Milk of Magnesia, and cinchona bark. Noted natural physician Hakim Chishti suggests the powder of myrrh gum, applied directly to the ulcer. The gel side of an aloe leaf can also be applied to soothe the sore.

Probably the most outstanding herbal remedy for mouth sores is licorice root, a potent anti-inflammatory and tissue healer. Put a pinch of powder on the sore, or suck on a lozenge made from DGL (de-glycyrrhizinated licorice).

Cardiovascular Conditions

The heart, of course, is the stuff of poetry. But when we say, "Eat your heart out," we don't really mean it literally. Yet it seems that in America, we're doing just that. As a people, we gobble such huge quantities of animal fat that our arteries are clogged like the L.A. freeway at rush hour. The bad news: According to The American Heart Association, 1.5 million Americans will have a heart attack this year.[677] Heart disease is the nation's No.1 killer. The good news: preventive measures can reduce your risk.

One cause of cardiovascular disease is high blood pressure, and this condition is so common that one in five Americans adults has it.[678]

Follow a heart healthy diet

Our bodies produce cholesterol from dietary fat. Saturated fats (animal fats and margarine) increase clotting, raise LDL, and lower HDL cholesterol. Every 1 percent decrease in total blood cholesterol reduces a person's risk of coronary heart disease by 2 to 3 percent. So, the primary goal of diet is to lower cholesterol by reducing the intake of cholesterol and fat.

Eat your fruit and veggies, and your heart will thank you for it. At least, that's the indication of a study in *The American Journal of Clinical Nutrition.* Women who ate between four and 10 servings of fruits and vegetables per day reduced their risk of cardiovascular disease by between 20 percent and 30 percent.[679] Women without any cardiovascular risk factors, such as diabetes or hypertension, fared even better. This news shouldn't surprise you. The researchers said that the 20 to 30 percent reduction in risk associated with increased intake of fruits and vegetables might be a conservative estimate, due to measurement techniques.

Herbal Heart Medicines

"The results I got were phenomenal. I tell everybody I talk to about the great effect," says Guruchander Singh Khalsa, D.C., of Espanola, N.M.

Dr. Khalsa, a successful chiropractic physician, has had total cholesterol numbers of over 300 for 20 years. He comes from a family with genetically high cholesterol. On his mother's side, one brother died at age 42 of a massive heart attack, and all the remaining siblings have had quadruple bypass surgery, along with heart attacks. Dr. Khalsa has managed to avoid serious disease with diet and yoga, but the cholesterol numbers were becoming seriously worrisome. His thyroid function was depressed as well with the thyroid stimulating hormone reading at triple the normal value. After a bit of professional consultation, we settled on having him try guggul gum at 6 grams per day, to quickly lower blood fats, and a combination of gotu kola leaf, saw palmetto berry, scullcap leaf, elder berry, and willow bark, to increase thyroid function. Four months later, the cholesterol had dropped a whopping 180 points, and the thyroid blood test was exactly normal.

Treatment by Dosha

Remedies for balancing heart problems caused by kapha in general include vacha, neem and pipali.

Remedies for balancing heart problems caused by pitta in general include honey, raw sugar, ghee, bala, and licorice.

Remedies for balancing heart problems caused by vata in general include asafoetida, rock salt, cardamom, ginger, and triphala.

Ayurvedic physicians use arjuna in a wide variety of cardiovascular conditions-it is virtually a panacea for cardiac failure, hypertension, angina, endocarditis, pericarditis and edema.[680]

Our colleague, Alan Keith Tillotson, PhD, author of The One Earth

Herbal Sourcebook, says "Arjuna bark is one of the most important heart tonics in Ayurvedic medicine, used to treat all forms of heart disease. It reduces the heart-damaging culprits of inflammation and mucus." Use it with guggul for high cholesterol. This herb is particularly effective for congestive heart failure.[681] Arjuna also benefits cardiomyopathy and the treatment of heart attack. It works for a wide range of related symptoms (angina, pumping strength, enlarged heart)[682] and protects the tissue of the heart from damage. [683]

Garlic reduces blood pressure levels by about 5 to 10%.[684 685 686] We see larger reductions with higher doses.

Guggul gum is a standby for lowering cholesterol, rivaling any natural substance. Guggul has lowered total cholesterol by over 20 percent, while increasing good HDL cholesterol by 36 percent.[687] It can assist in managing overall body fat. It exerts its effect at least partially through the thyroid.[688 689 690] Guggul can be taken in a dose of 1,500 mg, three times daily. Triphala Guggul lowers body fat as well.[691]

Cataract

Cataract, the opacification of the lens or its capsule, is called "*timira*" or "*linga nasha*" in Sanskrit. Eye conditions, particularly cataract, are quite complex, and can arise from many possible variations of *multi-dosha* imbalance.

Cataracts are a clouding of the inner structures of the eye. If you live long enough, this might be inevitable. Then again, it might not. Signs of cataract formation typically begin after age 50. Very common in older adults, cataracts cause about one-third of all severe eyesight problems in this age group. One large study in the U.S. found a visually significant cataract in at least one eye in approximately 39% of men and about 46% of women age 75 years or older.[692]

This particular area of the eye doesn't need a blood supply to receive toxins or accumulated excess waste; it comes straight in from the lymph. If the lymphatic system is not being pumped adequately or draining properly—either because it is overwhelmed with its processing tasks or because of insufficient breath or muscular activity to drive its circulation—the backup can show here.

Make no mistake- cataracts can be treated nonsurgically about 85 percent of the time in our estimation. Dr. Abel concurs, citing a figure of 80%. The average time necessary to improve this condition sufficiently to reverse the need for surgery is six months.

Cataracts caused by pitta will produce visual symptoms of images which are bright and circular, vibrating, and with rainbow-hued emanations. Since pitta regulates the overall function of the eyes, antipitta botanicals may have a generally beneficial effect.

Kapha is responsible for the production, deposition, and accumulation of all sticky, tissue clogging wastes, especially lipids. Thus, the actual material on the lens could be considered an accumulation of excess kapha, and treated with antikapha therapies.

Cataracts caused by kapha will produce visual symptoms of images which are white, greasy-looking, enlarged, wet looking, as if underwater, and resemble puffy clouds. Diabetic cataracts should be treated with ant-kapha botanicals and diet.

Primarily, however, *timira* is regarded as an aggravation of vata. A fundamental property of vata is to cause dryness in tissues. Ayurveda considers the loss of lubrication and softness of the lens and its capsule to be a result of this accrued vata in the eye.[693]

Vata predominates in the nervous system generally, so the eyes, as part of that system, are subject to vata derangement. Cataracts caused by vata will produce visual symptoms of images which are unsteady, dusty, reddish and irregular.

Diseases of the eye, ear, nose, and throat, primarily problems of vata, can be caused by rapid changes in environmental temperature, such as a cold both after hot sun, overuse of the eyes at a particular focal point, such as long distance, exposure of the eyes to atmospheric contaminants, suppression of natural urges, such as urination, emotional excesses, sexual overindulgence, or staring at close distance.[694]

Triphala nourishes the eyeball, and strengthens the nerves and other tissues.[695] The dose is 500 mg to 2 grams per day, as a general tonic, possibly for a lifetime.

Amla is a strong rejuvenative, and the primary anti-pitta medicine, and is the most frequently used cataract medicine. Amla generally benefits the eyes, and is known to improve eyesight.[696] Amla is a potent inhibitor of free radicals, which are one cause of cataracts. The dose is 250 mg to 1 gram per day for one to two years or as needed.

Haritaki nourishes the nervous system and promotes vision. The dose is 250 mg to 500 mg per day.

Bibitaki regulates kapha. Like amla and haritaki, it improves the vision. The dose is 250 mg to 500 mg. per day.

Mahasudarshan (literally "the great formula for good vision") contains bitter herbs that cool and cleanse the eyes.[697]

Yashtimadhu (licorice root) is anti-inflammatory and has a generally beneficially effect for cataract. Chandana (sandalwood) controls the two doshas commonly involved in cataract. Ashwaganda root has a similar effect. Bringraj herb is a tridoshic medicine that cools pitta in the eyes. Sevanti (Chrysanthemum flower) has an affinity for the head, and cools pitta.

Turmeric has been shown to prevent cataract formation.[698]

The foremost treatment objective is to control vata, by moistening, warming, mobilizing, and detoxifying the affected tissue. Ghee controls vata, and is considered the most important remedy for the eyes. The older the ghee, the more therapeutic the effect.[699] The dose is 1-2 tsp twice daily.[700]

Ghrita, medicated ghee, is used in cataract. The preparation Maha triphala ghrita, which includes ghee and triphala, among other ingredients, is used in the early stages of cataract. The medicated ghee is used at a dose of 2 teaspoons twice daily, one hour before meals, with a cup of warm milk.

Shigru leaf is prophylactic for those at risk of cataract. The dose is 5 grams per day.

Anise seed, coriander seed, and almonds are used together to benefit cataract.[701]

Netra basti, or eye washes, are popular in Ayurvedic ophthalmology. Several herbs are administered in this manner:

- Triphala water - add 1 tablespoon triphala powder to 10 oz water. Cover and let sit for 12 hours. Filter and apply with an eyedropper or eye cup.[702] A cold infusion of amla only may be substituted.[703]
- Shigru juice - Mix with honey and apply and apply to the eyes daily. Shigru leaf is rich in vitamin A,[704] as well as vitamin C.[705]

Eyewashes can also be made from infusions of chamomile flowers, chrysanthemum flowers, or rose petals.[706]

Netra Basti is often done with ghee. This low technology procedure involves making dough of wheat flour and water. The dough is formed into a ring about the size of a doughnut and placed around the eye. (The patient is lying on her back.) The dough ring is filled with liquid ghee that has been heated to a comfortable temperature (test it first). The patient allows the ghee to soak the eye for about 20 minutes, and then repeats the process on the other eye.

Ayurveda uses herbal pastes applied to the entire head to balance the doshas in that area. A typical formula for the paste includes mung bean flour, minced fresh ginger, raw cream, ghee, sesame oil, mustard oil, and water.[707]

Amla fruit decoction mixed with buttermilk may be poured on the forehead in a thin, continuous stream.[708]

The buildup of a thick, sweet, accumulated ama is comprised of advanced glycosylation end products, or AGE's, which stick to the surface of the lens and cross link the proteins, binding them into a web-like formation.

Ayurvedic herbs which can assist in this process include the following, all of which have primarily anti-kapha and anti-ama action:

Bitter melon - 2 ounces of fresh juice, per day, or the equivalent
Gurmar herb - 10 grams per day
Asana bark - 3-6 grams per day [709] [710]
Tulsi herb - 10 grams per day
Ginger root - 5 grams per day
Neem leaf - 5 grams per day
Guggul gum - 3-10 grams per day
Kutki - 5 grams per day
Diet

The dietary strategy should be based on the primary underlying dosha imbalance, usually vata. If vata is the dosha to be controlled, the diet should be warming, moisturizing, nourishing, easy to digest, and primarily consist of cooked foods.

Specific foods that benefit cataract are cow's ghee, milk (warm with digestive spices such as clove and cinnamon), butter, rice, wheat, mung bean, banana, spinach, okra, grapes, pomegranates, apples, and oranges.

Pungent, bitter, sour, and salty foods promote cataracts and should be minimized.[711]

To underline this, one study found that people who eat the highest amounts of butter and salt double their cataract risk compared to those who consume the lowest amounts of these foods. Spinach, peppers, melons, tomatoes and citrus fruits reduce the relative risk of needing cataract surgery by half.[712] Folks who eat less than five servings of fruits and vegetables per day are 5 to 13 times more likely to develop cataracts. Vitamin C deficiency increases cataract risk 4 to 11 times.[713]

A Harvard Medical School study surveyed 50,828 nurses and reported that women who had spinach five or more times per week, and those who took vitamin C supplements for 10 years or more, reduced their risk of cataract surgery by more than 45 percent.[714] Presumably the dietary lutein and zeaxanthin were responsible.

Cold and flu

Herbal medicine regimes for infection include three fundamental steps. We must boot out the invader, nourish the tissue (in this case, the respiratory system) that allowed the infection to take root and support the immune system to prevent relapse.

Cooling diaphoretics are used to reduce fever and inflammation. Chrysanthemum flower and honeysuckle flower are also strongly antimicrobial. Warming diaphoretics, taken hot, also treat the flu. Use them when the main symptom is chills. Basil leaf is favored for reducing mucus in the lungs and nasal passages.[715 716 717 718] Basil kills bacteria and stimulates the immune system.[719 720] Cinnamon bark is a very effective warming diaphoretic, used at a lower dose, say one half ounce, or in medicinal beverage mixtures.

Gokshura, a soothing, slimy herb, is used internally for sore throats.

Kalmegh is a very widely used medicine for upper respiratory infection. It is sometimes now being used in combination with echinacea, lemon balm, slippery elm bark, cinnamon bark and Chinese frittillaria bulb. Take 10-15 grams per day for an acute cold. Guduchi is a standby folk remedy for cold and flu. Use up to 20 grams per day, in capsules, or stirred into ghee, in an acute situation.

Yogi Bhajan recommended 10 peppercorns boiled in a cup of milk to release congestion. A good general tea includes dry ginger, cinnamon, tulsi, peppercorn, lemon grass and raw sugar. Trikatu tea or pills will loosen congestion.

Application of dry ginger paste over the sinuses helps.

For the brave hearted, try this one. Heat two tablespoons of mustard oil over medium heat. Add one half teaspoon of asafetida or 5 garlic cloves. Cook the oil until the herbs turn brown. Cool, filter, and add a pinch of salt. Use this oil for massage.

Constipation

There are several ways to gently handle constipation. One method is with herbs that promote bowel movements. These include Shatavari and Gokshura.

Shatavari and Gokshura are similar in action and can be used together or by themselves. Both are mucilaginous agents (demulcents). They create a slimy, gelatinous mass which is nourishing and healing to mucous membranes, including those of the digestive tract. Two to four heaping tablespoons of powder a day, mixed with water (or yogurt, oatmeal, applesauce or maple syrup) to make a paste will increase stool motility.

Senna leaf makes a pretty decent-tasting tea, but can also be used in capsules, one or two a day.

Rhubarb Root, also called Asian rhubarb or turkey rhubarb, is milder than and two to four capsules a day would be appropriate.

Aloe Vera juice will provide the soothing effect of the gel and the liquefying effect on intestinal contents.

Cooling rose petal is also very mild, so use one to five capsules per day.

Demulcent licorice root is still another mild option at one to five capsules per day.

Senna, rhubarb and aloe vera all contain anthraquinones, which cause contractions of the bowels. In higher doses or stronger preparations, this can cause cramping or "griping." For this reason they are often mixed with carminative herbs (those that prevent gas or soothe the digestive tract).

Triphala is a very gentle light laxative. Most folks will have an easy bowel movement in about 12 hours from a dose of around 5 grams.

Psyllium seed, a common bulk fiber laxative, balances bowel function and relieves pain in irritable bowels.[721] Psyllium's capacity to absorb fluids means that it is useful for treating diarrhea. As it travels through the gut, the mucilage in psyllium creates a soothing benefit, which may relieve cramping.[722] A study to determine the optimum dose recommended 20 grams per day.[723]

Baba Hari Dass proposed to take a number of large manuka raisins, remove the seeds, skewer with an iron rod and roast. Mix this with a little black pepper.[724]

Depression

An estimated 19 million American adults are living with major depression.[725] Most everyone has the occasional attack of "the blues" or a "down in the dumps" funk, short periods when things don't seem to go well and life isn't looking too rosy. Feeling a bit depressed is a normal reaction to struggling loss or bruised self-esteem.

Clinical depression is different. If the feeling of sadness becomes intense, lasting for long periods of time and preventing a person from leading a normal life, it is characterized as a treatable medical condition called major depressive disorder, one of a number of depressive illnesses. It is a medical disorder characterized by persistent and sometimes severe feelings of worthlessness, guilt, sadness, helplessness and hopelessness.

Natural Treatments for Mild to Moderate Depression

Depression is a complex condition. Herbal medicine can be very effective for depression, especially mild forms of the disease. Shwaganda is one of the most promising herbs for mental health. It a "grounding" herb that stabilizes mood.

Gokshura promotes mental clarity, and in fact, we recommend it for its exceptional clinical effect in depression. It may be taken with ashwaganda as a tonic nervine.

Shankhapushi helps restore clear quality of the mind and relaxation. This herb is a tonic for the mind and nerve tissue, especially effective for anxiety and fear. Often taken with or prepared in ghee, it promotes tranquility without dulling the mind. In depression, it uplifts.

Brahmi has been used in medicine for anxiety, emotional stress, mental exhaustion and forgetfulness.

Cayenne and other chilies, especially red varieties, are excellent treatments for depression. Although the mechanism is not yet known, it is proven that chilies enhance production of endorphins, the mood elevating brain chemicals responsible for the "chili eater's high."

Use cayenne in gradually increasing doses, in capsules or as a food spice, as your stomach tolerates it.

Don't take brain function decline lying down. Get up and exercise. Aerobic workouts can improve high-level brain functions in those over 50, maintain Duke University researchers.[726]

Detoxification

To treat the symptoms of excess ama, and the underlying toxin accumulation that causes them, herbalists use a broad spectrum of remedies that assist the body in removing the waste products from the tissues.

When it comes to detoxifying the liver, few herbs are more widely used than burdock root. It is specific for eruptions of the head, face and neck. Dandelion root acts to increase bile flow. Dandelion root can be taken as tea, tincture, or capsules. Three thousand milligrams per day is a good dose. Roasted dandelion root is brewed as a delicious coffee substitute.

Used mainly as an exotic vegetable, artichoke is a thistle-like plant in the daisy family. However, this plant is used herbally as an excellent detoxifier of the liver and gallbladder. It also reduces blood fats, like cholesterol and effectively treats gallstones and obesity.

One study showed a significant lowering of elevated cholesterol (12.2%), triglyceride (5.7%) levels and body weight with artichoke extract.[727] The raw globe can also be juiced.

Sarsaparilla has a history of use, in Asia and Europe, as a blood purifier, dating back to the 16th century. Several saponin compounds in sarsaparilla have been shown to be effective in treating psoriasis. Take 3-12 grams of sarsaparilla root per day as a tasty tea, or the equivalent in capsules.

Besides being a general tonic, triphala is a light laxative, skin, eye, and liver nourisher, and a general detoxifier. It is used as a cleansing throat gargle, and as a dry massage powder.

Amla is the frontline anti-inflammatory herb, and is used for a wide variety of inflammatory conditions, including hemorrhoids, gastritis, and colitis.

Bibitaki is the best single herb for generally controlling excess fat toxins. It excels at removing stones and accumulations of toxins (mucus, cholesterol, mineral deposits) in the digestive, urinary, and respiratory tracts. It is unique in being both laxative and astringent, so it purges the intestines, while simultaneously toning the tissues.

Haritaki is the best single herb for generally controlling dryness and constipation. The gentle laxative qualities of haritaki are perfect for easy detoxification.

To keep the bowels open during a gentle cleanse, start triphala at 3 grams per day, and increase by one gram per day until the bowels are comfortably regular.

Bhumy amalaki is the standby for liver detoxification. Use it whenever a general hepatic is indicated. In our experience, it increases bile flow in a very mild way, so is well tolerated by people for whom a stronger cholagogue is contraindicated. Use up to 10g per day in capsules.

Radish (*Raphanus sativus*), a member of the cabbage family, is known the world over for liver and gallbladder detoxification. The black radish is regarded as a stronger remedy, but the common red radish also works. Other radishes, including daikon (called "mooli" in India), are used in their respective cultures. Radish is not a true cholagogue, but rather a choleretic. According to European sources, it does not promote bile flow, instead relaxing the smooth musculature of the bile ducts, allowing freer bile flow. Radish is good in cases of chronic constipation. Use as a food, raw or cooked, or as juice, depending on tolerance. Mooli pranthas are popular in Ayurvedic cuisine.

Diabetes

Diabetes, *madhumeha*, has been known for thousands of years. Diabetes and similar diseases form a group of twenty conditions, *pramehas*, which are characterized by changes in the urine. The ten kapha types are easily cured. The six pitta types are curable with difficulty, while the four conditions caused by vata are incurable but treatable.

Ayurveda mentions these preliminary symptoms of diabetic condition: accumulation of tartar on the teeth, burning sensations on the palms and soles, stickiness of the skin all over the body, thirst, and a persistent sweet taste in the mouth.

Noninsulin Dependent Diabetes Mellitus (NIDDM), or type II, usually is diagnosed after forty years of age. Ninety percent of diabetics in our culture are type II. NIDDM is a disease of loss of sensitivity to insulin. Typically, insulin levels in the blood are actually increased, but the tissues have lost their ability to respond to the hormone.

The typical NIDDM patient is a classic example of kapha derangement- fat, slow, greasy, cold- even the urine is sweet. Getting kapha under control makes this type of diabetes easily curable.

Of course, we know that atherosclerosis is a major complication in diabetes. Therefore, lifelong maintenance of proper cholesterol levels is essential. Recent studies have shown that lowering cholesterol levels retards the progression of diabetic nephropathy, or kidney disease. Not only do dietary measures affect cholesterol levels, but, as we shall see, many herbs are quite successful in this area.

Green and black teas, powerful antioxidant plants containing catechin and epicatechin, compounds belonging to the flavonol category, have been shown to aid in diabetes.

The bark of the asana is one of the few remedies that is thought to have an effect on type I diabetes. Dr. Svoboda says that asana bark has been reported to regenerate the insulin producing cells of the pancreas, but only if the disease is of recent origin. Drs. Pizzorno and Murray confirm this and suggest that asana is the only substance, drug or otherwise, that is known to have this effect. Asana is another rich source of epicatechin.

The name *gurmar* means *killer of sweet*. When chewed, these leaves block sweet taste on the tongue, reducing the appeal of sugar foods. Gurmar is a very promising remedy for diabetes. In use for centuries in India, it is now being recognized by modern science.

Gurmar is truly a revolutionary herb. Its benefits extend to type I and type II diabetes. It significantly improves cholesterol and triglyceride levels, as well. It certainly could be the backbone of a natural diabetes program.

Fenugreek is an effective blood sugar lowering herb. Since fenugreek actually tastes good, it may be more practical for people to use on a daily basis. One study used fenugreek seed baked into flat bread, which proved effective.

It is not known whether the active principle in fenugreek lies in the high soluble fiber content, or in another unknown compound. Fenugreek is effective in both types of diabetes, is cheap, well tolerated, and at 28% protein content, a favorable food source. While demonstrating significant anti-diabetic activities, fenugreek has one disadvantage - the dose. One recent successful study used 100 grams (about 3 1/2 ounces) per day. The typical diabetic may have resistance to the large amount of herb required. Commonly, fenugreek seeds would be eaten after being soaked in water overnight.

Karela is widely known as a folk remedy in diabetes. Doses as small as 2 ounces of juice per day are effective. The juice is difficult to make palatable, so plug your nose, and take a two ounce shot - down the hatch!

Jambul fruit, or seeds alone, is used in Ayurvedic medicine as one of the most powerful hypoglycemic herbs. Doses of as little as one gram of powdered dry herb per day can be effective. Jambul is thought to be particularly synergistic with okra. Chakravarti explicitly recommends this combination, mentioning that you should be able to see large blood sugar reductions in ten days.[728]

Neem is one of the most useful plants grown in Asia, and one of the most widely used. It stimulates insulin secretion in the pancreas, as well as possessing actions that support the immune system, which is often damaged as a complication of diabetes.

Whether consumed as a delicious food, or as a potent medicine, ginger acts in diabetes both by stimulating pancreas cells and by lowering lipids (cholesterol, triglycerides) in the blood.

Tulsi increases uptake of glucose in the peripheral tissues of the body. Therefore, tulsi potentiates the action of all other diabetes medicines, including insulin, bitter melon, and neem leaf.

Stress is a major cause in diabetes, and a major effect, as the tissues respond to the damage from high blood glucose. This *vicious stress cycle* is resolved with holy basil, as it has demonstrated anti-stress action.

Guggul is an effective herb for managing all fats in the body. In diabetes, it normalizes cholesterol, triglycerides, and body fat, thus reducing the chance of arterial deposits. Guggul also prevents abnormal blood clotting. This combination of actions is dynamic for reducing retinopathy (eye damage), neuropathy (nerve degeneration, usually starting in the feet), and gangrene, which are secondary to atherosclerosis, and common, very serious complications of diabetes. Myrrh gum is an herb, more well known in the west, which is related to guggul, and may be substituted for it.

Kutki contains a wealth of medicines for diabetes. The main properties stimulate digestive secretions, which in turn stimulate pancreatic insulin secretion. Kutki also enhances immune functions.

A unique action of this herb is to normalize the function of the liver, which is obviously a key to proper healthy living. Kutki assists the liver in storing blood sugar in the form of glycogen, which is essential in diabetes management. It is sometimes used to protect the liver from the toxic effects of anti-diabetic drugs.

Amla has proven useful in diabetic treatment.

Shilajit is a general detoxifier and rejuvenative, and is particularly useful in diabetes.

The leaves of bilwa, the *stone apple* tree, stimulate the pancreas to secrete insulin. One teaspoon of fresh leaf juice per day is the typical dose.

Diabetics, as we have seen, often experience cardiovascular symptoms. Death from cardiovascular disease is 60-70% in diabetics, versus 20-25% in non-diabetics. Arjuna is the herb of choice. The most significant dietary fiber for diabetes comes from legumes, such as kidney beans. Legumes are beneficial at least in part because they contain a water soluble, gel - forming fiber which has been shown to enhance diabetic control.

In addition to a well crafted diet, diabetics can make therapeutic use of certain foods to adjust blood sugar levels.

Okra is an Ayurvedic remedy for blood sugar. Many American patients who have tried this food have success with the juice of okra pods added to their diet. Okra is delicious as a steamed vegetable, also.

Dandelion greens have been quite successful for many diabetics. Again, the most practical form is freshly squeezed juice. For winter, the greens can be frozen and juiced daily as needed. Of course, fresh dandelion greens are delicious in a salad.

Other foods that have been helpful for diabetics include cinnamon, nutmeg, turmeric, bay leaf, cashew, celery, cayenne, ginger, coriander seed, lettuce, cabbage, turnip, papaya fruit, cranberry, Jerusalem artichoke, millet, oats, barley, and buckwheat.

While well known as common foods, the bulbs of onion and garlic are significant hypoglycemics. The active properties are thought to be sulfur containing compounds (disulphides), such as allicin. Evidence suggests that these compounds lower glucose levels by competing with insulin (also a disulphide) in the liver. The well known cardiovascular benefits of these herbs alone (regulating blood pressure, cholesterol, and platelet aggregation) justify their use in diabetes. However, even at moderate dietary levels, these herbs have potent effects. Diabetics should use these herbs liberally.

Every authority in diabetes stresses the role of exercise in effective treatment. Every factor of diabetes is benefited by exercise. Obese diabetics are encouraged to gradually build up the intensity of their exercise program, and then to go for the maximum they can possibly do. Thin types (usually IDDM) may have to be a bit more moderate, with the focus on brisk walking.

Also we should note that exercise reduces insulin resistance. The more fit the person is, the more muscular tissues and other tissues respond to insulin. Several studies of strength training in older people have recently proved that they can change their insulin levels with exercise alone.

Yoga has been used to treat diabetes for thousands of years. For obese people, very vigorous exercises with aerobic benefit should be encouraged, leading to normalizing weight. Deep cleansing breathing (pranayama) practices can be helpful.

Recommended yoga exercises are:

Sarbangasana (shoulder stand)
Shirshasana (head stand)
Yoga - Mudra (front bend lotus)
Matsyasana (fish pose)
Janu - Shirasana (one leg front stretch)
Matsyendrasana (spinal twist)

Fibromyalgia

Fibromyalgia (FMS) is characterized by chronic, generalized muscular pain, usually in specific well known areas, and fatigue. After osteoarthritis, it is the second most common arthritis disorder, more common even than rheumatoid arthritis.

Turmeric root is a standby for the musculoskeletal system and greatly improves FMS. For acute episodes, the dose might be as high as one ounce (4 tbs) per day. For ongoing use, its 1 gram per day as a spice, or in capsules. Standardized extract is available. The dose is 1500 mg of total curcumin content per day.

Willow bark is nature's remedy for joint pain. Use a tea brewed from up to 1 oz., dry weight, of the raw herb, per day, or an extract containing 240 mg total salicin per day. Willow can be used for as long as necessary.

Many other herbs are candidates for FMS treatment. Consider these:

Ginger root - increases circulation to muscles - 1-10 grams per day.

Cayenne - increases circulation, relieves pain - 1-3 capsules per day (caution - spicy).

Boswellia gum - reduces inflammation – (standardized to 65% boswellic acids)- 300-1200 mg per day

Guggul gum - the main herb for arthritic diseases - 2-10 capsules per day

Many FMS patients gain tremendous relief from massage therapy with the addition of herbal ointments. Massage increases flexibility and oxygenation of the muscles, bring fresh blood and lymph to the sore areas.

The herbal salves that have the greatest effect, say FMS patients, contain either menthol, or cayenne extract. Cayenne plasters reduce non-specific low back pain substantially.[729]

The herbal treatments are rubbed on the sore muscle, or sometimes just on the tender point. Patients have told us they were the difference between walking or not walking on any given day.

Gallstones

A gallbladder attack is a horrible experience. Usually the patient has just finished a nice, filling, probably high fat, meal, and is relaxing, lying down, in the evening after dinner. Then the wrenching pain starts. Many people who have gone through this say that it is the worst pain they have ever felt, comparable to childbirth. Then the nausea and sweating begin. After seemingly endless hours of this, the symptoms eventually subside. Never wanting to feel even a fraction of that again, the patient runs to the doctor. Usually the gallbladder is removed as a matter of course.

Gallstones are lumps of solid matter that form in the interior space of the gallbladder, and may be as small as a grain of sand, or become as large as an inch in diameter. Over time gallstones may grow in size and/or numbers.

Gallbladder treatment will use herbs of these types:

- Anti-inflammatory herbs will reduce swelling.
- Anti-spasmodics will reduce constriction.
- Hepatics will generally benefit the liver.
- Immune enhancers may be necessary if there is chronic infection.
- Nervines will ease pain and stress.
- Cholagogues will be necessary to thin the bile, and to increase bile production, but must be used with caution, as they may increase contractions.

Cholagogues will be the first line of attack. Remember, they must be used carefully. As a general rule, cholagogues tend to be nauseating, and to cause loose stool. Since constipation is characteristic of this condition, however, this can be a benefit. In fact, many of these cholagogues are listed as purgatives. Inducing bile flow is a typical way of promoting bowel action. Also, causing an unwanted sudden contraction of the gallbladder may cause, at the least, an acute attack, and, at the worst, may lodge a stone in the duct, which ends the patient up in the hospital.

Dandelion increases bile flow, benefiting liver congestion, bile duct inflammation, and gallstones. Burdock has a long history of use as a biliary detoxifier. The high levels of lignans and inulin have shown proven anti-inflammatory activities, explaining its use in pitta conditions.

Similarly, turmeric increases bile flow and is useful in jaundice. Increases in liver inflammation, measured by the blood tests SGOT and SGPT, are prevented by turmeric.[730]

Radish (*Raphanus sativus*) is known for liver and gallbladder treatment. The black radish, red radish and daikon (*mooli*), are effective. Use radish as a food, or as juice, depending on tolerance.

Asian rhubarb root is another cold, bitter bile promoter, which cools and eliminates pitta. We see that these qualities again make it suitable for jaundice. Generally considered to be widely well tolerated, rhubarb root can be used for a broad range. Use 3-12 g, to bowel tolerance, per day in capsules.

Use bhumy amalaki whenever a general hepatic is indicated. It increases bile flow in a very mild way, so is well tolerated by people for whom a stronger cholagogue is contraindicated. Use up to 10g per day in capsules.

Menthol and related terpenes (menthone, pinene, bornoel, cineole, and camphene) has shown promise for gallstone treatment. This safe preparation can be used for extended periods, up to several years. These terpenes reduce bile cholesterol levels, while also increasing bile acid and lecithin levels in the biliary system. Khalsa has had very good clinical success in reversing gallstone symptoms in cases diagnosed by ultrasound using peppermint powder in capsules, oral peppermint oil, and encapsulated camphor. In particular, the peppermint is very effective for the aggravating chronic burping that often accompanies this syndrome.

In the diet, apple juice has been shown to be a benefit. Members of the cabbage family, especially raw (radish, Brussels sprouts), can help. Vegetarian diets show benefit. High fiber content in the diet binds fats in the gut and lowers cholesterol in the bile. Adequate water is essential to keep the stool moist, and the bile thin.

Topically, use castor oil packs with heat.

Gastritis, Heartburn and Ulcer

The *hot* type of indigestion, caused by pitta, known medically as *gastritis*, involves inflammation or irritation of the inner lining (mucosa) of the stomach. Gastritis can be caused by many factors and, in some cases, may precede ulcer. Heartburn is a burning sensation caused by stomach acid regurgitating into the esophagus. These people often suffer from diarrhea. Remedies include cooling, soothing herbs.

Ulcer, the next step in the degradation of the intestinal mucous lining, can be caused by vata or pitta.[731] Vata ulcer responds to the demulcents licorice, shatavari and comfrey. Pitta ulcer calls for cooling amla or red coral pishti.

Chanchal Cabrera sees a lot of heartburn and esophagitis in her practice in Ashland, Oregon. She sees a lot of cancer patients who have just undergone chemotherapy. The powerful cancer drugs damage the stomach lining cells, and reduce gastric mucus flow. She recommends coating liquids- milk, soy and nut milk and yogurt, with small, frequent meals. Aloe vera inhibits gastric acid secretion and soothes the stomach lining.

Turmeric stimulates gallbladder contractions, promoting better digestion.[732 733] Turmeric increases the production of several important secretions in the digestive tract. Turmeric is widely use for indigestion, and there is some scientific evidence that curcumin treats dyspepsia. A double-blind placebo-controlled study with 106 patients measured the effects of 500 mg curcumin 4 times daily against placebo. Seven days into the study, 87% percent of the curcumin group experienced full or partial dyspepsia symptom relief, compared to 53% of the placebo group.[734] With its ability to suppress inflammation, increase mucin content of the stomach, and stop bleeding, turmeric prevents and treats ulcerations of all types, including gastritis, peptic ulcer,[735] irritable bowel syndrome and colitis.

Licorice guards digestive mucous membranes. Peppermint is a well-known herb for tummy troubles.

Demulcent marshmallow is used for inflammation of the stomach membranes.[736]

Tasty, aromatic ginger is a time-tested remedy for stomach upset. It is used by nearly every culture in the world. Ginger's effect on nausea has been thoroughly proven. It reduces spasm, absorbs and neutralizes toxins in the gastrointestinal tract and increases the secretion of digestive juices, including bile and saliva.[737] Ginger contains ingredients that soothe the gut and aid digestion by increasing peristalsis that moves food through the intestine.

Cinnamon bark is a mild but useful remedy for sluggish indigestion. The

German Commission E, the European standard for herbal medicines, recommends cinnamon for loss of appetite, dyspeptic complaints, mild gastrointestinal spasm, bloating and flatulence.

To promote jathar agni, we use herb medicines. Tikshnagni responds to Triphala, Avipatikar, kumari and licorice. Mandagni is benefited by Triphala, trikatu, cayenne, ghee, ginger, pipali and rock salt. Vishamagni improves with triphala, trikatu, ghee, ginger, licorice, pipali and rock salt.

Glaucoma

Normal eye fluid is a clear fluid that comes in and out through lymph vessels but if these fluids flow too rapidly into the area and/or flow out too slowly, there can be big problems. Inside the eye, this pressure buildup damages the optic nerve and causes glaucoma. Victims have reduced peripheral vision. Glaucoma is the second most common cause of legal blindness in the United States.

Glaucoma can have elements of derangement of any of the three doshas - kapha, pitta, or vata. The classic open angle glaucoma patient is presenting a kapha dosha excess. If an inflammatory constituent is involved, it is necessary to treat pitta.

The objective in anti-kapha therapy is to normalize body weight and lipids, warm the tissues, and dry the body, possibly with diuretics.

Many Ayurvedic botanicals are used to generally strengthen the eye and enhance vision. Triphala is the most widely used formula for general eye benefit. Also consider Mahasudarshan ("the great formula for vision"). Primarily an anti-pitta remedy, it is widely applied in eye disease, as pitta dosha regulates the eyes generally. This formula contains herbs which cool and cleanse the eyes.

Another well known formula for general eye conditions is "Saptamrita lauha," containing the triphala herbs, licorice root, iron, honey, and ghee. Research has shown it to be successful in reducing hemorrhage in the eye in diabetes and hypertension.

Neem leaf is a bitter detoxifier used in eye diseases generally, particularly with ama. The dose is five grams of powder per day.

Sala wood (Shorea robusta) is also used for general eye benefit, especially with diabetes. The dose is ten grams per day.

Coleus (Coleus forskohlii) is quite effective in glaucoma. This herb is a general cardiovascular remedy which increases cyclic adenosine monophospate (cAMP) in cells. This action has far reaching application in healing. [738] Increase in cAMP results in inhibition of platelet activation and degranulation, inhibition of mast cell degranulation and histamine release, increased force of contraction of the heart muscle, relaxation of the arteries and other smooth muscles, increased insulin secretion, increased thyroid function, and increased lipolysis, all of which benefit hypertension and diabetes, and secondarily, glaucoma. Applied directly to the eyes, it increases intraocular blood flow and reduces intraocular pressure.[739]

Black pepper is a superlative herb for warming and drying the tissues, exactly the objective in glaucoma involving kapha. The dose can be increased to two heaping tablespoons of powdered peppercorns with food or water throughout the day, as tolerated.

Topical treatments with herb decoctions or oils are common. They are administered with an eyedropper or eye cup. Solutions of chamomile flowers, chrysanthemum flowers, and rose petals reduce inflammation. Gurmar leaf as a wash treats diabetic eye conditions. Aqueous preparations of palasa leaf and root (Butea frondosa) show substantial benefit in reducing intraocular pressure.[740] Ghee, clarified butter, is used as a soaking application for the entire eye and orbital region.

Honey is highly valued as an eye application, particularly in early glaucoma. Applied and retained with a closed lid for five minutes twice daily, it acts as a vasodilator and lymph circulation enhancer in non-inflammatory conditions.

Control of the doshas in the head can be benefited by applying the medicine directly into the nostril. Nasal medicines include infused oils or juices of higru, vidanga and long pepper. Ghee, applied as a nasal medicine is generally healing to the balance of doshas in the head.

Diabetes is strongly linked with glaucoma. Diabetes is the quintessential kapha condition: the entire body is big, wet, cold, sweet, and fat. Herbs which treat kapha and ama reduce lipids and blood glucose. All are used to treat glaucoma.

For typical glaucoma caused by kapha, the diet should be warm, light, dry and low fat. Pungent, bitter, and astringent tastes should be emphasized. Foods and beverage teas which promote diuresis should be encouraged.

Hair

Notice that many famous yogis seem to do special things with their hair? Grown long, shaved off, tied in a knot- everyone seems to do something exceptional. That's no accident, because hair has a lot of energy. Just look at how much attention goes to caring for hair in modern life. It's likely the first place our eyes are drawn when we meet someone.

The hair reflects the internal condition of the body. Healthy hair comes from a healthy body. The hair is the extension of the shushumna, the energy spine. It acts as an energy antenna and prana regulator to consolidate the energy coming through the chakras. It connects us energetically to the environment. Renunciate yogis shave it off to disconnect from the day-to-day world. Householder yogis grow it long, to capture energy, and keep them grounded and engaged in the life of the world.

Yogis who grow long hair sometimes cover it with a turban to keep it clean and organized. Left to grow long, and covered by a porous cloth, hair will accumulate some natural scalp oil. This oil, exposed to the filtered sunlight, is a major source of vitamin D for the body. A hair covering will also help disciplined yogis stay modest and make it easier to remember to remain graceful in social situations.

Hair is a tissue, so the body never stops producing it to replace lost strands

When it reaches the proper genetic length for you body, it will get no longer, but only replace individual hairs. Think about- the hair on your arms isn't three feet long, is it?

Gathering that long hair at crown of the head keeps it contained and the energy concentrated, aligned with the chakras. Yogis and yoginis tie it in a "rishi knot," or "joora," that sits atop the head.

If you use remedies to help your hair stay healthy, remember that the changes will happen in the base of the hair shaft, and that hair grows slowly. You may not see the results of your efforts for months! In the world of hairy things, patience pays.

Damaged, falling or prematurely graying hair is a sign of too much pitta in the head. To keep your hair healthy, avoid anything that promotes heat, inflammation, or extreme intensity and stress. Engage in cooling activities, such as moonlight walks by the lake, and eat cooling foods like cucumber, celery, spearmint and melon.

Bringraj is a master tonic for the hair- an herb that cools the metabolism. Use up to 5 grams per day as capsules or tea. Chinese medicine has a related remedy, Han Lian Cao (*Eclipta prostrata*), that also cools the body and treats premature graying of the hair at a similar dose.

Amla fruit, in Chyavanprash or other forms, is considered to be the prime general herb to treat premature gray hair. Use 1-2 grams per day in capsules.

Mandukaparni stimulates the growth of hair and nails, increases blood supply to the skin. Two or three cups of tea per day increases keratinization in the skin and hair.

Oiling the hair daily is a basic yoga lifestyle practice. Vata resides in the brain, so tends to collect in the head and is the main element that causes disturbed sleep. Controlling vata will reduce that overactive mind that plagues us when we most want to slumber. At bedtime, apply a little oil to your scalp. Ayurveda suggests a drop of castor oil for this, but it's a little messy. Almond works well. The anterior fontanel is the best spot.

Oil is the main general remedy for controlling the air tattva. To keep your mind on track through the day, use cooling oils for daily scalp care, including coconut and ghee Pumpkin seed hair oil helps the memory along similar lines. Sesame and almond are also good general choices for keeping the scalp soft and moist.

Hair oils are usually made form cooling herbs. Use prepared Ayurvedic hair oil made from amla fruit, madukaparni leaf or bringraj. Buttermilk head massage is a traditional treatment used to treat dry hair, dandruff and hair loss.

Try this. Combine bringaraj oil, shikakai oil and sesame or coconut oil, in equal parts. Leave the oil blend on overnight. Shampoo out in the morning.

Hay Fever

Hay fever (allergic rhinitis) is the sixth most common condition in the United States, surpassing cardiac disease.[741]

Yogi Bhajan taught a unique use for triphala.[742] To use triphala churna as a rapid-acting expectorant, cold infuse 5 g of the churna in 10 ounces of water overnight. Consumed first thing in the morning upon arising, a dramatic expectoration follows within minutes.

Guduchi is an anti-inflammatory herb and potent immune system support medicine. In a 2005 study, 75 patients with hay fever took guduchi or a placebo. Eighty-three percent of the guduchi group reported total relief from sneezing, but only 79% of the placebo patients reported no relief at all. Similar results were obtained for drippy nose, congestion and itchy nose.[743]

Nettle is a modern day anti-inflammatory allergy miracle [744] [745] Many people take up to 3,000 mg of specially processed nettle leaf powder in capsules per day to relieve the temporary symptoms of hay fever and other allergic reactions, including animal allergy. [746] [747]

Headache

Yogi Bhajan had an experience with headache. "There is a lady we treated, who for all her life, her headache would never go away. We have put her on a parantha which is made from the ginger- bread ginger parantha- and now, with the God's grace, she never has a headache. Because we know ginger affects the nervous system. Actually pain and disease in the body is disease in the energy, and pain is the signal, a call where the body wants help."

Willow bark is rapid acting and effective for relieving headache pain. Use 1 ounce, brewed as tea.

Godanti Bhasma is used for headache at 250 mg, 2-3 times per day with warm water. Coral powder or bhasma at 500 mg thrice daily can complement the Godanti Bhasma, or act alone.[748]

On a more prosaic note, Baba Hari Dass proposes tying a string around the arm above the elbow.[749]

Herpes and cold sores

What's a sore more painful than a scrape or bruise, uglier and more embarrassing than a big pimple, and caused by a virus so contagious that it's spread simply through kissing? A cold sore.

This disgusting malady, seemingly put here just to ruin tonight's party or this weekend's big date, is in fact a viral disease.

Don't confuse cold sores with *canker sores*, correctly called *aphthous ulcers*, which are small ulcers that form on mucous membranes of the digestive tract, including the oral cavity. They are not caused by virus.

Mints have general antiviral properties. While Melissa is widely regarded as the foremost herb for cold sores, most other mints will work almost as well. Mints are all rich sources of antiviral constituents, including caffeic acid, quercitin, tannic acid, and thymol. James Duke, Ph.D., a widely respected herbal medicine authority, recommends using several strongly brewed cups of a tea made from an assortment of good tasting mints- hyssop, lemon balm, oregano, rosemary, sage, self-heal, and thyme.

Licorice is an herb with a long history of benefit for the immune system. This powerful herb can be taken internally, or used in the form of an ointment. It is a strong anti-inflammatory medicine, with actions comparable to cortisone. Taken internally, the dose would be 3,000 mg per day, stirred into an anupan, or in capsule form. This herb can be a little stool loosening, so work up gradually. Make sure the effective dose is comfortable. The ointment will contain the active ingredient *glycyrretinic acid*, or the related compound, *glycyrrhizic acid.* Topical glycyrretinic acid has been shown in clinical studies to reduce pain and healing time. Apply the cream directly to the blister as necessary.

Impotence and Erectile Dysfunction

Each of us is unique. But, as Yogi Berra (well, he was a yogi) might say, some of us are more unique than others. Men have simpler plumbing, and they don't go to the doctor as much, but they still need care and attention.

Men's health is actually a particularly challenging area. For a generation, clinicians in the United States have seen women as the vast majority of their practices, perhaps as high as 95%, even in a general practice setting. Men just don't visit alternative practitioners (or any other practitioners, for that matter). But men's needs are just as serious. They die earlier. And while they are still alive, they are just as miserable, or perhaps more miserable, if they don't seek help.

One in four men over the age of 50, or some 20 million American men, experience some form of impotence. It strikes up to half of all men between the ages of 40 and 70.[750]

Apana vata controls the downward movement of energy in the pelvic area. Erectile Dysfunction (ED) is caused by a disorder in apana vata. Root causes include exhaustion, lack of sleep, strong negative emotions and relationship difficulties. Organic causes abound, including diabetes, nerve diseases and circulatory insufficiency. Smoking worsens ED.

Essentially, ED responds to a coordinated program of vajikarana therapies. Home remedies that Ayurveda promotes for ED include garlic, onion, asparagus spears, okra, ginger and raisin.

Yogi Bhajan recommended banyan tree milk (sap) for ED. He said, "These men should ask for banyan milk. The man should take it for seven or eight days. For those eight and the ten days following, he should abstain from sex. If necessary, he should repeat the whole process. It works. Banyan tree milk also cures the condition in which semen is passed with the urine because a membrane ruptures. This sometimes happens to athletes. My grandfather taught me this formula. He put banyan tree milk on a sugar cane; with that he gave me yogurt containing sugar cane juice. I had to do that for one week. I never had trouble thereafter."[751]

Shilajit is a widely used beneficial remedy for the genitourinary tract in general. Many men's remedies include it. One such is Shilajit Vati, a blend of shilajit and triphala powder, processed in the juices of the fresh triphala fruits. Yogi Bhajan recommends taking shilajit daily with equal parts black pepper, boiled in milk.[752]

Safed musali tuber is an aphrodisiac remedy, containing stigmasterol derivatives. Nutritive and demulcent, it teats urinary disorders, increases semen volume and bumps up total sperm count. Clinical trails also showed it to increase stamina.[753] It is sweet, hot and heavy, so it pacifies vata and pitta. For general sexual weakness and impotence, cook safed musali in milk. It is often used at a dose of 1-2 grams per day.[754] For acute low libido, use 10 or more grams per day.

I (Khalsa) would have to rank garlic as the number one aphrodisiac herb. I use it consistently, and it produces consistently. It has all the qualities you would want in a sexual enhancer. It increases circulation and promotes erectile force, as well as increasing desire. Related onion has a similar, milder effect. Garlic is so good at increasing libido that celibate people don't use it.

Garlic is hot, so it can aggravate pitta and the sex organs. It increases semen. For Americans, deodorized garlic might be a better choice. Use a large dose- 10 grams per day. Expect to see sexy results in about a month, and then- watch out.

Pipali peppercorn is a powerful, rejuvenating, warming alterative rasayana remedy, which moistens the tissues and offsets the drying action of the other herbs. It is often combined with black pepper to offset the opposite moisture characteristics.

Ashwaganda is a sexual tonic. Jodi O'Neill, an herbalist colleague of ours, owns a retail herb apothecary in Kent, Washington. She relates a story that reflects ashwaganda's benefits. Jodi consulted with a couple about the husband's serious erectile dysfunction. After suggesting ashwaganda and cautioning not to expect results before the one month mark, Jodi went about her other tasks, until a dozen red roses arrived at the store two weeks later. The enclosed note told the story. I guess you can guess what had happened the night before.

Studies show that extracts of ashwaganda increased production of sex hormones and sperm, presumably by exerting a testosterone-like effect.[755] Ashwaganda improves the cardiovascular aspects of ED.[756] In the long run, in some individuals, it increases sadhaka pitta in the head and heart. To counteract this possibility, combine ashwaganda with cooling herbs or foods, such as licorice, ghee, raw sugar, milk and rice.

Gokshura is outstanding for sexual building, and has a particular affinity for the urogenital tract. It is sweet and cold, so it is appropriate for pitta conditions. For spermatorrhea and impotence, use equal parts powdered gokshura, sesame seed, kapi kachu and ashwaganda. Take 6 grams of this mixture with honey, ghee or milk.

Amla is the basis for "Chyavanprash," the most famous Ayurvedic rejuvenating jelly. The formulator, the sage Chyawan, designed this medicinal food supplement to enhance sexual functions and fertility.[757] [758] For sexual rejuvenation, stir chyavanprash into warm milk or spread on toast, and consume 1-2 tbs every day.

Licorice is used to improve sexual potency, libido eyesight and physical strength. Cloves are mildly aphrodisiac and stimulating. Saffron, a very powerful and expensive herb, is an acclaimed vajikarana.[759] Not a tonic in itself, it synergizes with other tonic herbs. It is often used in milk preparations. Yogi Bhajan used a remedy, which combined saffron with camphor, for male rejuvenation.

Bala is a sweet, cold, heavy vata tonic herb for ED.[760] Use 1 gram or more as tolerated, per day, as powder, decoction or milk decoction.

Proprietary and classical impotence formulas often center on a combination of ashwaganda, shatavari and kapi kachu. Kapi kachu seed is considered to be one of the best male reproductive tonics. It contains l-dopa. For impotence, powder 2 seeds (about 2 grams) and take with warm milk daily at bedtime. It increases libido and erectile function. A traditional aphrodisiac (*Vanari Vatika*) is made by boiling the seeds in milk. Then the seeds are pounded, fried in ghee and mixed with raw sugar. This mass is soaked in honey and rolled into a bolus.

External Preparations

To keep the body young, massage daily with a combination of the infused oils of ashwaganda, shatavari and bala. Leave on to absorb for 2 hours before bathing. This program is antiaging (vayasthapan), as it treats excess vata. A simple oil of ashwaganda infused in sesame is a basic penis massage oil.

Herbs are infused into sesame oil and used for genital massage as a general treatment for impotence. Ingredients include ashwaganda, shatavari, karanj (Pongamia glabra), saffron (kesar) and sandalwood.[761] Many other similar formulas are used.

Ten Lifestyle Tips for Erectile Dysfunction

1. Practicing yoga and meditation to manage stress
2. Get some sleep- at least for 8 hours a night for a while
3. Massage with an appropriate aphrodisiac and antistress herbal oil
4. Say no to alcohol, tobacco, drugs
5. Daily exercise
6. Avoid hot, pungent and bitter foods
7. If not overweight, consume sweets, milk products, nuts, urid dal
8. Use ghee in rejuvenating beverages
9. Slow Down. Wait four days to make love again
10. Use appropriate herbal preparations to rejuvenate the reproductive organs

Figure 25 Ten Lifestyle Tips for Erectile Dysfunction

Insomnia

Balanced sleep, balanced diet and balanced sexual life are the three key areas, that, taken together are the base foundation of Ayurvedic lifestyle and therapeutics. Sleep is the time when the body is able to repair and heal itself.

Deep sleep is what we need to rejuvenate, and most of that restorative deep sleep is experienced in the first 3 hours. After four-and-one-half hours in bed, we alternately wake up and dream. Yogis say that all you need is one to three hours of sleep if you are, in fact, getting the restorative deep sleep. Most of us can learn to function well with six to seven-and-a half hours of sleep if we train ourselves to get deep rest.

Start with a few basics: go to bed and wake up at the same time each day (even on the weekends) and get regular exercise during the course of the day. Create an inviting sleep atmosphere (using your bedroom only for sleep and sex); keep your room at a comfortable temperature (not too hot or too cold); and to do something relaxing, play soothing music, or meditate, before bed.

The primary cause of insomnia is excessive thinking and sensory stimulation, which ultimately disrupt our inner clock. People who live out-of-doors find their rhythms closely entrained by the rising and setting of the sun. But most of us live cut off from the natural world. Sunrise and sunset mean nothing to us. Inside our offices and homes we are surrounded by artificial stimulation in the form of etc. In fact, we are bombarded with sensory stimulation- lights, TVs, computers- all day long.

To recover your slumber, get your life regulated. Establish times to wake up, go to sleep, eat, exercise, and enjoy quiet relaxation. Exercise, along with light, initiates the active cycle of the day, so it's pretty important. But no strenuous exercise after dinner. Most people do well with the conventional breakfast, lunch and dinner, but be finished dinner by 8 o'clock, or even better, earlier. Having a light, early dinner at least two hours before bedtime to reduce insomnia caused by digestive problems. Eat your main protein of the day at lunch, and avoid caffeine, alcohol, tobacco, sugar, fried foods and strong spices.

For many people, the best plan is to begin winding down the day by 8:00 p.m. That means turning down the lights, the TV and the computer.

Pitta Problems

For people with excess pitta, one of the most important ingredients in a good sleep is to fall asleep before 10:00 p.m., when the pitta phase of night begins. If you stay awake past 10:00, your sleep will have the active, restless qualities of pitta, and it will be tough to rest deeply. Pitta conditions, such as heartburn, tend to increase between 10:00 and 2:00, so it's better to snooze through them.

Vata Variations

If increased vata is your dilemma, get to bed when you are tired, but certainly before 2:00. Creative vata types tend to get a second wind as the night rolls on, get immersed in the latest project, and then prowl the halls, "too tired to sleep." Going to bed during the slow kapha time, between 6:00 and 10:00, will help. To balance vata, a regular routine is important.

Oil decreases vata. Have a warm foot bath, followed by oiling and massaging the feet with sesame or almond oil before bed.

Conquering Kapha

The kapha man has a large body build, a problem with weight control, and an easy-going personality. Like a slumbering bear, he sleeps all too well- nine or ten hours every night. But come the morning, he feels tired, and stiff. He has to drink three cups of coffee just to wake up. A lethargic, dull feeling often continues throughout the day.

For the kapha bear, the key is to sleep little, and to rise early. If he gets going before 6:00 am., during the vata time of morning, he'll feel infused with the light, alert, energetic qualities of vata dosha, and will feel more alert and energetic throughout the day. Sleeping past dawn, into the kapha time of the morning (6:00-10:00 am.) causes toxins to accumulate and creates a dull, tired feeling.

Vigorous exercise is essential for balancing Kapha. The best time to exercise is during the Kapha time of the morning (6:00 am. to 10:00 am.), when it will help wash away some of the dullness of the night and make you feel more energetic all day.

The Sleep Herbs

Tierra likes a combination of mandukaparni and amla for pitta, and vacha for vata. Use 3 teaspoons of a powder of the combination, with warm milk or water, during the day, to regulate sleep patterns. Use the same combination as shirodara oil.[762]

Ashwaganda regulates sleep cycles over time, facilitating more refreshing sleep.

Tagara is a relaxant herb that has a calming effect on the autonomic nervous system. It is a good short-term sedative that works quickly, offering a healthy, nontoxic alternative to strong prescription drugs. [763] [764]

For insomnia, tagara is taken right at bedtime to help induce sleep quickly.[765] It is best for insomniacs who have trouble falling asleep, because it decreases the amount of time it takes to fall asleep, but doesn't necessarily work on the length of sleep.

A typical dose of valerian root, powdered in capsules, would be 1,000- 3,000 mg, as necessary, several times per day, for anxiety, or 5,000 mg or more, as necessary, as a one-time dose, before bed, to relax for sleep. Jatamansi is a related plant, and is a possible alternative to tagara. Shankpushpi is a cooling sleep herb. The use and doses of both are comparable to tagara.

Nutmeg is appropriate for sleep sustain insomnia. The sedating action of nutmeg begins after a predictable delay of 3 and one half to 5 hours, depending on the patient, and results in a prolonged somnolence of a predictable 8 hours. For insomnia, begin with a dose of one capsule at 6:00 pm. The next night, increase the dose to two capsules. Continue increasing incrementally. Adjust the time of administration slightly to promote proper time of initiation of effects. The patient should feel profoundly drowsy at bedtime. Adjust the dose for the desired depth of sleep. Allow adequate time for the sleep effects, as patients will still be sedated if awakened before the full duration of action (8 hours). A typical dose for insomnia, given as one unit in the evening, is 3 grams.

Many sources[766] recommend taking small doses of nutmeg upon retiring, but this is problematic. The medicine will not take effect for 4 hours, so it is not appropriate for sleep onset insomnia when taken at bedtime. Since the duration is a solid eight hours, the patient will be sedated upon arising if taken at bedtime.

Poppy seed is a warming sleep remedy that acts immediately. Brew 4 tbs as decoction. Drink the tea one half hour before bed. The effect typically lasts for about 4 hours.

Administering nutmeg at bedtime with poppy seeds will produce 12 hour of sound sleep. Poppy takes effect immediately, so the patient is already asleep fours later when the nutmeg becomes active. This can be of great value in convalescence.

Sleep Symptoms

Pitta sleep symptoms

Intense mental activity, heat, heartburn, insomnia between 10:00 pm and 2:00 am.

Vata sleep symptoms

Body exhausted, mind won't stop, cold hands and feet, insomnia between 2:00 am and 6:00 am.

Kapha sleep symptoms

Sleeps like a log, but trouble waking up, dullness upon awakening, wakes full of mucus.

Figure 26 Sleep Symptoms

Conquering Sleep

Pacifying Pitta for Sleep

Eat a large enough evening meal, so you don't feel hungry before bed
Before bed- enjoy a blender drink of milk, dates and cinnamon
Keep the bedroom cool
Fall asleep before 10:00 pm (pitta aggravation time)
Diet: Use sweet, bitter and astringent foods
Avoid less sour, salty and pungent foods (especially chilies)
Sweet, juicy fruits
Cool temperature food

Vanquishing Vata for Sleep

Have a bedtime snack, to balance blood sugar (warm milk with sesame seeds is good)

Stay warm in a cozy bed, in a dark, clean, and uncluttered bedroom

Fall asleep when you are tired- don't stay up (Kapha dominates from 6:00 pm to 10:00 pm, when it's easier to fall asleep)

Diet: Warm, cooked, moist, easy-to-digest foods such as asparagus soup, lentils and rice

Eat foods with the sweet, sour and salty tastes.

Minimize pungent, bitter and astringent foods, and raw salads

Watch the caffeine, even early in the day

Clobbering Kapha for Sleep

Enjoy teas of basil, mint and clove

Gradually decrease coffee consumption. Green tea is a good substitute.

Diet: Spicy foods invigorate the body and energize digestion.

Eat cooked food, served hot.

Light, easily digestible foods such as soups, beans and spiced cooked vegetables

Eat bitter, astringent and pungent foods

Avoid desserts and heavy, cold sweets, such as ice cream, fried foods, leftovers, and aged foods

Figure 27 Conquering Sleep

Irritable Bowel Syndrome

Irritable Bowel Syndrome (IBS) is known by many names--colitis, mucous colitis, spastic colon, spastic bowel and functional bowel disease. But none of these terms really describes IBS properly. IBS doesn't involve inflammation and should not be confused with ulcerative colitis.

Triphala, in a dose that normalizes daily bowel rhythms, is the base for starting treatment. Once agni is normalized, generalized tonic therapy can be helpful. A nourishing diet, plus herbs such as ashwaganda, shatavari and bala will help.

One formula from *Sharangdhara Samhita* for IBS is a decoction of equal parts of bilwa fruit, coriander seed, nutgrass root and Vertivert grass.

Peppermint is a relaxant for the muscles of the intestinal wall. In one double blind trial from Taiwan, four out of every five IBS victims experienced reduced symptoms when given enteric-coated peppermint oil.[767] Caraway has similar properties.[768] A German study confirmed that a combination of peppermint and caraway oils effectively reduced the speed of intestinal movement.[769]

Psyllium seed balances bowel function and relieves pain in IBS.[770] Psyllium's capacity to absorb fluids means that it is useful for treating diarrhea, a common IBS symptom. As it travels through the gut, the mucilage in psyllium creates a soothing benefit, which may relieve cramping. An English study revealed that constipation significantly improved in patients taking psyllium. Eighty-two percent of the subjects had IBS symptom relief.[771] A study to determine the optimum dose recommended 20 grams per day.[772]

For some, eating a restricted diet reduces IBS symptoms. The diet must be individualized, depending on the individual triggers. Fiber usually helps. Clinicians usually recommend just enough fiber so that you have soft, easily passed, and painless bowel movements. More frequent, smaller meals usually work better.

Macular Degeneration

The retina is about the size of a postage stamp and is the site of millions of light receptor cells. In normal retinas, we can see a yellow spot in the visual center- the macula, which provides the best visual acuity of the human eye- the clear, sharp, central vision that you use for focusing on what is in front of you.

Macular degeneration is a degenerative disease of the elderly in which retinal function declines, destroying central vision, but it turns out that it is very treatable with herbs and diet. "The majority of clinicians tell people with macular degeneration that there is nothing they can do—go home and wait to go blind," says Dr. Dever. "But this is a progressive disease, so there is the possibility of halting the progress, and then there is the issue of dealing with the damage already done. Both are possible."

Herbs used for this condition include amla fruit or triphala and ashwaganda. Also, says Dr. Dever, "The retina loves the B vitamins, and vitamin A (not just carotenes)." The amino acid taurine is excellent for tissue regeneration, and seems to have an affinity for the retina.

A formula called *Saptamrita Lauha* ("sevenfold nectar") is presented in an Ayurvedic formulary from 1893 for the treatment of blindness. Composed of licorice root, triphala, purified iron, ghee, and honey, the efficacy of Saptamrita Lauha was assessed in a clinical trial of 48 retinopathic eyes. The formula was found to be highly effective, with the rapid clearing of retinal hemorrhaging, observed in both diabetic and hypertensive subjects. In three eyes the hemorrhage was cleared completely. The recurrence of a hemorrhagic episode was found to be statistically lower in eyes treated with Saptamrita Lauha.[773]

Turmeric is a classic Ayurvedic treatment for all "leaky" conditions. An astringent, it helps curb bleeding or other fluid excesses, and pulls in tissue that's prolapsed, so it's appropriate for "wet" macular degeneration. Its also a very effective anti-inflammatory, and works well for inflammatory conditions in the eye. A typical dose of turmeric to control active inflammation would be about ½ ounce of the powder per day, and for prevention, a teaspoon, or 2 capsules, would do.

Memory

It can happen to the best of us. You head into the other room for that important something. By the time you arrive, you forget what we came in for. You scratch your head and chalk it up to the normal aging process.

Yet those "senior moments" may not be unavoidable. As it turns out, there are herbal treatments that can be helpful. Here's what you can do to boost your brain power.

Gotu kola is a mainstay of herbal medicine. Widely considered a superior herb for the nervous system, gotu kola has a host of benefits. This herb is used as an aid to meditation, and it is considered to be the most spiritual of all herbs. It is used to promote circulation, especially the blood vessels of the skin and mucous membranes, and is a rejuvenator for the nerves and brain.

Gotu kola strengthens memory, concentration and intelligence, promotes longevity, improves the voice, physical strength and the complexion. This medicine is used to treat diseases as diverse as epilepsy, senility, hair loss and psoriasis.

A 1992 study in rats showed an impressive improvement in memory. The treated rats were able to retain learned behavior 3 to 60 times better than the control rats.[774]

More recently, a new study out of Korea shows that components in gotu kola show potential for treating Alzheimer's disease, a very promising conclusion.[775]

Brahmi (Bacopa), or water hyssop, has been used in medicine for uncounted centuries for the treatment of nerve diseases, mental exhaustion and to improve memory.

In particular, brahmi shows promise in the treatment of cognitive and behavioral disorders. In 1990, Indian researchers conducted an open trial with Bacopa, conducted in India on 35 adult patients with anxiety neurosis. Concentration and immediate memory span were both significantly increased. On-the-job mental fatigue also was improved.

In 1987, scientists performed a single-blind trial in India, administering brahmi to 40 schoolchildren, aged 6-8. Maze learning improved, immediate memory and perception and reaction/performance times all improved.

An experiment on mice in 2000 demonstrated that Bacopa reduced the cognitive decline caused by a powerful anticonvulsant drug.[776]

Menstrual cramps, PMS, Menopause

Shatavari root is the main Ayurvedic sexual rejuvenating tonic for women, with much the same role as the famous Chinese tonic, dong quai. Considered a builder and balancer for the female reproductive organs, it increases milk and sexual juices in general. This herb is said to increase fertility, and balance female hormones, making it valuable in treating menopausal complaints, such as vaginal atrophy.

This cooling herb acts as a blood cleanser, supports the immune system, improves the intellect, and enhances digestion and physical strength. A recent study found that a medicine containing shatavari reduced stress effects substantially.[777]

Women in Asia may start shatavari at puberty, and may take 1-2 grams per day for a lifetime. In many ethnic groups in Asia, menopausal complaints are almost unknown. To treat a wide variety of female hormonal symptoms (PMS, menstrual cramps, mood changes, menopausal hot flushes, etc.), higher doses can be used. Work up gradually to the dose that is effective, to about 7 grams per day.

Amla is a tonic for the blood, bones, liver, and heart. It enhances production of red blood cells and strengthens the teeth, hair, and nails, as well as improving eyesight and regulating blood sugar. Amla is the basis for Chyavanprash, the most famous Ayurvedic rejuvenating jelly. As a mild all around health tonic, chyavanprash can be used by people of all ages. For sexual rejuvenation, stir Chyavanprash into warm milk or spread on toast, and consume 1-2 Tbs. every day.

Called "kumari" ("virgin") aloe is said to restore the energy of youth and to renew the female nature. It is a main tonic for the female reproductive system, and it also nourishes the liver, spleen and blood.

Aloe balances blood sugar and fats [778] and promotes digestion. You may use aloe to encourage a menstrual period and balance the menstrual cycle.

Aloe can be used by anyone, as it balances all three doshas. Since it is sweet, bitter and cooling, it especially benefits pitta dosha. This valuable herb combines well with Shatavari.

Ginger promotes menstrual blood flow, and eases cramps. To reduce excessive blood flow, sauté 8 almonds, skins on, in ghee, stir in a tablespoon of astringent honey and eat them for breakfast on bleeding days.

The good news about PMS is that you can find help through many effective treatments. According to Yogi Bhajan, "In Ayurvedic medicine, betel (sopari) was used for menstrual problems. If you are having heavy cramps or leucorrhea, blend powdered betel nut with ginger, sesame seeds and honey to form a paste. To use, mix one tablespoon with five or six ounces of milk. Either just before or during menstruation, twice a day, have one tablespoon of sesame seed oil mixed with honey. Have it as a paste or mixed with milk. To alleviate menstrual problems in general, take vitamins B, C and E regularly."[779]

Dandelion is a standout for the water retention that often accompanies PMS.

Dysmenorrhea and amenorrhea often come along with digestive disturbance, lower back and pelvic pain, anxiety, mood swings and general debility. Vata is the main cause. The lower pelvis is the seat of apana vata, which is responsible for the elimination of menstrual blood, stool and urine. Herbs that promite apana will reduce cramps and promote menstrual blood movement. Use garlic, aloe vera, triphala and cumin seed tea with raw sugar. Sesame oil massage of the pelvis, followed by a hot water bottle will bring blood to the area and enhance apana Betel nut treats menstrual cramps. Blend powdered betel nut with ginger, sesame seeds and honey to form a paste. Just before, and during menstruation, twice a day have one tablespoon as a paste or mixed with milk.[780]

With amenorrhea or cramps, stay away from greasy, fried food, sour food and gas producing food. Take food warm. Avoid vata promoting food such as the cabbage family. Use cooked squash and warming spices. Take light exercise, including walking.

Premature Ejaculation

Premature ejaculation (PE) is one of the most common and stressful sexual problems experienced by men. It is an inability to delay ejaculation until a time when it is mutually desirable for both partners. It could occur due to being very excited, anxiety, fear, or alcohol or drug use. Lifestyle stress or severe depression could also lead to this problem.

PE is caused by an imbalance in pitta and vata. Pitta thins body fluids and increase the outflow of, in this case, semen. Vata can be influenced by anxiety or large intestine dysfunction. These aggravated doshas can result in hyperactivity of the muscles in the penis and reproductive tract, leading to early ejaculation.

PE is generally treated with a long term strategy. Modest doses of medicines are given daily for several weeks or months, as opposed to shortly before intercourse.

Nutmeg gets Khalsa's vote for the best remedy for this condition.[781] This calming pungent herb regulates the function of the large intestine, which is key in treating this disorder. Fresh medicine is essential. Nutmeg is sedating, but small chronic doses for PE should not be problem in this regard. Use about 1 gram per day. Start with 500 mg, and increase the dose to tolerance of the sedating effects. Expect PE benefits in about 2-4 weeks. Continue a small daily dose as necessary.

Safed musali tuber, a relative of shatavari, is a potent Ayurvedic aphrodisiac plant that has been used since the 11th century A.D. It contains various stigmasterol derivatives. It is nutritive and demulcent, so suits urinary disorders. It is also been shown significant effect in increasing semen volume and total sperm count. Clinical trails also showed it to enhance working capacity.[782] Similar to ashwaganda, it imparts strength. Safed Musali in traditionally used for male lack of libido and impotence and is well known for PE. It is also widely used as a general health promoting, anti-aging tonic, with an affinity for the pelvis and rectum.

For general sexual debility and impotence, it is cooked in milk. It is often used in combination with other similar herbs, in a dose of 1-2 grams per day.[783] For acute current sexual problems, use 10 or more grams per day.

Amla fruit is used for PE.[784] It tends to work slowly, so the effects will be cumulative over up to several months. The speed of effect can be hastened somewhat by using doses in the 5 gram range. Chyavanprash, a special Ayurvedic medicinal jelly, is a general remedy for enhancing and balancing sexual functions, and is used for slow but steady treatment of this condition.

Shilajit is a general detoxifier and rejuvenator, and is beneficial for the genitourinary tract in general, so is widely employed for impotence and long term treatment of PE. The dose is 1-2 grams per day, usually with milk. Practitioners often recommend taking shilajit daily with equal parts black pepper, boiled in milk.[785] Shilajit Vati is a mixture of shilajit paste and triphala powder, processed in the juices of the fresh triphala fruits.

Shatavari and kapi kachu also get the nod for PE.

Various Ayurvedic combination formulas are used for PE. One such proprietary combination includes the herbs shatavari, gokshura, trikatu, ashwaganda, and musali, along with an assortment of minor ingredients.

PE is benefited by longer, more gradual foreplay. Deep breathing will stabilize vata. Keeping cool will reduce pitta. Avoid spicy foods that aggravate pitta and provoke PE.

Skin Cancer

Vata cancer includes emotional symptoms of fear, anxiety, depression, and insomnia. The skin is gray or brown, with the growths being dry, hard, and variable in size, shape, and consistency.

Pitta cancer includes emotional symptoms of anger, irritability, and resentment. The growths are inflamed, infected, burning, and bleeding, and the skin is hot, oily, and spotted. Most skin cancer is pitta type.

Kapha cancer includes emotional symptoms of depression, lethargy, and fatigue. The skin is cold, pale, and oily. The growths are often benign at first, becoming malignant over time.

As cancer is fundamentally a disease characterized by material that should not be there, detoxification is paramount. Herbal detoxification relies primarily on bitter tasting herbs, which have alterative qualities. Pungent herbs are thought to be particularly beneficial in the resolution of skin growths. The combination of bitter herbs with pungent herbs is ideal for detoxification generally, as both are detoxifying, and the heat of the pungency offsets the cold and catabolic effects of the bitter taste.

Ayurveda uses alteratives to remove toxins, and reduce infections. Alteratives are particularly indicated for skin cancer, as the pitta type people who typically develop this disease can often withstand radical detoxification. Very high doses may be necessary, up to 2-3 ounces per day. Red clover leaf, dandelion root and sarsaparilla root are often used.

Being a pitta organ, skin is usually treated with anti-pitta herbs. Herbs which act on pitta are cold, dry, and heavy, with the tastes of sweet, bitter, and astringent, all of which have a cooling action.

Gotu kola leaf has a special role in the treatment of all connective tissue. It is used extensively in treating wounds of all types, including inflammatory skin lesions. Gotu kola also has anti-cancer effects. In a recent in vitro study, gotu kola destroyed 100 percent of cultured tumor cells. More importantly, almost no toxic effects were detected in human white blood cells. Gotu kola appears to have selective toxicity against tumor cells.

Guggul gum is an excellent alterative for skin conditions. Guggul is highly anti-inflammatory, and is widely used in leprosy. Five grams per day or more would be a typical dose for acute conditions.

Saffron is a special herb for nourishing the skin, particularly taken as a milk decoction.

Turmeric is probably the most often mentioned anti-cancer Ayurvedic herb. It is strongly anti-inflammatory, antioxidant, hepatoprotective, and antimicrobial. Turmeric is cytotoxic, promotes healing of skin cancers, and inhibits recurrence of melanomas. Many recent studies have confirmed these benefits. Turmeric constituents (curcumins) inhibit cancer at initiation, promotion, and progression stages of development. Of course, in pitta-associated skin cancer, controlling inflammation is critical. Doses of up to an ounce per day are not uncommon.

Aloe leaf is a detoxifier and rebuilder. Animal studies show it to be powerfully immunostimulant. Studies have revealed many biologically active substances in the plant. It seems to be a nonspecific booster of the immune system, possibly by stimulating macrophages.

Coptis root is a berberine containing herb. It is very cold, and strongly detoxifying. Several studies support the use ofberberine, and the related berbamine, in cancer, and specifically skin cancer. Berberine promotes macrophage activation.

Guduchi is an immune enhancer, sometimes called "Ayurvedic quinine," which is widely used to treat infections and fever. It is particularly effective in treating immune suppression resulting from toxicity.

Amla fruit is called the "fruit of rejuvenation" and is the most widely used general tonic herb, and it is also the most generally pitta suppressing. As the richest natural source of vitamin C ever discovered, it is obvious why it would benefit cancer. In addition, amla contains high levels of superoxide dismutase, making it a useful antioxidant in cancer treatment. Amla increases the secretion of interferon and corticosteroids. Amla is an ingredient in the famed revitalizer triphala, along with bibitaki fruit, and haritaki fruit, all of which are superb alteratives and skin rejuvenators. Amla is often prepared as a medicinal jelly, known by many names, but traditionally called "Chyavanprash." Many studies have shown this amla jelly to be potent in treating cancer.

Ashwaganda root is valuable in rebuilding after acute cancer treatment. It is also strongly hepatoprotective and anti-tumor. Ashwaganda is not directly cytotoxic, but is rather an immune booster, increasing natural resistance against tumor cells.

Other Ayurvedic anti-cancer herbs include:

- Gentian root (Gentiana spp.) - bitter detoxifier, anti-pitta
- Black pepper (Piper nigrum) - a powerful detoxifier and hepatoprotective

Turmeric, in various paste-like preparations, is frequently applied to the skin. It is cytotoxic, antioxidant, and skin healing. In one impressive study, 62 patients, with either ulcerating oral or cutaneous squamous cell carcinomas who had failed to respond to standard treatments, were given topical preparations of curcumin. After 18 months, the treatment was found to have been very effective in reducing the smell of the lesion (90% of patients), itching, exudate (70%), pain (50%) and the size of the lesion.

Castor oil is a widely used skin treatment, primarily for controlling vata. Castor oil packs placed over the involved area increase blood supply, as well as increasing immune activity in the area, apparently via a counterirritant effect. The Gerson treatment for skin cancer includes the use of castor oil internally as a detoxifier, particularly for the liver. This use parallels the Ayurvedic indication.

Aloe vera is widely used in natural healing in several systems as a general skin healer. It is also strongly immune enhancing.

Bala root is a generally beneficial topical for wounds, ulcers, and other skin lesions. It is often used as an infused oil.

Ghee is the primary Ayurvedic topical for controlling pitta. For pitta skin cancers, daily message with ghee is indicated. Ghee is considered to be cooling and anti inflammatory. Saffron paste serves as a general treatment for skin conditions. Gotu kola is also applied as a paste for tumors of the skin and underlying tissue.

When skin cancer is pitta-involved, purgation is indicated, provided the patient has the required stamina. Purgation is generally beneficial in skin diseases.

Ayurveda recommends a detoxifying diet, tailored to the patient, for treating cancer. Meat and dairy products are to be avoided. The diet should focus on raw vegetables and juices, particularly green juices. As these foods are cold, warming herbs may be added as necessary.

Weight Loss

Improper diet is the main underlying physical factor that induces disease. So, when we modify the diet, we also get at one of the underlying problems. Ayurveda recognizes that each of us is unique, and emphasizes the correct diet for each individual.

To balance excess kapha, which is the most common in overweight individuals, avoid cold, oily, heavy food. Focus on the reducing tastes- pungent, bitter and astringent- in your diet. Eat less total food, include low fat and low calorie foods and hot spices. Fasting occasionally is good. Eat less frequently, with the largest meal at midday. Use dry and astringent fruits (apple, raisin), vegetables (especially raw), dry grains (rice cakes), hot spices (black pepper, chilies), cooked beans with warming spices, and spicy herbal teas (ginger). Stay away from sweet fruits, nuts, milk products and oil.

Thermogenesis is the production of heat in the body when you burn food. But thermogenesis slows down as we age. Probably the leading theory in metabolic weight control today involves the upping of food burning to use up excess calories through body heat. Many leading herbal candidates for weight loss work in this way. One such herb is green tea.

Several pungent Ayurvedic herbs, including cayenne and ginger, have been demonstrated to promote thermogenesis. Now add another to this list. Researchers fed rats high fat diets, but added garlic. After four weeks, the rats had lost weight, and had lower levels of triglycerides, as well as increased sympathetic nerve function. They concluded that garlic assists in burning fat through increasing metabolism.[786] Use pungent herbs as comfortable in your food- the more the better.

Fiber is critical to many functions in the intestinal tract, including digestion and waste elimination. It also has a mild cholesterol-lowering effect. Many new studies propose that water-soluble fibers may also help individuals lose weight. Taken with a meal, they produce a feeling of fullness. The other anti-fat benefits of fiber include reducing the absorption of total calories, promoting blood sugar control, and enhancing the effect of insulin. In clinical studies of weight loss, fiber reduced absorbed calories by 30-180 calories per day, the equivalent of 3 to 18 pounds of fat loss over a year.

A double-blind placebo-controlled study looked at 97 mildly overweight women on a strict low-calorie diet. Patients who took 7 g of an insoluble fiber daily for 11 weeks lost 10.8 pounds compared to 7.3 pounds in the placebo group.[787]

Psyllium seed looks especially promising. A triple-blind experiment done last year in London with non-dieting subjects revealed that the participants felt much fuller than normal one hour after the meal, and ended up eating 15 grams less fat per day than usual.[788] Use 2 grams of psyllium seed powder, stirred into water three hours before each meal, and another 2 grams with each meal. It is best to gradually work up to these doses, allowing your body to gradually adjust, to avoid any gas or intestinal discomfort.

The typical dose of fiber used in such studies is 5 to 7 g per day.

Slimming Ayurvedic Herbs

Guggul is a standby medicine for the management of body fats. Particularly valuable in lowering cholesterol, guggul rivals any natural substance. Without dietary adjustments, guggul has lowered total cholesterol by over 20 percent, while increasing good HDL cholesterol by 36 percent.[789]

Like its effect on blood lipids, guggul can assist in managing overall body fat. Guggul seems to exert its effect at least partially through the thyroid, which could account for its fat loss benefit.[790] [791] [792] Another placebo-controlled study from 1999 combined guggul extract with *Garcinia cambogia* extract and tyrosine. Over six weeks, twenty obese persons had a significant decrease in body fat mass and average body weight. The subjects lost body fat, but not lean mass. Fatigue went down, and there were no adverse effects.[793] Guggul can be taken in a dose of 1,500 mg, three times daily.

Triphala has a light laxative effect and is well studied as a supreme general detoxifier and antioxidant. The combination of guggul and triphala recently showed a surprising effect in controlling body fat. When 48 obese subjects took this combination three times a day for three months, with no attempt to control their food intake, the resulting weight loss averaged almost 18 pounds, along with a drop in total cholesterol of 18 points. The dose used in the study was only 500 mg of the combination, three times per day.[794]

Gurmar has been proven in study after study to increase the production and activity of insulin produced in the body. This insulin increase is thought by many experts to be the primary successful method of promoting fat burning. Gurmar will also lower blood fats. Recently this herb demonstrated a startling ability to lower all types of lipids in the blood.[795]

So it seems that we have an ideal herb for treating the diabetic/obesity syndrome that is so common in America. Gurmar is available as an extract from the health food store. The typical extract dose is 1,200-1,500 mg per day.

When Natural Healing Should Give Way to Modern Medicine

Are drugs ever better than herbs and other natural medicines? For most conditions, only as a last resort. While drugs sometimes are actually a better choice, natural healing is much more sophisticated, effective and powerful than most people think it is. Natural methods can treat just about any health problem you can come up with, from acute issues to long-term chronic conditions to tricky, challenging puzzles.

We often see posed the question, "Do these natural remedies really work?" First of all, why not? Why don't we ever see an article that asks, "Do these drugs we take all the time really work?" In most of the world it would simply not be posed, for why question the obvious? Even scientific inquiry in cultures with established natural healing systems focus on the *how,* not the *if.*

Only 5% of the pharmaceuticals in common use have met the world standard of safety and efficacy.[796]

Since the dawn of humanity, when people got sick, their food was their medicine. Before the first pharmaceuticals came into being 100 years ago, practitioners were their own pharmacists, and their pharmacies consisted of herbal and other natural substances. Health practitioners would treat people from cradle to grave with those procedures and medicines. Natural preparations were available in a vast range of forms, for kids, adults and elderly.

According to Dr. Tillotson, "Western diagnostic methods (imaging, blood tests) can often reveal hidden problems, such as leukemias, cancers, protein deficiencies, liver enzyme elevations, etc., all of which are of great importance to the herbal practitioner to know sometimes."[797]

When the contest between so called natural and conventional western medicine lets up, there will be a great place for an integrative approach drawing on the best of all systems.

Furthermore, the kind of situation in which drugs really are most appropriate can frequently be avoided in the first place. That's what this book is about. Even when total prevention is not achieved, problems in early stages can be easily handled using gentle, mild methods.

Herbal medicine doesn't always work instantly or dramatically, for the most part, although it can. But mostly, herbal medicine works by gentle nudging. By comparison, drugs may be unnecessary overreactions.

The choice of whether to use a drug or an herb, or a combination, in any given case, depends on a lot of factors, some of them quite subjective. Often the main issues have nothing to do with therapeutic effectiveness, but with compliance considerations, including economic concerns, convenience, insurance, legal issues, family opinions, and perceived risk tolerance.

In any case, herbal medicine and natural medicine should be the first not the last choice for most problems. When they seem to produce the desired results then drugs can be used and the focus on the use of herbs and natural medicine to counteract the adverse effects of the drugs as well as to foster a healthy immune system and promote the health of body and mind.

· THIRTEEN ·

INTEGRATING AYURVEDIC HERBS AND FOODS INTO DAILY LIFE

Ayurveda keeps the body in balance with the environment. Ayurveda aims to give us the tools to adapt our lives to the changes that always come with the environment.

When it's hot, we need to keep cool. When it's dry, we need to stay moisturized. As the years pass, we age, and need to stay rested and nourished. Ayurvedic science has established techniques to help us adjust every facet of our lives to the changes that occur around us. The teachings include diet, lifestyle scheduling, herbal medicines, clothing, yoga methods and a host of other procedures to keep us physically and mentally balanced and happy.

One of the most significant changes we experience is the cycle of the changing seasons. As the temperature shifts, the days and nights change length and the rains come and go, our bodies have to deal with the stress of the changes. Ayurveda helps us predict these cyclic changes, and ma

The doshas don't fluctuate and battle for center stage only inside our bodies; their dance is evident in the environment around us. In the cycles of the day, the season and the length of a lifetime, vata, pitta and kapha take turns "driving the bus." It's helpful to know how the dosha that dominates during a particular season can affect you, so you can adjust as much as possible using factors that are within your control.

During spring, kapha increases; it has accumulated all winter. Then, with summer, everyone deals with pitta; diseases of heat become more common. In autumn, vata increases; pitta becomes more disturbed, as well. During cold winter, we tend to be sedentary, and kapha accumulates.

As an example, summer is the unhealthiest season in most places around the world because of the heat and humidity, but in Seattle it's the healthiest because it's about the only time we get to dry up at all. Seattle is a very kapha promoting climate- cold and wet. This type of climate aggravates kapha more than the other doshas. People with kapha constitution who want to thrive through winter in Seattle need to pay special attention to warming and drying strategies. Likewise, pitta constitution folks will do better during hot humid weather if they emphasize cooling and drying; vata constitution individuals in the desert can intervene with moistening foods and herbs.

Ayurveda is all about balance- how to know if we have it, how to achieve it and how to keep it. One of the most important things we can do to stay in balance is to keep an eye on the calendar. As the seasons slide from one into another, our body's needs also slowly change. Ayurveda has come up with a scheme to adjust our diet and lifestyle practices to stay in tune with the changes in nature. Ritucharya, the science of seasonal rhythms, is based on the weather outside the window and the effect that will have on the body's patterns of health.

To understand the effects of the seasons on our health, and to appreciate the whys and wherefores of the food we ought to eat in each season, we must look at the waxing and waning patterns of the three doshas. After all, the doshas are the supervisors of the body and their moods govern the well being of an individual at all times.

Ritucharya (seasonal programs) is based on an awareness of the climate, not on to calendar months or dates. If spring comes early, your program will change to the spring routine a little early, too. For example, if the weather is warming up, we can gradually increase the amounts of cooling foods in our daily meals to compensate.

On the other hand, the routine suggested for the spring season should not be adopted just because it is March, if there is still a nip in the air and the nights are cold enough to make you think about a blanket.

So, one does not switch off one season and switch on the next, overnight. One season blends progressively into the next, merging gracefully into it, and so also should our dietary and living habits slip from one to the other without a hitch.

DOSHA CYCLES

Cycle	Kapha	Pitta	Vata
Climate	Spring (Accumulated all winter)	Summer	Autumn/ winter
Day	6:00 am-10:00 am	10:00 am- 2:00 pm (Time to eat)	2:00 pm- 6:00 pm (Sunset)
Night	6:00 pm- 10:00 pm	10:00 pm- 2:00 am	2:00 am- 6:00 am Sadhana (Kapha accumulates)
Digestion	Stomach (mucus)	Small intestine	Large intestine
Life	Early (before puberty)	Midlife (peaks age 40)	Elderly (last 1/3)

Figure 28 Dosha Cycles

Spring

Spring is a time of changes- in like a lion, out like a lamb. In fact, the transition from winter to spring is one of the most difficult and stressful shifts we go through during the year. Winter, with its cold weather, gradually gives way to the increasing warmth of summer, so we go from a time of excess kapha energy to the increasing heat of the pitta season.

And all this doesn't always happen quite as easily as we'd like. During the unpredictable beginning of spring, our bodies don't know who to believe- Old Man Winter or the green grass of spring. Does our immune system still have to guard us against colds, or do our adrenal glands have to get us up and out the door?

Just like the plants that start poking out in spring, we need to gradually start to poke our noses out into the world.

Your goal in spring will be to stabilize your health and make sure you are detoxified from the stored products of our sedentary winter metabolism. Your health strategy will be to stay warm, get moving, dry out, and lighten up your life.

Spring is a time for warming exercise, gradually getting back into shape. Add to that some invigorating massage, to get the blood circulating, and nice warm baths, saunas and warm herb rubs to revitalize and stimulate the tissues.

A Little Spring Cleaning

During spring, concentrate on cleansing foods and teas. After all, you've been hibernating all winter, you old bear. Now, like it or not, it's time to get up, get cleaned out and get active. Mucus tends to accumulate in the winter (remember all those miserable days at home with a cold?), and that same mucus likes to flow in the spring, like the sap rising in the trees.

Milk tends to increase mucus, so limit milk products in the morning during the spring. To counteract this tendency for excess morning mucus, drink a cup of warm water with a teaspoon of honey instead.

Pungent, bitter and astringent tastes assist in cleaning out the tissues. Leafy green vegetables, leeks, lettuce, okra, parsley and spinach are bitter cleansing foods. Artichoke is an excellent detoxifier of the liver and gallbladder. Turmeric detoxifies and reduces inflammation. Root vegetables, including beets, carrots, radishes and turnips- raw, cooked or juiced- help keep the liver clean while it does its extra spring cleaning.

Split peas and navy beans are good sources of protein for this season, because they stick to the ribs but are easy enough to digest that the body still detoxifies easily.

Astringent foods, like berries and grapes, especially green ones, are detoxifying.

A good lunch for a warm spring day would be a soup of mung beans and rice, with ghee, cilantro, and grated coconut.

The warming herbs green tea, basil, ginger, cloves and coriander keep the later chill away. Pungent onions, garlic, ginger and chilies help speed up circulation, bringing cleansing blood to all the organs.

Many folks develop some joint and muscle pain over the long winter. Detoxifying vegetarian diets have been studied in chronic muscle pain, to good effect in general. A Norwegian study tested the effects of a three week vegetarian diet for people with chronic muscle pain. Serum peroxide, plasma fibrinogen, total cholesterol and high density lipoprotein cholesterol all reduced.

The panchakarma therapies of theraprutic vomiting and nasal medicines can help, if monitored by a professional.

Clean Out all the Pipes

Spring is the allergy season, and what a misery it can be for those who suffer! In excess, the wet and heavy energy of kapha contributes to this bane of spring for those who are susceptible.

During the spring, use the neti pot daily, just like brushing your teeth. A warm saltwater and herbal rinse of the nasal passages takes just a few seconds a day, but it can save days of misery from sick sinuses.

In the neti, triphala will shrink swollen membranes, eucalyptus will thin mucus and goldenseal will kill bacteria. Gotu kola, scullcap and calamus are traditional nasal application herbs for sinus conditions. For inflamed sinuses, add a teaspoon of ghee to the neti.

Summer

With the strongest sun of the year, summer is hot, and pitta dosha is getting high.

People tend to have respiratory problems as the season changes from spring to summer, so cooling respiratory herbs and foods are in order. Diseases of fever tend to increase, as do those of inflammation. All are signs of heat.

Since people in temperate climates are more active in summer, they tend to succumb to athletic injuries and accidents. Be careful while you enjoy your fun, and get your fitness up before those weekend softball games.

Your seasonal strategy at this time is to stay cool, prevent water retention and stay balanced and even in your activities. Don't overdo it if you have a tendency to heat up.

During this hot season, use cooling foods. Stay cool. Get up early in the morning when it is cool. Avoid working in hot environments and be careful not to get overheated. No arguing.

Wear cooler clothes, like cotton or silk. Ayurveda suggests cooling massages with coconut oil during hot weather. Cooling aromas, or essential oils, including sandal or rose, help to quell the fire.

Bitter taste, which is cooling, is composed of air and ether elements, the same elements that predominate in the mind. Herbs with cooling bitter taste generally open the mind, increase the sensitivity of awareness and improve mental function. Bitter tasting herbs are cooling, calming and mind expanding, so they combat mental dullness. Bitter mind herbs are chamomile and gotu kola.

Sweet taste, composed of earth and water elements, is grounding, cooling and calming. Sweet herbs for the mind include ashwaganda and licorice.

Use cooling, bitter and astringent herbs to brush your teeth, and rinse your mouth with cool herbs, including neem and mint.

In your diet, concentrate on sweet, bitter and astringent tastes. Focus on the fresh, sweet, fruits and vegetables that grow in this season. Use more raw foods, like salads.

Cucumber, watermelon, non-acidic fruits and juices, grains, wheat, rice, and milk are ideal summer foods. Add to the list for summer meals a few more cooling foods: coconut, sweet fruits (grapes, pineapple, apricot, cabbage, black olives, squash, wheat, white beans, sprouts and sweet potato.

A delicious mid-summer drink is a lassi made with cilantro and cumin, or lime water with cumin or coriander powder. As a cooling drink in the evening, use cool milk, with raw sugar, rosewater and blanched almonds.

Eat fewer foods with pungent, sour and salty tastes. Foods to minimize in summer include yogurt, cheese, tomatoes, vinegar and hot spices.

To stay fit, healthy and maintain your stamina, use mild tonic herbs during the summer. Ashwaganda is a good choice.

Good cooling herbs for summer teas include cumin seed, spearmint, chamomile, chrysanthemum and honeysuckle.

Cooling diaphoretics are used to reduce fever and inflammation. Cooling chrysanthemum flower and honeysuckle flower are also strongly antimicrobial. Elder flower, yarrow flower and boneset leaf are cooling Western diaphoretics.

Traditionally, Ayurveda uses many cooling herbs to help us become more accepting of ourselves and others, and to open the heart, manage anger and enhance communication.

Mandukaparni awakens the crown chakra and balances brain hemispheres. It is a cooling herb- it helps to cool down anger. Hibiscus flower is a sweet cooling herb that purifies the heart and the blood, both physically and spiritually. It promotes wisdom.

Rose flower is a cooling herb that opens the heart and the mind. Use rose water as a refreshing drink. It combines well with hibiscus.

Scullcap leaf reduces jealousy, hatred and anger, calms the heart and reduces overabundant desire. Scullcap assists awareness and detachment from negative emotions.

Mints, such as spearmint, contain large amounts of ether element, which is mentally soothing and clarifying.

Jasmine, sandalwood and rose are cooling scents to use during the summer heat. When cooling peppermint and eucalyptus oils are swabbed on the temples, the oils increase cognitive performance and have a muscle-relaxing and mentally relaxing effect. Peppermint oil mixed with alcohol has a significant analgesic effect with a reduction in sensitivity to headache.

Fall

Fall season if a time of transition.

We transition from hot weather to cold weather. We transition from vacation time back to school. It feels like a new beginning for many people. For our bodies its a time of adjustment, and sometimes, confusion. Its a time when its easy to "fall" into ill health.

Hot, pitta summer begins to transition into cool autumn and bring out vata dosha. During this change of season, often a difficult time, it is a good time for a last detoxification program before the sedentary winter season sets in.

And the fall season is a good time to fortify your immune system, in preparation for the winter colds and flu. Stabilize transition to winter by sticking to your health program and living a disciplined, consistent life.

Your autumn routine will vary a bit, depending on where you live. As the weather gets gradually colder, vata dosha gets more aggravated, and our attention will be turned more and more toward keeping vata from becoming excess.

If it's still hot in autumn where you live, pitta can still be aggravated, so remain cautious about getting too hot, and watch the spicy foods until the weather cools down.

According to Ayurveda, we should get up early during the fall, when the world is calm, to prepare the mind for the day.

After going through your wake up routine and cleansing procedures, brush your teeth and rinse your mouth with a warm mouth rinse.

During the autumn, concentrate on a diet that is warm, moist and nourishing. Well cooked steamed vegetables, rice with ghee and soft, mushy soups fit the bill, especially as the weather gets colder. Other warming and nourishing fall foods are radish, fenugreek, soy milk, almond, walnut, Brazil nut, tortillas and whole wheat. Onion, garlic and ginger keep the body warm and the endocrine and immune systems supported.

Eat lots of sweet, sour and salty foods in the fall. Keep your meals moderate in size and well balanced with a food variety of foods.

Sweet taste is grounding. Examples include avocado, cherries, grapefruit and carrot.

Sour and salty tastes, like pickles, in moderation, promote digestion.

To top off your meal, Ayurvedic cuisine suggests a dessert of sweetened cream of wheat with almonds. And before bed, how about a delicious nighttime drink for the fall, made from half water and half milk, boiled with ginger, cardamom and nutmeg?

Warming herb teas are perfect for the fall. Use licorice root, cinnamon bark, ginger root, basil, cardamom seed, black pepper and clove.

Lead a stable life. Stick to your routine. Be kind to your immune system- you'll need it soon enough.

Constipation tends to worsen in the fall, so make sure you use herbs, high fiber cooked foods and lubricating foods like vegetable oils to keep things moving.

Soaked raisins keep the bowels moist and moving. Triphala, ayurveda's most famous herbal blend, does wonders to keep the digestion moving.

If fall is dry where you live, massage your skin with oil daily to prevent dryness. Good massage oils for the fall are sesame and almond.

To avoid aggravating vata during the fall, avoid loud noise, fast driving and chaotic activities. Don't stay up late, and get a good night's sleep.

Immune herbs can play a role in fall season health. Isatidis and astragalus are all purpose Chinese herbal tonics, while echinacea can help if you feel a bug coming on.

Some climates have a rainy period in the first part of the fall. Use haritaki as a rejuvenating remedy. For kapha, take it with honey. To control pitta, use ghee with the herb and to pacify vata, drink some warm milk with the haritaki.

Fall can be a time of exciting new projects and a time to get serious and, maybe, artistic. Enjoy your fall and make the most of the season with your healthy routine.

Winter

In winter, the thermometer plummets. We get deep into the hibernation time of kapha, the cold and wet dosha. We feel sluggish. We may get mucus diseases. We need to warm up and dry out- especially our respiratory tracts. We need to save our strength to fight the cold.

In some areas, winter is also dry. In a cold, dry climate, people are more prone to nervous system diseases. In this environment, warm and moisten, and avoid wind and cold.

During winter, avoid getting exhausted. To maintain your good health, eat a nutritive diet that will build good healthy tissues, and stabilize your routine and food habits with consistency and regularity in your schedule. Promote a calming atmosphere. Prevent constipation. Right nostril breathing will speed up your metabolism and help keep you warmer.

Exercise with mild activities, to your capacity. Have regular massage with warm, moistening oils (castor, sesame, mustard, olive).

Your winter food choices should be easy to digest. Eat warm, dry food, like rice cakes, millet, corn bread and barley. Drink hot beverages to stay nice and warm. Use mild warming spices, including garlic, cinnamon and cloves.

Avoid high fat food, as people tend to put on weight during the winter. A little light oil, such as ghee or sesame oil, is essential to keep the tissues moist if winter is a dry season where you live.

Concentrate on foods with pungent taste, like ginger or radish, to keep warm. Add bitter taste, like leafy greens or dandelion root, and astringent taste, like cranberry or apple, to maintain the body's detoxification during the sedentary season.

If winter is dry where you live, add sweet, filling foods, including figs, carrots, tomatoes, dates and warm milk products.

Outstanding winter foods are apples, prunes, beets, broccoli, buckwheat, dry oats, rye and beans (pinto, garbanzo, etc.).

To your list of satisfying winter foods, add cabbage, carrots, cauliflower, tofu (in warm dishes), corn and pumpkin seeds.

Warming winter teas include sarsaparilla root, ginger root, juniper berry, cinnamon, cardamom, clove and black pepper.

How to live it day to day

As the doshas go through their cycles during the day, we can adjust our activities to best take advantage of the opportunities to treat them and maintain balance. Subtle changes in the daily routine can have profound lasting effects over years.

During the cold and slow kapha dominant time, for example, we want to stay warm and be active. During vata times, we want to be stable, solid, safe, warm and secure.

And making all these changes isn't always easy. For some, they are pretty radical, so they need to be gradual. Start with one change that you can cope with. If it's a commitment to gradually hot spices over a couple of months, until you are not using them at all, great. If its a plan to transition to cooking with whole grains over 3 months, while you get the hang of the new ingredients, that's progress.

AYURVEDA DAILY ROUTINE

Arise (before the sun, if possible)

Excrete wastes

Brush teeth and gums, scrape tongue
Tooth powder: alum, salt, black pepper, turmeric

Clean eyes (cold water, etc.)

Shower (cold, if desired)

Spiritual practice ("sadhana"- yoga, prayer)

Ointment to eyes

Clean elimination systems:
Nose- sniff: black pepper, ginger
Throat- gargle: astringent (triphala, etc.) or oil (i.e. sesame, etc.)
Chest- inhale: eucalyptus oil, menthol, turmeric smoke

Fragrance- flowers, incense

Breakfast as appropriate

Work portion of day

Exercise- before- massage with oil, after- with medicated powder (triphala, etc.). Bathe.

Lunch as appropriate

Remainder of activities (work, etc.)

Supper as appropriate (light)

Prepare for bed (meditation, etc.)

Wash feet, hands, apply oil to feet and head

Bed

Figure 29 Daily Routine

Daily Lifestyle Tidbits

Getting up in the morning

- Awaken gradually and slowly.
- With eyes still closed, stretch your spine.
- Stretch each knee across the other leg, twisting the spine to each side in turn.
- Place your palms over your closed eyes.
- Open your eyes to stare at your palms. Slowly gaze at your palms as you lift your hand 18 inches from your face.
- Massage your face, neck, and ears.
- Stretch pose: Lift heels six inches off the bed; lift your head to focus your eyes on your toes. Hold with "breath of fire" for one minute.
- Pull your knees to your chest and your nose to your knees with breath of fire for 30 seconds.
- Take a few deep breaths and gracefully arise.

Cold shower in the morning before yoga (adjust to your constitutional tolerance)

- Let the spray splash your face, elbows, ears, chest, low back, feet.
- Stay in until you are warm and tingly.
- Towel off briskly.
- You'll be warm, alert and energized.

After eating, sit in "rock pose" (sit on heels) for seven minutes to enhance digestion.

Washing your hair (Hair is the physical manifestation of the Sushumna.)

- Oil your head with a pure vegetable oil like almond or sesame.
- Massage your scalp vigorously.
- Add a mixture of oil, yogurt, and any fragrance you desire.
- Wrap hair in a towel for 12 hours.
- Wash the yogurt/oil out with clear water.
- Sun dry your hair.

If you feel yourself getting angry and upset, drink a tall glass of water to readjust your blood chemistry

Personalize Your Lifestyle with Ayurveda

As each person is viewed as an individual in the ways we've mentioned, so, too, can we understand how each person should conduct their life, according to the dosha they are seeking to balance. Your schedule, your relationships, your choice of exercise, all can be calculated using Ayurveda.

When Kapha dominates, people are slow and lethargic. They like a lot of sleep, and tend toward obesity. When Pitta dominates, people are hot, intense, aggressive and demanding. When vata dominates people are spaced-out, flighty, erratic, anxious and insomniac. Through Ayurveda, the ultimate self-care system, we can adjust all these factors with careful lifestyle choices.

	To Balance Kapha	To Balance Pitta	To Balance Vata
Keywords	*Be Active*	*Be Calm*	*Be Moderate*
Activity level	Stimulating activities	Cut down the schedule	Disciplined schedule
Physical work	Physical labor	Rest and relax	Mild physical effort
Temperature	Stay active	Stay cool	Stay warm
Weather	Sunbathing	Take in cool breezes	Take in the sun
Climate	Avoid cold and damp	Avoid the sun	Avoid wind and cold
Light	Sunshine	Moonlight	Dusk
Sleep	Less sleep (shorter nights rest, no naps)	Sleep only as needed	Adequate sleep
Sleep schedule	Get up early	Midday rest	Get to bed early
Professional life	Mental stimulation	Cut down striving	Avoid overwork
Daily life	Mix it up (variety of activities)	Simplify your life	Consistency
Recreation time	Cultivate physical challenges	Gardens, gardening, flowers	Avoid excess stimulation (TV, etc.)
Love life	Bring variety to sex	Cool romance, poetry	Sexual moderation
Travel	Promote travel	Moderate travel	Avoid intense travel
Stress	Avoid "couch potato" behavior	Avoid angry confrontation	Avoid all types of stress
Emotions	Motivation	Forgiveness	Persistence
Environment	Enthusiasm	Contentment	Coziness
Daily routine	Variety in schedule	Alternate rest and work	Regular hours

PERSONALIZE YOUR EXERCISE ROUTINE WITH AYURVEDA

For Balancing Kapha	For Balancing Pitta	For Balancing Vata
Get hot	Don't overheat, cool air	Stay warm
Sweat	Don't be fanatical - take a break	Mild only - don't overdo
Vigorous aerobic	Drink plenty of water	Regular routine - stick with a program
Work up to pushing your limits	Vary the routine to avoid boredom	Slow, gradual progress
Discipline	Varied overall fitness program	Walking
Powerful calisthenics	Moderate intensity	Stretching, mild yoga

Personal Ethics

In the interest of holistic approach to sustaining health, Ayurveda prescribes certain rules of conduct for maintaining a vigorous mind and life. The mind and behavior have a great effect on the doshas, perhaps as great as diet and herbs. Here are the lifestyle rules:

- Always speak the truth
- Speak pleasant words
- Do not lose your temper under any circumstances
- Do not harm anyone
- Be straightforward and kind
- Act courteously and politely
- Observe self control
- Do not get addicted to sensory pleasures
- Control your passions
- Control your sense organs
- Be patient
- Do not expose yourself to hardships
- Meditate every day
- Observe cleanliness in all things
- Distribute knowledge, good advice and money
- Devote your services to God, the wise, the respectable and the elderly
- Keep daily activities regular
- Avoid excess in eating, drinking, sexual activity and little sleep
- Behave according to the time and place where you are residing
- Do good, avoid bad

Personalize Your Love Life with Ayurveda

Your relationship can improve if you understand the doshas. Ayurveda suggests a spouse of a different constitution. This helps you balance each other in the relationship, and prevents your offspring from being too extreme in anyone dosha. Two vatas produce a child who is doubly vata, for example.

	For balancing Kapha	For Balancing Pitta	For Balancing Vata
Spouse	Marry vata	Marry kapha or vata	Marry kapha
Family Life	Active family life	Balance work with family	Commitment in relationship
Conversation	Stimulating conversations	Soothing conversations	Less thinking, more acting Don't overtalk & overanalyze
Communication	Encourage talking	No confrontation	Slow and Steady
Touching	Energizing massages	Cooling massages	Relaxing massages
Social Life	Go out and get interested	Take "cool off" breaks	No wild experimental lifestyles
Money matters	Be more creative with options	No impulse buying	Careful managing money
Romance	Encourage sexual interest	Slow down and cool off to take time and care for sex	Consistent and supportive, caution with sexual experimentation

Sex and Rejuvenation with Ayurveda

The goal of life is to experience and master four complementary areas, which, taken together, make up the totality of fulfillment.

Dharma, or the path of righteousness, is the complete collection of virtuous, religious works and practices. Artha is the accumulation and enjoyment of material possessions and earthly well-being. Moksha is spiritual liberation. The fourth area may be the most misunderstood. Kama is romantic and sexual love and all its associated pleasures of the senses. Everyone has heard about *The Kama Sutra*, which is an extensive treatise on the subject.

According to the Kama Sutra, all of these aspects should be of equal importance, without any of these areas taking precedence over the others. For a fulfilled and meaningful life, the striving after one goal shouldn't inhibit striving after others. Neglect of any one of these spheres leads to a diminished stability and to imbalance in men. Practicing dharma, artha and kama makes it possible to lead a meaningful and joyous life in this world and to move on to spiritual freedom.

Sexuality and the erotic life are important, integrated elements of the human life, and are as important as eating. The sensual pleasures increase the joy of life and maintain psychological balance, and actually aid further mental and spiritual development. Sexuality and erotic practices contain the secret of life within them.

Ayurveda identifies three key areas that are, taken together, considered to be the base foundation of Ayurvedic lifestyle and therapeutics- balanced diet, balanced sleep and balanced sexual life. We should indulge in sex such a way so as not to have any adverse effect on health. Ayurveda advises moderate sexual activity during midlife, according to personal constitution and other traits. Being alert to avoid excess or deficiency in food, sleep or sex goes a long way toward keep the doshas in balance.

The companion sciences of rejuvenation (*rasayana*); and aphrodisiacs, or virilization, (*vajikarana*) are well researched, practical areas of health maintenance that anyone can use to stay well and sexy throughout a long life. ("Vaji" is a stallion. You get the idea.)

Ayurveda places special emphasis on maintaining excellent health well into elderhood. Over time, practitioners have developed excellent therapies for keeping the mind and body young. Of course, sex is an important part of that life. Most people enjoy sex and would love for their romantic life to continue indefinitely. In our culture, though, there's a general sense that sexual desire, performance, and pleasure will unavoidably wane, much to our disappointment. While no one will literally be the same at eighty as they were at twenty, the physical degeneration can be much less than we might think.

Literally translated as "the path of juice," this branch of Ayurveda aims to nourish, restore and balance the body functions which have been taxed by the wear and tear of daily life. Signs of aging are all marks of lack of "juice," from arthritis with lack of joint fluids, to fatigue with lack of endocrine hormones, to menopause difficulties with vaginal dryness.[798]

Ayurvedic rasayana practices are directed toward strengthening, purifying and nourishing body tissues to bring back the glow of youth - replacing that "juiciness." Rasayana is intended to improve overall health, generate high quality tissues, eradicate senility and diseases of aging, lengthen life, boost memory and improve intelligence, youth, skin luster, voice quality, strength of body and senses, and beauty. Rasayana regimes act to augment tissue mass, digestive capacity, hormone function, elimination systems, brain function, immunity and homeostasis.

Modern science tells us that calorie restriction and the reduction of body temperature will extend life span, at least in experimental animals. Ayurveda teaches that the body ages and dries out in proportion to the metabolic rate. Any practice that will slow down the metabolism and calm the body and mind will retard age-related degeneration and reduce the loss of plumpness and lubrication. The loss of juice is closely related to increased vata dosha. Vata increases naturally with age. Ayurvedic antiaging remedies are essentially a fight to control the catabolic actions of vata for as long as possible.

Rejuvenation comes in two forms - lifestyle and medicine. "Hot" activities, such as passion and anger, age the body more rapidly, so calming behavior is suggested. To live longer and have better sex, speak the truth, avoid becoming angry, practice meditation, avoid conflict, and steer away from drugs and alcohol.

Rasayana practices can be based on diet, lifestyle or medicine. Rasayana medicines are classified as to their function. *Kamya rasayanas* promote normal health- vitality, intelligence and complexion. *Naimittika rasayana* medicines treat specific diseases.

Rasayana medicines include a large array of herbs and foods. Sweet taste, contained in carbohydrates and good quality fats, is the most rejuvenating, so sweet food, including milk, ghee, and especially honey, is recommended to rebuild body tissues and restore sexual juices.[799] Ideally, a patient will undergo vigorous detoxification before undertaking serious rasayana therapy.

Closely related to rasayana, vajikarana, virilization, including the use of aphrodisiacs and sexual rebuilding tonics, aims to support sexual pleasure, fertility, and performance. Sexual fluids, including semen, are the most important concentrated essence of all the body's tissues. Ayurveda recommends retaining some of it to use in the rest of the body for renewing body and mind. Since sex depletes the body's juices, vajikarana, like rasayana, also focuses on replacing tissue nutrients and fluids.[800] Vajikarana practices improve sexual activity, and can be used for such, but they also help direct sexual energy inward for renewal. Visualize the body as a tree, with the reproductive system as the roots. Vajikarana therapies start at the roots, but continue to feed the entire body with tonic energy over time. Producing more and better quality semen, if it is retained to a certain extent, regenerates the mind and the immune system. Vajikarana deals not only with increasing sexual vigor, but also psychosomatic disorders. Vajikarana is valuable for all around health. The influence of the mind is the origin of momentum for sexual desire, so virilization must consider mental health. Vajikarana therapies can be utilized for treating disorders of the mind, including depression. Vajikarana therapies are for mentally balanced, sexually active people between 18 and 70.

Overall, vajikarana therapies promote happiness, daily stamina, fertility and improved erectile function.

Sex is an integral part of our daily habits, and should be given as much attention as diet or exercise. Ayurveda says that human sex is not simply physical mating but is the union of two bodies, minds and souls, and that it can be a transformative and healing experience if managed correctly. For people who want to rebuild sexually, Ayurveda proposes a one month interval of absolute sexual chastity, allowing the body to relax and balance. After this readjustment period, you may use detoxification remedies and diet to clean out old accumulated wastes, followed by the actual foods and herbs to enhance sexual function.

If extensive vajikarana therapy is necessary, the deep cleansing practices (panchakarma) of Ayurveda are usually employed as a preparatory measure. Interestingly, Charaka says that the female is the greatest of all vajikarana medicines!

The actual sex act is important in maintaining sexual pleasure and potency. The atmosphere should include sweet music, sweet fragrance and flowers. Wait a while after eating. Ideally, partners should be physically, emotionally and spiritually involved with the other.

An absolutely satisfying sexual union confers health and vitality upon you and your partner. It is essential that both partners are satisfied. Deviant or unsatisfying sex has adverse effects on mental and physical health. It aggravates the doshas and reduces immunity. Afterwards, urinate to balance the energy in the pelvis, and relax, perhaps with a warm bath. Finish with a special drink of hot milk or almond milk with ghee and honey or dates and saffron.

The evening, especially after two hours of dinner, is the ideal time for intimacy, as it is kapha time.

The frequency of sex depends on constitution. Kapha types may engage in sex more frequently than vata & pitta types thanks to their innate extra stamina. Vata types may seek satisfaction in changing partners. Pitta types are usually on a quest for more sexual intensity.

Those who regulate their sexual energy will have increased memory, physical stamina, intelligence, health and longevity.

For good sex, turn to some Ayurvedic suggestions:

- Both partners must want to engage in sex
- Both should be good in physical and mental health
- Mensturating women should not engage in vaginal intercourse
- Avoid partners who are devoid of passion, not clean, too old, too young or sick
- Pregnant women should not be sexual after 120 days of gestation, with certain exceptions
- Both partners, after enjoying sexual activity, should take a cool bath, and drink cool water, milk or juice, or eat food containing natural sugar

Ojas

Central to the Ayurvedic idea of sexual rejuvenation is the concept of *ojas*, which is the most concentrated essence of nutritional substances in the body, roughly comparable to semen and/or cerebrospinal fluid. Ojas is a conceptualized as a very fine biological substance that comprises the most concentrated essence of nutrients and energy in the body. It is the essence of all the types of tissues and the physical expression of consciousness in the body. The basic biological strength of the tissues depends on it. It is strongly correlated with vitality and our immunity.[801] Ayurveda maintains that food, once consumed, is progressively concentrated into ever more distilled categories of tissue building nutrients.[802] It is said that one hundred bites of food will produce one drop of blood, and that one hundred drops of blood will produce one drop of ojas.[803] Modern scholars have linked the concept of ojas to the blood protein albumin. Others have hypothesized that it may parallel essential fatty acids. Ojas is especially concentrated in the heart (a total quantity of 8 drops worth), but is pervades the entire breadth of the body, as the essence of honey is present in a flower. So, as we can see, starting with good quality food is essential to maintaining good health, especially sexual health.

When ojas has become deficient, we see a syndrome consisting of a collection of clinical signs:

- Vibheti- Fear
- Durbalo abhikshanam- Physical and mental weakness
- Vyathit Indriya- Discomfort in sense organs
- Duschhaya- Abnormal colors
- Durmana- Impaired mental functions
- Ruksha- Dryness
- Kshama- Abnormal complexion
- Precious ojas can be destroyed by pretty much any health defeating factor. In particular, these causes are identified:
- Abhighatat- Trauma
- Kshayat- Loss of other refined tissue essence (Dhatus)
- Negative Emotions - Anger (Kopat), grief (Shokat)
- Dhyanat- Mental stress
- Shramat- Physical hard work
- Kshudha- Hunger

The diet that promotes ojas and sexual rejuvenation is a highly nutritive program, emphasizing whole grains like wheat and rice, seeds, nuts, milk products, and natural sugars, such as honey.[804] Cooked, moist foods (soups) and meat juice will help. The diet should be balanced to contain a broad range of tastes - sweet, sour, salty, spicy, bitter, astringent. Generally, use food that is sweet, oily, cold, light and easily digestible. Use less dry or raw food, and include a good quality raw vegetable oil (almond, sesame) and ghee. Onion, garlic, ginger, eggplant, figs and dates are aphrodisiac.

Ojas is stored in muscles, fat and organs- throughout the body. Most of it is made at night during restorative sleep. The production of ojas comes after the production of sexual fluids (shukra). Thus depletion of shukra channels body resources toward shukra production and ojas production is curtailed. Ojas is used for immunity and procreation, so it is easily depleted by either use. With a thorough and disciplined program, it takes thirty days to replenish the ojas reserves in the body. Sexual abstinence during this time will help ojas accumulate.

Rejuvenating Ojas Drink (especially for after sex)

8-10 oz milk
1-3 tsp grated fresh ginger root
1-3 tsp black sesame seed (or white sesame seed)
1-3 tsp ghee
Cinnamon and clove to taste.
Honey to taste if desired.

Warm milk to comfortable drinking temperature. Blend ingredients in blender. Drink after sex, especially men, or daily as a restorative for sexual function.

General Mouth Care

Brush your teeth upon arising. Ayurveda does not, as a general rule, recommend toothpaste. Typical toothpaste is cold, heavy, slimy and sweet- just the qualities that increase the very accumulated kapha you are brushing your teeth to get rid of. Modern Ayurvedic toothpastes do exist, as a compromise for those who are used to brushing with paste. You will find them to be drier, astringent, and pungent.

Many ingredients have been included in Ayurvedic tooth powders, including alum, salt, black pepper and turmeric. Students of Yogi Bhajan use a finely ground mixture of 2 parts potassium alum and 1 part salt.

Daily tongue cleaning to remove the accumulated ama (tongue fur) is a critical part of maintaining oral health. Brush your tongue while brushing your teeth, or use a tongue scraper, available from Ayurvedic suppliers.

Many scrapers are now made from plastic, but authentic Ayurvedic models are made from metal, and will last a lifetime. Stainless steel makes a hardy scraper, while gold and copper models will be warming and a silver one will be cooling.

Tongue cleaning reduces bad breath, and helps prevent plaque.

Use of warming, astringent, connective tissue healing herbs will generally enhance and maintain oral health. These herbs can be applied as packs (a pinch of powder, wetted to a mush with a liquid such as water or vitamin E, and tucked next to the teeth), or as a rinse.

Ayurvedic herbalist Melanie Sachs suggests a gum massage with this mixture: 5 parts alum powder, 2 parts rock salt powder, 3 parts black pepper powder, and 1 part turmeric root powder.

Unani herbalist Hakim Chishti suggests a pack for the gums, made from rose petal, oak leaf, and carob powder. The rose petal is cooling and anti-inflammatory, the oak leaf is astringent, and the carob powder is coating and soothing.

Rinses are made by preparing an herb as tea in the usual way, or by simply stirring herb powder into water. Hold the rinse in the mouth for a few seconds or up to several minutes, gargle, and spit out. Barberry root is a very good choice for an oral rinse, as it is astringent, tones the mucus membranes, and is antibacterial.

Amla is used as a general rebuilder for oral health. Amla is the highest known natural source of vitamin C, which has been shown to stabilize the collagen in the gum structures. Use amla as a mouth rinse, or 1-2 grams per day in capsules can be taken as an oral dose of for long-term benefit to the teeth and gums.

The gums are connective tissue. Herbs that support the healing and development of connective tissue when taken internally will always benefit the gums. Since they must saturate the whole body as well as the gums, the healing effect tends to be slower, but more permanent.

Bilberry fruit and hawthorn berry, both rich sources of proanthcyanidins, the red pigments in plants, known to be highly anti-inflammatory, stabilize collagen, strengthening the gum tissue. Licorice root is a gem for the mouth, as it acts to suppress dental caries, reduce plaque, and has an antibacterial effect.

The tooth sockets, of course, are joints, and the teeth are essentially bones. Herbs that treat the skeleton and the joints, taken orally are good bets for long-term tooth health. Standouts include yellow dock root, alfalfa leaf, cinnamon bark, and turmeric root. Lad recommends chewing a handful of calcium-rich sesame seeds every morning.

· FOURTEEN ·

AYURVEDA, KUNDALINI AND YOGA

Kundalini yoga is appropriate particularly for people who live in the world - those who marry, have families, and jobs, and who need efficient yoga practices to enhance their busy lives. Kundalini yoga methods are quick and powerful, and produce their effects fast - no need to sit for years in a cave.

All yoga systems stress that each style of practice leads eventually to the same goal - spiritual union with our infinite nature. However, we all are different - different bodies, different personalities, different challenges, so different paths of yoga are suitable for different people.

Kundalini yoga is vast in scope, yet practical in day-to-day use, it requires dedication, focus, and intensity to practice, but is ideal for modern American yoga students, who demand fast, noticeable results and who have little time to devote to spiritual practice. After a one hour kundalini yoga class, you know you've done something!

In the words of Yogi Bhajan, "Kundalini Yoga is the science to unite the finite with infinity and it's the art to experience infinity in the finite. This is it. It is straight. It is simple."

Swami Sivananda Radha, the first western woman to be initiated into the sacred order of Sanyas and to become a swami, characterizes kundalini yoga as "a foundation for character building, courage, and awareness."

Kundalini, the Mother of all Yogas includes:
Hatha ("Sun/Moon") Yoga - physical body
Laya Yoga - yoga of sound and vibration
Raja ("Royal") yoga - meditation and discrimination
Mantra Yoga - yoga of mental focus
Karma Yoga - yoga of good works
Pranayam - yoga of breath

Tantra and the History of Kundalini

Kundalini is a key concept in the broader science of Tantra. The word, "tantra," is from a Sanskrit root tan-, "to expand." It is often translated as "warp and weave," referring to the crossfibers in woven cloth, implying a new structure, a diagonal, which could not exist without the originals. Practically, tantra means knowledge of an experimental scientific system, designed to expand consciousness, awareness, and the mental and physical abilities. In other words, tantra aims to assist the human to reach his full inherent spiritual potential.

The term tantra is also more broadly used to refer to any form of literature or philosophy involving "expanding" consciousness.

Tantra is mystery in action. The teachings mobilize us to transmute our every thought, action, and mundane task evermore into inner awareness. Tantra teaches, not withdrawal, but transformation - the transformation of our activities of daily life into creative evolution.

Tantra teaches that spirit and matter are one - consciousness pervades everywhere, and it is this synthesis of spirit and matter which provokes the person to achieve excellence in all things - to reach the full natural and spiritual potential. Renunciation is not the way of tantra. Detachment and asceticism, designed to free one from the bondage of existence, to connect with the infinity of the spirit, is not the goal. Rather, tantra teaches the complete acceptance of life as a human, with all its feelings, desires, thoughts, problems, and joys. In fact, one of my teacher Yogi Bhajan's favorite sayings is, "If you can't see God in all, you can't see God at all."

Tantra heals the schism between the inner and the outer, between the physical world and the inner reality. Spiritual life, according to tantra, is the fulfillment of the organic life. The goal of tantric practice is not to discover the unknown, but to realize the known, at every moment, moment after moment. From the *Visvasara Tantra* text: "What is here, is elsewhere. What is not here, is nowhere."

Scholars debate the exact time the term tantra was first used, and likewise are unsure when tantric practice and philosophy were originally introduced. Tantra is an ancient school, however - it is closely associated with the time of the Vedas, about 2000 B.C. In fact, some tantric practices are based on Vedic principles.

We can safely say that tantric teachings and practices are ancient and have been developing for centuries. We find the impact of these Indo-Aryan concepts traveled widely, and was felt in Nepal, Tibet, China, Japan, and South Asia.

Above all a practical system for realization, for awareness, tantra has developed a cornucopia of techniques, methods, and approaches to suit the different spiritual seekers, considering each one's condition and abilities. Based on the same fundamental tenets as conventional Indian philosophy, tantra is little concerned with abstract speculations, but is focused exclusively on practical ways and means to the goal. Since tantra developed largely outside the Indian establishment, as a school it had the unique opportunity to acquire its own perspective. Tantra, being so concerned with demonstrable experience, developed very little rigid dogma or clichés. Each seeker has great freedom to follow the path in her own way. Practitioners of all the schools and offshoots of tantra are great experimenters - they are the scientists of consciousness. Tantra keeps alive and fresh as the years go by - it incorporates all new experience into the pursuit of awareness.

We have these tantric experimenters to thank for the concept of "chakras," the psychic energy centers so valuable in the study of yoga.

Success with tantra can come from working on the self at many levels. Kundalini yoga uses the body as the tool. Meditation engages the mind. Mantra harnesses the voice. The diverse methods of tantric yoga invoke every sense - physical, mental, spiritual - singly or harmoniously.

A pivotal concept in tantra is the concept that all reality, seen and unseen, is one, a whole without division. Called Shiva-Shakti, or Cosmic Consciousness, it is the union of all apparent opposites. Shiva is pure consciousness. Shakti is creative power. The two are forever joined - like two lovers they can never be separated. One cannot be differentiated for the other. To intuit and experience this Cosmic Consciousness is the purpose of tantra. Since the spiritual seeker is an integral part of this cosmic scheme, self realization cannot be achieved by escape or negation - only by merging; by blissful union with the Divine.

All existence is, according to tantra, based on two primal forces. Purusha (Cosmic Consciousness) is the male principle, while prakruti (Creative Nature) is the female. Tantric yoga stresses meditating on this polarity, in every form, cosmic and earthly, to realize the integrated wholeness of all. Achieving this integration, the practitioner *becomes* Shiva-Shakti, united as one. The bliss of this cosmic union ("ananda") is indescribable ecstasy.

Tantra is the ultimate support for the diversity, dignity, and equality of women. God is usually described in feminine terms in tantric systems. Shakti, is, after all, the source of each and every aspect of life -the power to create or destroy, the power of sensuality or mystical subtlety, the power to grant a life of ease or a life of horror. Shakti is the prime mover in the universe, the source of all energy. The process of self-actualization, the highest goal, the arousal of the kundalini, is but an individual reflection of the ultimate Shakti.

Arousing the Inner Energy

Liberation, merging with Infinite Consciousness, whole still alive in the human body is the highest goal of yoga. The manifested individual personality in a body is the finite spark of the infinite cosmos. Tantric practitioners assert that the complete drama of the universe manifests in microcosm in each human body. That very body, with its material processes, is a channel for the cosmos to display itself.

The connection between the Cosmic Consciousness and the human body is yoga. That yoga can have as many styles and nuances as there are people practicing. Bhakti-yoga seeks union through devotion and love of God, Raja-yoga is the yoga of meditation, Karma-yoga is the yoga of proper work and worldly action,

Jnana-yoga uses discernment, and Hatha-yoga conditions the body to use as a tool for self-realization.

To these elements, the tantric tradition adds Kundalini yoga. In Sanskrit, Kundalini means "coiled up," a reference to the form this energy takes in the body.

Kundalini is the female creative energy of the universe, latent in every human being, but also in every atom in existence. The goal of kundalini yoga is to awaken this cosmic force (Shakti), allow it to unite with Infinity (Shiva), and to experience the bliss of oneness.

Kundalini Shakti (Yogi Bhajan calls this "the coil of the hair of the beloved") is the primordial potential of psychic energy in the being - the total and ultimate force of creation. The goal of raising the kundalini is, in fact, the basis of all yogas, whatever their particular discipline. The energies of Kundalini an ahamkara are the same energy. When our energy is limited and connected to your limitations, we know it as the ego. When your energy is universal, we call it Kundalini.[805]

Mother Kundalini is so beautiful and special, she is described poetically in a thousand ways. "She is beautiful as a chain of lightning and fine as a fiber, and shines in the mind of the sages. She is extremely subtle, the awakener of pure knowledge, the embodiment of bliss, whose true nature is pure consciousness."[806] Kundalini yoga is the joining of the separated lovers, the resolution of duality into unity.

The kundalini shakti, lying dormant in the body, sits coiled in three and one-half circles at the base of the spine in the energy body. When awakened, the energy ascends the spine, to merge into pure consciousness at the crown of the head. Of course, this process happens in the energy body, not the actual physical body. As the various bodies are linked, however, the physical body is also somewhat affected.

As the kundalini uncoils and rises up the subtle spine, she passes through seven distinct "chakras" ("wheel" in Sanskrit - due to their spinning form), or energy centers. As the energy ascends, energizing each chakra in turn, consciousness begins to change. As the awakening continues, step by step, awareness grows. Finally, through the disciplines of yoga, kundalini reaches full bloom - merging with the absolute in the bliss of cosmic awareness.

The great yogi, Swami Vivekananda, said, "Wherever there was any manifestation of what is ordinarily called a supernatural power or wisdom, there a little current of kundalini must have found its way into the sushumna. Only, in the vast majority of such cases, people had ignorantly stumbled on some practice which set free a minute portion of the coiled up kundalini. All worship, consciously or unconsciously, leads to this end."

Prana and Pranayam

Prana is the creative energy of the breath. Says Dr. Svoboda, "You live your life well when you live it at the right rate."[807] How true. If you live too fast, you burn out. If you live too slow, you bog down.

Patanjali, the foremost proponent of yoga, said that yoga is restraint of the fluctuations of the mind. Management of prana is central to yoga. Well cultivated prana is the key to dosha balance. Prana facilitaes meditation, and meditation regulates the breath. Singing and chanting control the breath.

Apana is the counterpoint to prana, the eliminative energy of the breath, which regulates the area below the navel. When muscles lock, "bandhs" are applied in the rectum, navel, and sex organs, ("muhlbandh") the apana is directed upwards, where it mixes with prana in the region of the navel. This intense mixing of prana and apana raises kundalini, causing the latent life force to move upward through the chakras.

Pranayam infuses the body and mind with prana. That surplus of energy can substitute, to a certain extent, for sleep. There is a saying in yoga,

'Alap ahaar sulap see nindra.'
'Eat little and sleep little.'[808]

Probably the most important factor in yoga, breathing practices create a direct connection with the vital energy of the cosmos. Hundreds of variations of breathing processes are used, depending on the desired result.

The left nostril is connected to the lunar channel, Ida, and has a relaxing, cooling effect on the mind and the body. Conversely, the right nostril connects with Pingala, the solar channel. Breathing through the right nostril stimulates and energizes the mind and body.

Kundalini Yoga Today

The goal of all yogas is union - union with the Infinite, with the Divine.

The total science of yoga is vast - encyclopedic - and covers every aspect of what it is to be a human. All yogas, actually, all spiritual practices, raise kundalini. It's just a matter of taste which form you pick. While today there is often great emphasis on asana, yoga is not about physical perfection - you don't have to be a pretzel.

Every aspect of yoga works, and every aspect is important. While perfection of asana is desirable, so is perfection of every other aspect of yoga.

Kundalini yoga was, until recently, a secret science, passed on from master to student as a closely guarded jewel. Certainly it was not taught to non-Indians.

Now it is being taught openly and widely for the first time in history. Yogi Bhajan began teaching kundalini yoga in 1969, out of compassion for the needs of Americans, and the speed we needed to get results we were after.

Sometimes people practicing kundalini yoga experience visions, sounds, or unusual physical sensations, which can at times be quite impressive. These experiences are not the goal, and can be a time consuming distraction. These phenomena are not the sign that kundalini has risen. They are the "glitter at the bottom of the ladder," according to Yogi Bhajan.

Kundalini Yoga has been developing for several thousand years. It is a finely tuned, practical technology for householder spiritual seekers. The fastest of all yogas, it is ideal for people with busy lives. It brings awareness to all aspects of daily life.

Kundalini Shakti is the energy of creation. She's the Divine Mother of us all.

· FIFTEEN ·

CONCLUSION

Our failures should be stepping stones to our success.
- Swami Satchidananda

Ayurveda and yoga teach us the way to self realization, and how to become healthy, happy and holy.[809] The final goal of life is spiritual liberation, which, of course, is nothing more than realizing that "I am a soul." So long as we think we are bodies, we are bound, and we go on carrying out schemes for the pleasure of mind, senses and body. When we remember, there is harmony.

When you perform only good actions (karma), and receive good reactions (fruit) in return, you will be always happy. Only the soul is conscious. The mind, body and senses are material, and they always want to do material activities. But the soul, being conscious, will never become happy by material activities. In theory, this is easy to understand, but we need some reminding. Ayurveda is the science that explains the process- a roadmap. Life is journey back to the source. Following a map just makes it a little quicker to reach the destination.

Now that we've looked at Ayurvedic herbalism from all sides, how should you actually proceed with managing your health?

Ayurveda is to be used. According to Yogi Bhajan, "To know and not to do… is to not know."[810]

Ayurveda is practical. Experiment. Use what you can and work it out.

Ayurveda has something for everyone. From small adjustments to balance your diet to align with your constitution, to a full blown Ayurvedic life makeover, you can use these techniques to become more healthy, happy and holy.

First, be aware. Take a moment every day to assess how you are feeling. Use the principles of Ayurveda, systematically evaluate what's going on in your body and mind. Do you feel energetic? Are you free from pain? Are you sleeping well?

Over time, check in and test your self daily for many days, to get a consistent feeling of your state of health and recognize a pattern. Once you get a sense of how Ayurveda works in your individual body, begin to notice changes from your lifestyle practices. The way you feel today is a pretty good measure of what you did and ate yesterday. Notice any changes from day to day, and think about what happened the day before the change. A weekend sugar binge? A couple bowls of 5 alarm chili? No, not you, Mr. Pitta. A dietary diary (be honest, now) might help.

Now begin to experiment. Purposely attempt to adjust your dosha balance.

Choose and follow a program for a week. Any difference? Be aware, subtly, of how you feel. Most people will not notice much at that point, because their body is working overtime already to keep you humming, but subtle changes may already be starting.

Next, dive into a more intensive regime for a similar time. Note changes. Once you get the hang of what will make a difference in you individually, zero in on a proportion that keeps you in the healthy zone.

It takes many months (or for some people, years) for all these adjustments to fully balance. Make it a habit to honestly assess how you are feeling as the years go by. Filling out a symptom questionnaire every so often, say once a year, is a great way to put on paper how you are feeling, and to remind yourself of any changes. Rating each symptom with a 1-10 scale will give you some perspective. You may be surprised at how slowly, yet extensively, your chronic illnesses will improve. Of course, checking in with a professional Ayurveda practitioner may help speed up results.

Making all these changes isn't always easy. For some, they are pretty radical. These changes need to be gradual. When we see someone who becomes an Ayurveda fanatic, and goes home, cleans out all the cupboards, and dumps it all in the garbage, we see someone whose cupboards will soon be filled right back up with the very same products. They don't know anything else to do, anything else to eat. How do you prepare mung beans, anyway?

Start with one change that you can manage. If its a commitment to add ashwaganda and triphala to your life, great. If its a plan to transition to cooking according to your constitution over 3 months, while you get the hang of the new ingredients, that's progress.

Its all about getting in the habit of thinking the Ayurvedic way, and letting that mindset become your lifestyle. Start thinking about your new regime before you go to the store. Make a list and stick to it. Add a few new items each time, and gradually switch over.

You need to plan. The moment you arrive home late, after a grueling day at the office, is not the time to start the kicharee boiling on the stove for the first time. Instead, fill your refrigerator in advance with healthy foods that you know will balance your dosha needs. Select foods and herbs that are reasonable to use with your schedule. Do some prep work on the weekend. (That's the time to have the garbanzo beans boiling- while you're cleaning the garage on Saturday afternoon.)

Perhaps an herbal food is to your liking. Zucchini is a simple vegetable that cooks quickly, and tastes good. When you get home, already exhausted, simply slice them and put on the stove to steam. Go hit the shower. By the time you're out, dinner will be ready. Spice it with condiments that balance you body, and enjoy.

Perhaps you will start with herbal teas that you can cook quickly and simply. Drink herbal teas every day. Check our herbs lists for good suggestions. Select one or more mild medicinal teas that match your long term health needs, or a selection of herbal beverage teas that appeals to you. Brew a strong pot in the morning and savor several cups during the day. Take herb tea to work with you as a substitute for soft drinks.

Use yogi tea regularly. This special Ayurvedic blend is used by yoga practitioners to maintain stamina, good digestion and support the immune system. In the Khalsa house, we make this tea in large batches and drink it every day. Its also available in every health food store and grocery store, in teabags.

Exercise every day. Movement helps the muscles and other tissues shed their acid burden. Increasing your breathing dumps wastes and purifies the cells. Check out your Ayurvedic constitution and adapt your program to compliment your body's ideal exercise needs.

Ayurveda is systematic and user friendly. You will find the methods in this book easy to understand and logical to apply. As we proceed, Ayurvedic balancing will come through as systematic, consistent and eminently useful.

There's much to learn- and it can be easy, fun and most importantly, effective beyond even what you might imagine. You will become more deeply committed to your health – and will have powerful new tools with which to do something about it. Ayurvedic herbs will help Americans change the way they see health, disease, medicine and healing. And it will tangibly impact what can do about it day to day.

Generate, organize and deliver your prana, and your life will flow with grace, power, tranquility, effectiveness and joy.

APPENDIX
SYNOPSIS OF THERAPY

Ayurveda is the ultimate holistic system for treating disease, regaining body balance, and antiaging therapy. When this system is followed, it works. Use this chart as a master plan to summarize bringing the doshas into balance. Here's Ayurveda in a nutshell: treat kapha like an enemy. Treat pitta like a lover. Treat vata like a flower.

Dosha	Vata	Pitta	Kapha
Therapeutic Strategy	Warm, moisten, build	Cool, dry, reduce	Warm, dry, reduce
Therapeutic Settings	Warm blanket, hot water bottle, cozy, homey, soft light, gold color, relaxing, slow, silk fabric, quiet sound, music, flowers- deep, rich colors	Cool, open, luxurious, elegant, lightweight sheets, light blue, silver colors, green plants, flowers- white and pink rose, cool eye pillow	Warm, stimulating, exciting, lively, red sheets, bright colors, light wool fabrics, copper vessels, etc. flowers- red, bright
Aromas	Geranium, juniper, lavender, myrrh, sage, patchouli, basil	Gardenia, jasmine, rose, lavender, lotus, sandalwood, vertivert	Basil, camphor, eucalyptus, frankincense, lemon, peppermint, rosemary, sage
Massage Technique	Mild, nurturing, no pain	Relaxing, cooling, cool environment	Dry, warm, stimulating, rough
Oils	Warm, heavy- castor, sesame, almond, olive	Cooling, sweet, ghee, coconut, pumpkin	Light, mustard, corn, jojoba
Main Therapy	Castor oil	Ghee	Honey
Yoga and Exercise	Sitting, lying, backbends, inverted, deep breathing, low intensity	Sitting, lying, shoulder stand, cooling breathing, medium intensity, cool	Strong aerobic workouts, hot, breath of fire

Digestive Herbs	Salt, garlic, ginger, cinnamon	Aloe, gentian, turmeric, fennel, mint	Cayenne, black pepper, pipali, clove
Elimination Herbs	Bulk laxative, triphala, castor oil	Cascara, rhubarb, senna, rose petal, ghee, psyllium	Generally not necessary
Energy Herbs	Ashwaganda, shatavari, amla, ginseng	Licorice, guduchi, dandelion root	Garlic, cinnamon, guggul, myrrh
Mind Herbs	Valerian, nutmeg, chamomile	Gotu kola, sandalwood, hibiscus	Basil, sage, skullcap
Lifestyle	Adequate sleep, regular hours, sun, mid activity, moderation	Cooling, gardens, flowers, contentment	Vigorous activity, warmth, exercise
Therapy	Enema (often dashmula tea)	Strong laxatives	Therapeutic vomiting
Diet	Nutritive, satisfying, Sweet, sour, salty, warm, heavy, moist, frequent small meals	Strengthening, reducing Sweet, bitter, astringent, raw foods & juices, cool, heavy, dry, no hot spices	Reducing, pungent, bitter, astringent Warm, light, dry, hot spices, fasting

APPENDIX VEGETABLE JUICES TO FOR A GENTLE DETOX

Herb	Common Uses	Other Preparations
Artichoke globe	Liver	Steamed, juice, powdered
Asparagus stem (vegetable)	Increase lactation, cough, skin rash, diuretic	Juice, steamed
Basil leaf	Antimicrobial, menstrual cramps	Soup, cook with ginger, green onion and protein for crams caused by cold
Beet root and greens	Liver detoxification (high doses encourage rashes to completely exit the surface)	Steamed, soup, juice, congee, powdered
Berries (Raspberry, blackberry, strawberry, black raspberry, cherry, blueberry, huckleberry, bilberry)	Polyphenol antioxidant rich	Soup, jelly, cobbler, chutney, stewed, pudding, sorbet, muffins, pancakes
Bitter greens (kale, mustard, dandelion, etc.)	Digestive	Steamed, juice
Burdock root (gobo)	Liver detoxification	Sushi, Steamed, juice
Cranberry (also related blueberry and similar)	Urinary, polyphenols	Juice, sauce salad, baked goods
Dandelion leaf	Cooling, diuretic, bitter	Steamed, salad
Dandelion root	Liver detoxification	Coffee substitute, steamed vegetable
Elder berry	Immune	Soup, jelly, cobbler, chutney, stewed, pudding, sorbet, muffins, pancakes
Garlic bulb	Immune, cardiovascular, aphrodisiac	Soup, broth, garlic toast
Ginger root	Digestive, joint, cardiovascular	Dice-sautéed until crunchy, use as garnish, juice, ginger toast

Lettuce	Relaxant	Juice or steamed (high dose)
Mung bean sprout	Nutritive, cooling	Congee
Mustard greens	Cough	Saag, (as congee for cough)
Nettle leaf	Tonic, nutritive, respiratory	Soups, etc.
Onion bulb	Immune, cardiovascular, aphrodisiac	Steamed, salad
Parsley leaf	Diuretic	Pilau rice dishes, juice
Peppermint leaf (fresh)	Digestive	Chutney, salsa, juice
Plantain leaf (fresh)	Demulcent, cooling	Juice
Prickly pear cactus	Diabetes	Salad, tacos
Radish	Expectorant, liver detoxification	Congee, juice
Rhubarb stem	Laxative	Pudding, juice
Rose flower	Laxative, cooling	Jelly, honey preserve
Thyme leaf	Antimicrobial	Grain and vegetable dishes
Turmeric root	Inflammation, astringent	Paste, golden milk, sandwich
Watercress leaf	Sinus	Salad, steamed, juice
Watermelon	Moisturizing, cooling	Decoct in water, use as broth base for congee or soup
Wild cherry bark	Cough	Lozenge, syrup, candy, pudding
Wild yam (Chinese or North American)	Liver	Congee (decoct with lichee fruit and schisandra fruit, use as broth base)
Yucca root	Detoxification	Shredded and fried in patties

APPENDIX OF SELECTED AYURVEDIC RECIPES

Main Dishes and Soups

MUNG BEAN STEWS

Mung Bean Stew (kicharee), a one pot meal, is the renowned nutritive and convalescent food of Ayurveda. A soft gruel of grain and bean, it easily digested and nutritious- a perfect combination of life sustaining protein and carbohydrates. Kicharee provides vegetarian amino acid balance with beans and grains. This dish can be used for a deep cleansing monodiet.

There are many simple recipes for kicharee. Mild spices often include all the six tastes to balance the recipe. For example, coriander and cumin seeds have warm, spicy energy and benefit the lungs and spleen for better assimilation and transformation of food into energy. Turmeric, with its bitter and pungent tastes, is well known for its liver detoxifying and blood and energy circulating properties that help to prevent stagnation and relieve pain.

MUNG BEANS AND RICE

1 cup mung beans
1 cup basmati rice
9 cups water
4- 6 cups chopped assorted vegetables (carrot, celery, zucchini, broccoli, etc.)
2 onions, chopped
1/3 cup minced ginger root
8-10 cloves garlic, minced
1 heaping t. turmeric
1/2 tsp black pepper
1 heaping tsp garam masala (curry powder)

1 tsp crushed red chilies (to taste)
1 tbs basil
2 bay leaves
Seeds of 5 cardamom pods
Salt or soy sauce to taste

Wash beans and rice. Bring water to boil, add rice and beans, and let boil over medium high flame. Prepare vegetables. Add vegetables to cooking rice and beans. Heat oil (about 1/2 cup) in large frying pan. Add onion, ginger and garlic. Sauté over medium high flame until browned. Add spices (not salt or herbs). When nicely well done, combine onion mixture with cooking beans and rice. Stir often to prevent scorching. Add herbs. Continue cooking until totally and completely well done, over a medium high flame, stirring often. The consistency should be rich, thick, and soupy, with ingredients mixed. Serve with yogurt, or with cheese melted over the top. Prepare less spicy for elderly or small children. Serves 6-8.

MICHAEL TIERRA'S KICHAREE

1 cup whole mung beans
2 cups brown rice
4 and one quarter cups cold water
1-2 tbs ghee
3/4 tsp sea salt or rock salt
1 Tbs cumin seed, ground
1 Tbs coriander seed, ground
1 Tbs turmeric

Place mung beans, rice and water into large covered pot. When it boils, lower temperature to low and cook for 45 minutes. After 35 minutes, place ghee, salt, cumin, coriander and turmeric into a frying pan, with the heat on low, for ten minutes or so... just to fuse all the spices. When rice/mung beans ready, spoon about half the rice/mung bean mix into the frying pan with the spices and thoroughly mix. Serve topped with chopped ginger root, plain yogurt and squeeze of lime. This kicharee is great with some yogurt and banana in the morning, or with almond milk, cinnamon, raisins and maple syrup.

ORANGE PEEL DIGESTIVE KICHAREE

Here is another somewhat unusual bean and rice dish. Orange peel is an excellent sour digestive remedy. Sauted or steamed, it can be added to foods to enhance agni and facilitate digestion. Yogi Bhajan taught about the basics of this recipe. He described it as balancing metals and vitamins in the body.

1 cup rice
2 cups water
1 onion, medium, coarsely chopped
1 peel from medium orange (include white strings inside), finely chopped
1 cup previously boiled chick peas
1 tbs red chili, crushed, or to taste
1 cup assorted green vegetables, coarsely chopped
2 tbs Sesame oil

In large soup pot, combine rice and water. Bring to boil. Add onion, cook until soft. Add orange peel, chick peas, red chilies, green vegetables and oil. If desired, add ginseng broth to taste. Simmer until vegetables soft. All ingredients may be adjusted to taste.

URID DAL

The Urid (black) lentil is sweet, unctuous, heavy and warm. It is aphrodisiac, brighan (gives strength to body), laxative and stanyaganana (galactogogue). Urid increases pitta and kapha and pacifies vata. It is heavy and difficult to digest, so it is prepared with warming carminatives, such as ginger, garlic and asafetida.

1 cup split urud dal
4 cups water
1/4 tsp asafetida
1 tsp cumin seed
3 cloves garlic, chopped
1/2 tsp turmeric
2 tsp ginger, chopped
2-3 small green chillies (optional)
1 tsp mustard seed
1 tsp coriander powder
1 medium onion, finely chopped
1 tsp ghee
salt to taste

Wash urid dal well, drain. Boil dal in water in covered pan or pressure cooker with water, asafetida, garlic, ginger, turmeric, salt, coriander powder and green chillies until soft. Warm ghee in separate pan. Add cumin seeds and mustard seeds. Gently cook until slightly browned, without burning. Add ghee and spice mixture to daal. Serve warm with bread or chapati.

AJWAIN SEED IMMUNE PANCAKES

Ajwain seed is commonly used from northern India to Afganistan. Its essential oil is rich in antimicrobial thymol. Eat these pancakes during the cold and flu season. They are a main dish, not a sweet breakfast cake. They can be a little spicy, so start with lesser amounts of the herbs, and work up to taste.

1-2 tbs fresh ginger, finely chopped
2-3 tbs cauliflower, finely chopped
1-2 tbs ajwain seeds, whole or ground, or to taste
red chilies, crushed, to taste
black pepper to taste
Soy sauce or Bragg's Liquid Aminos (a liquid condiment similar to soy sauce)
Equal parts Bran and whole wheat flour, approximately one half cup each (Substitute besan, garbanzo flour, for some of the flour, as desired for more cohesive consistency)
1 jalapeno pepper, finely chopped, per pancake, if desired

In large mixing bowl, combine all ingredients. Drop batter onto griddle sprayed with vegetable spray or coated with lecithin to prevent sticking. Cook on low heat, flipping once, for about 1/2 hour total.

ENDURANCE PANCAKES

(Inspired by Yogi Bhajan)

This anti-kapha recipe warms the body, cleans out ama and supports the immune system. Yogi Bhajan says that mustard oil "kills everything that kills the body. Straightforward, right on."[811]

1 cup millet
1/2 corn flour or grits, optional, to taste
1 tbs ajwain seed
1 tbs black cumin seed
1 tsp black pepper, ground
cayenne, to taste
1 tbs mustard oil

In saucepan, boil millet, corn grits and spices unil it forms a batter consistency. In skillet, heat mustard oil. Cook batter in mustard oil to form pancakes, turning once. Adjust spices to taste.

CAULIFLOWER PARANTHA FOR MEN

(Inspired by Yogi Bhajan)

This stuffed flatbread is a sexual revitalizer for men. (Women will enjoy it, too.) Nutmeg is for premature ejaculation. The warming spices control vata. Bamboo manna balances the liver. Poppy is for anxiety.[812]

1 tbs nutmeg, ground
2 tbs cinnamon, ground
1 tbs cardamom, ground
8 tbs fennel seed, ground
15 cloves, ground
1 tbs poppy seed
1 tbs bamboo manna, optional
1 tbs cardamom seed, ground
1 tbs black pepper, ground

Mix spice mixture to taste with steamed cauliflower. Stuff a chapatti. Warm on hot grill with ghee.

Vegetables

KARELA SAUTÉ

8 ounces karela, coarsely chopped
2 tsp fennel seed, whole
1 medium Onion, chopped
1 medium tomato, chopped
4 tsp pomegranate seed powder (anar dana)
2 tsp coriander seed powder
1/2 tsp turmeric powder
fresh cilantro, chopped
salt to taste
vegetable oil or ghee

Wash karela with skin on. Heat oil in skillet. Add fennel seeds. When they sputter, add onion. Sauté until onion becomes clear. Add chopped tomato and spices. Stir. Sauté for 3 to 4 minutes until gravy consistency. Add chopped karela. Add water to cover. Simmer, covered, until karela is soft. Garnish with fresh cilantro.

KARELA COCONUT CURRY

1 medium bitter gourd, thinly sliced
1 tbs ghee
1 tsp brown mustard seed, whole
1 tsp urid dal beans
1/2 tsp cumin powder
1/2 tsp turmeric powder
6 curry leaves, crushed (optional)
1/2 cup coconut milk

Salt to taste

Blanch bitter gourd, drain. In separate skillet, sauté mustard seed and urid beans in ghee until it begins to sputter. Add bitter gourd, cumin, turmeric, curry leaves and salt. Stir. Mix coconut milk with equal quantity water. Add. Simmer until tender. Serve hot over rice. Serves 2.

OKRA CURRY WITH COCONUT-YOGURT SAUCE

Okra is aphrodisiac and a rejuvenator that increases semen. It increases kapha. It is sweet, astringent, hot, heavy and slimy. Somewhat paradoxically, it lowers blood sugar very effectively.

1 cup okra, sliced
1 cup yogurt
1/2 cup coconut milk
2 curry leaves (optional)
1/2 tsp black pepper, ground
1/4 tsp hing
1 tsp brown mustard seed
2 tbs ghee
Salt to taste

Heat ghee in skillet. Add hing and mustard seeds. When seeds sizzle, add okra and curry leaves. Saute okra slices, stirring, until slightly brown and crisp. Remove heat and cool. In seprarate bowl, combine yogurt, coconut milk, salt and pepper. Combine okra with yogurt sauce. Serves one.

Drinks

YOGI TEA

This is the original recipe given by Yogi Bhajan.

For each 8 oz cup, start with 10 oz. of water. For convenience, make at least 4 cups at one time.

For each cup of boiling water, add:

3 whole cloves
4 whole green cardamom pods
6 whole black peppercorns
1/2 stick cinnamon
Optional: 1 slice of fresh ginger root

Boil for 20-30 minutes, then add 1/4 tsp any black or green tea. Let sit for one or two minutes and then add 1/2 cup milk and reheat. Strain and serve with honey to taste.

Black pepper is a blood purifier, cardamom is for the colon (gas), cloves are for the nervous system and cinnamon for the bones. Ginger has a delicious taste and is helpful when suffering from a cold, recovering from the flu or for general physical weakness. The milk aids in the easy assimilation of the spices and avoids irritation to the colon. The black or green tea acts as an alloy for all of the ingredients, achieving a new chemical structure which makes the tea a healthful and delicious drink.

SHIKANJWI

Digestive Lemon Drink Lemon is Amla (sour), Guru (heavy), Ushna (warm), with an Amla (sour) vipak.This digestive lemon beverage has a special anuloma effect, restoring proper flow of apana, which relieves gas and bloating. It acts by enhancing the digestive fire and restoring appetite in cases of overeating. It is also good as a warming, soothing treatment for sore throat. This drink pacifies all the three doshas. Lemon should not be used by pitta people, as it increases acidic temperament of pitta dosha. The sour flavor of lemon is reduced by the raw sugar, ghee and water. Adding salt, black pepper and asafetida also benefits kapha and vata persons.

6 tsp lemon juice
10 oz water
3 tsp raw sugar
1/2 tsp salt
1/2 tsp ghee
a pinch black pepper powder

a pinch asafetida
1/2 tsp jeera (cumin seeds)

Warm the ghee in a pan. Add asafetida and cumin seeds and lightly sauté. Add water. Boil. As water begins to boil, add lemon juice, salt, black pepper and raw sugar. Boil for 1 or 2 more minutes. Drink warm.

GOLDEN MILK

A traditional Ayurvedic drink for arthritis
(Thanks to Yogi Bhajan for original recipe)
Part one, turmeric paste:
1) In saucepan, mix one-quarter cup of turmeric powder with one half cup water.
2) Bring to boil and cook until a thick paste is formed.
3) Store paste in refrigerator.

Part two, making the drink:
1) Mix 1 cup milk, one tsp almond oil, one half tsp turmeric paste, and honey to taste.
2) Stir on low heat. Bring just to boil.
3) Blend in blender to make a foamy drink. Serve.

FENNEL COOLER

(Sampf ka panak)
This is a good summer beverage. It nourishes the brain and nerves, increases vision, quenches thirst, helps dehydration from hot weather, improves digestive fire, is diuretic and strengthens the heart). It is especially good for those suffering from aggravated pitta. It is essentially tridoshic. Kapha persons can add honey in place of sugar.

8 oz fennel seed, coarsely ground (anise seed may be substituted)
2 cups rose water
7 oz raw sugar, to taste (substitute honey for kapha)

Soak ground fennel seed in rose water overnight. Completely dissolve raw sugar in 7 ounces boiling water. Reduce rosewater and fennel seed mixture to 12 ounces by boiling in covered pan. Add sugar syrup to rosewater mixture. Cool and serve.(If using honey instead of sugar, omit sugar in mixing stage. Add 8 ounces honey to cooled mixture. Do not add honey to hot liquid.)

SALTY MINT LASSI

(Pudina raita lassi)

Mint is katu (Pungent), light and dry. Many mints, such as spearmint, are cooling, while peppermint has a pungent taste. The vipak is pungent. Fresh mint juice, if available, can be gargled for bad breath. Mint also treats indigestion and gas. This beverage mainly balances pitta and to a lesser extent. Kapha, depending on the mint used. It may increase vata if the chosen mint is too cooling. Asafetida, salt and cumin seeds are included to pacify vata. Drink salty mint lassi in the afternoon.

1 cup yogurt (fresh thick homemade is best)
1 oz fresh mint leaves
1 cup water
1 tsp cumin seed
1/2 tsp vegetable oil
1/4 tsp asafetida powder
salt to taste

In blender, make a paste of mint with 2 ounces of the water. In a separate container, stir the yogurt with remaining water until smooth and thin. Add mint paste and salt to dilute yogurt. Mix thoroughly. Lightly sauté cumin seeds and asafetida powder in oil until light red, taking care not to burn. Add oil with spices in to yogurt mixture. Garnish with fresh mint leaves. Serve at room temperature with lunch or a mid afternoon refresher.

Snacks and Desserts

ROASTED FENNEL SEEDS

(Bhuni sampf)

Fennel seed is madhur sweet, katu (pungent) and tikat (bitter), laghu (light) and snigdh (oily). The temperature is arguably cold (some say warming). The vipak is sweet. It enhances digestive fire, improves digestion (pachan) and has the special effect of restoring proper flow of apana vata, called the anuloma effect, meaning that it reduces air element (gas) in the digestive tract. Raw fennels seeds reduce pitta and vata. Roasting them allows them to be good for kappa, as well. This snack is tridoshic.

Spread raw fennel seeds on a heavy warm pan on a burner. Roast fennels seeds on low heat until slightly brown, taking care not to burn. Try to make it fresh. Store in airtight container away from direct sunlight. Use one tablespoon after each meal to promote digestion and reduce gas.

ROASTED SWEET SESAME SEEDS

(Tilkutt)

Sesame seed is madhur (sweet), kashya (pungent) and titta (bitter), guru (heavy) and snigdh (oily). The temperature is hot, and the vipak is sweet. Sesame seed is a good warming winter food. It generally benefits skin and hair. Sesame is very useful in treating bedwetting. Sesame seed increases pitta and kapha, but pacifies vata. Roasting the sweet sesame seed make it tridoshic. Black sesame is superior, and has a more aphrodisiac quality.

3 oz raw sesame seeds
3 oz powdered raw sugar

Lightly brown sesame seeds and roast in a heavy pan on low heat, taking care not to burn. After cooling, grind seeds to coarse powder. Mix with powdered raw sugar, if desired, to taste. (The raw sugar suppresses pitta. Pitta people may also add ghee or butter.) Store in airtight container.

MUNG BEAN PATE

1/2 cup mung beans, split or whole
2 tbs nut butter (almond, tahini, etc.)
1 tbs olive oil
1 tbs lemon juice1 tbs fresh parsley, chopped
1 tbs fresh basil, chopped
1 tsp fresh ginger, minced
1/4 tsp cumin seed, ground
salt to taste
fresh ground black pepper to taste
1 medium clove garlic, peeled (optional)
1-2 tbs water as desired for consistency

Dry roast mung beans in skillet for 10-12 minutes, or until golden brown, stirring constantly. Grind to coarse powder. Combine the ingredients in food processor. Grind to smooth paste. Add water as necessary. Serve on crackers, or as vegetable dip.

GLOSSARY

Abhyanga- Ayurvedic massage with copious warm oil

Agni- Fire, light, heat (specifically, digestive fire, or collected power of digestion)

Agnimandya- Low digestive agni

Ahamkara- "I-former," self concept, egotism, pride, arrogance

Ahara- Food, that which goes in

Akasha- Ether element

Alterative- A remedy, such as an herb, that promotes detoxification, a "blood cleanser." Dandelion root is an alterative.

Ama- Totality of accumulated wastes, "toxins"

Amavata- Arthritis, specifically rheumatoid arthritis

Amla- Sour

Anuloma- Restoring proper flow of apana vata

Anupan- Vehicle in which to dilute the herb for ingestion

Ap- Water element

Apana- One of the five types of vata- goes downward, responsible for expulsion of faces, flatus, urine, menstrual blood- important energy in yoga, opposite of prana

Arisht- Medicated wine

Asana- (lit., "seat")- Posture, as in yoga posture

Asthi- Bone

Atma- Soul, spirit, true self

Basti- (lit., "bladder", from the original enema bag)- Enema (usually refers to medicated enema)

Bhringan- Strengthens and nourishes the muscular system

Bhumy (Bhoomi)- Earth

Brahmacharya- Routine followed during student life, and while studying sacred texts, often used to refer to celibacy or monogamy within marriage

Buddhi- Intelligence, intellect

Chikitsa- Treatment, a therapy to retain balance, medical practice (as in kaya chikitsa, treatment of body diseases, internal medicine)

Dal (or dahl)- Legumes

Decoction- A method of preparing herbs as "soups," or strong, concentrated teas. Decoctions are used for dense herbal parts, including roots and barks, which need longer cooking to release their active ingredients. They are usually prepared by simmering in a covered pot for 30-60 minutes.

Deepan- Improves digestive fire

Dharana- Concentration of mind

Dhyana- Meditation

Dinacharya- Daily routine

Dosha- Primal metabolic force

Dravyaguna- Ayurvedic pharmacology ("qualities of drugs")

Guna- Characteristic, quality, peculiarity, attitude, property

Guru- Heavy

Hridya- Heart tonic

Jal- Water

Jathara- Stomach, belly, abdomen

Jatharagni- Digestive fire, gastric juices, digestive enzymes

Jiva- Living soul, alive, life

Jivniya- Nourishing

Jwara- Fever

Kapha- Dosha formed from water and earth elements, stabilizing tendency

Kapha nissarana- Expectorant

Kaphaja- "Caused by kapha"

Karana- Doing, making, effecting, causing

Kas- Cough

Kasaswasahara- Relieves coughing and asthma

Kashaaya- Astringent

Katu- Pungent

Kaya- Body

Kleda- Subtle waste products

Kriya- Action, practice, as in applying a remedy

Laghu- Light

Lavana- Salty

Madana, or Madakari - Produces intoxication

Madhura- Sweet

Mahabhuta- "Great tendency," element, as in the 5 elements of Ayurveda

Mala- Bodily wastes (feces, sweat, etc.)

Manas- Mind

Mandagni- Digestive agni due to excess kapha

Mantra- Hymn, sacred or mystical verse, prayer

Medhya- Therapy for the mind, or brain tonic

Mutra- Urine

Mutravirechen- Diuretic

Nadi- Pulse, channel, tube, such as vein or artery

Nasya- Administering remedy through nose

Netra- Eye

Netrya- Increases vision

Nidra- Sleep

Ojas- Concentrated essence of nutritional substances in the tissues, vigor, strength, vitality

Panchan- Digestion

Panir- Fresh cheese curds

Pariksa- Examination, inspection

Pitta- Dosha formed from water and fire elements, metabolic tendency

Pittaja (or, paittika)- "Caused by pitta"

Prana- Universal term for energy, subdosha of vata
Prakruti- Original nature, natural form, in Ayurveda, "constitution"

Pranayama- Controlled breathing techniques

Prithvi- Earth, world

Pudia- Hand folded single dose paper

Purisa- Feces

Rajas- Active force

Rakta- Blood

Rasa- Essence (also- taste, sap, juice, appreciation, artistic delight, musical note)

Rasayana- (lit. "the path of juice")- Rejuvenative, rejuvenation

Ritucharya- Seasonal programs

Roga- Disease

Rogi- Patient

Sama- Balanced, equal, even

Samagni- Digestive agni from balanced doshas

Samhita- Encyclopedia, compilation

Sandhankar- Repairs joints

Sandhivata- Osteparthritis

Sandhigat vata- Arthralgia

Sattva- The energy of purity

Shirodara- Pouring oil on forehead

Shukra- Reproductive tissue

Snehana- Lubricating, annointing, unction

Snigdha- Sticky, viscid, unctuous

Sodhana- Cleaning, purifying

Srota- Channel, tube

Sthairyakar- Helps maintain balance and homeostasis

Takta- Bitter

Tamas- Inertia force, ignorance, darkness, illusion

Tattva- Element, as in the 5 elements of Ayurveda

Tejas- Fire, radiance

Tiksna- Sharp, hot, fiery, pungent

Tikshnagni- Digestive agni due to excess pittta

Tridoshasamak- Pacifies all three doshas

Trishna nigrahan- Thirst quenching

Unani-Tibb-(Unani- Ionian, "Greek)- Indigenous system of Muslim medicine in India

Ushna- Warm

Vaidya- Ayurvedic doctor

Vajikarana- (vaji- lit. "stallion") Sexually rejuvenation (make like a stallion)

Vamana- Vomiting

Vata- Dosha formed from air and ether elements, movement tendency

Vataja (or, vatika)- "Caused by vata"

Vayu- Air

Vyavayi- Facilitates the movement of vata

Vipak- Postdigestive effect

Vrishya- Aphrodisiac

Vishamagani- Digestive agni caused by excess vata

Yogavahi- An agent that facilitates delivery of a medicine to the desired tissue

BIBLIOGRAPHY

Agarwal, R.S., *Secrets of Indian Medicine*. School for Perfect Eyesight: Pondicherry (no year given)

Baker, Sidney MacDonald, *Detoxification & Healing*, Keats, 1997

Bartram, Thomas, *Encyclopedia of Herbal Medicine*, Grace Publishers: Christchurch, Dorset, 1995

Blumenthal, et al, *Complete German Commission E Monographs*, Integrative Medicine Communications: Austin, 1998

Brown, Susan E., *Better Bones, Better Body: A Comprehensive Self-Help Program for Preventing, Halting and Overcoming Osteoporosis*, Keats, 1996

Brown, Donald J., *Herbal Prescriptions for Better Health, Prima*, 1996.

Brown, Susan E., *Better Bones, Better Body: Beyond Estrogen and Calcium*, Contemporary Books: 2000

Chitale, P.K., *Comparative Study of Ayurveda and Treatment by Indian Drugs*, A, Sri Satguru Publications: Delhi, 1997

Dash, Bhagwan. A*yurvedic Cures for Common Diseases*, Hind Pocket: Delhi. 1995

Dash, Bhagwan. *Diabetes*. Jain: Delhi. 1986

Dash, Bhagwan. *Fundamentals of Ayurvedic Medicine*. Bansal: Delhi, 1980

Dash, Bhagwan. *High Blood Pressure and Sleeplessness*. Jain: New Delhi, 1993

Dash, Bhagwan. *Massage Therapy in Ayurveda*. Concept: New Delhi, 1992

Dash, Bhagwan, and Kashyap, Lalitesh. *Materia Medica of Ayurveda*. Concept: New Delhi, 1979

Dash, Bhagwan, and Junius, Manfred, *Handbook of Ayurveda*, A, Concept: New Delhi, 1987

Devaraj, T.L. *Ayurveda for Healthy Living*. UBS: New Delhi, 1992

Douillard, John, *Encyclopedia of Ayurvedic Massage*, The, North Atlantic-Books: Berkeley, 2004

Duke, James A. *The Green Pharmacy*, Rodale: 1997.

Erasmus, Udo, *Fats that Heal, Fats that Kill*, Alive Books: Burnaby, BC, Canada, 1986.

Feuerstein, Georg, *Sacred Paths*, Larson: 1991.

Frawley, David, *Ayurvedic Healing*, Lotus Press: Twin Lakes, WI, 1989, www.lotuspress.com

Gaby, Alan, *Preventing and Reversing Osteoporosis: What You Can Do About Bone Loss--A Leading Expert's Natural Approach to Increasing Bone Mass*, Prima: 1995

Griggs, Barbara, *Green Pharmacy,* Healing Arts Press: Rochester, Vermont, 1997

Hameed, H. Abdul. *Complete Book of Home Remedies, The*. Orient: Delhi, 1982

Heinerman, John, *Encyclopedia of Fruits, Vegetables, and Herbs,* Parker: New York, 1988.

Heyn, Birgit. *Ayurvedic Medicine*. Thorsons: Wellingborough, 1987

Holmes, Peter, *Energetics of Western Herbs,* NatTrop: Berkeley, 1993

Ingram, Cass, DO, *Supermarket Remedies,* Knowledge House: Buffalo Grove, Ilinois, 1998.

Kapoor, L.D. *CRC Handbook of Ayurvedic Medicinal Plants*. CRC Press: New York, 1989

Khalsa, Shakti Parwha Kaur, *Kundalini Yoga: the Flow of Eternal Power*, Time Capsule: 1996.

Krohn, Jacqueline & Taylor, Frances, *Natural Detoxification*, Hartley & Marks: 2000

Kumar, Abhimanyu, *Child Health Care in Ayurveda*, Sri Satguru Publications: Delhi, 1994

Jain, S.K., and DeFillips, Robert A., *Medicinal Plants of India, Reference Publications*, Algonac: Michigan, 1991, p.372.

Lad, Vasant, and Frawley, David, *Yoga of Herbs, The,* Lotus Press, Twin Lakes, WI, 1986, www.lotuspress.com

Lad, Vasant, *Ayurveda: The Science of Self-Healing,* Lotus Press, Twin Lakes, Wisconsin, 1984, www.lotuspress.com

Lad, Vasant, *The Complete Book of Ayurvedic Home Remedies,* Harmony Books: New York, 1998.

Lad, Vasant, *Textbook of Ayurveda*

Lad, Vasant, *Secrets of the Pulse*

Landis, Robyn, and Khalsa, Karta Purkh Singh, *Herbal Defense*, Warner Books: 1997.

Leung, Albert Y., Foster, Steven, *Encyclopedia of Common Natural Ingredients Used in Food, Drugs, and Cosmetics,* John Wiley & Sons: 1995

Lininger, Skye, et al, N*atural Pharmacy, The,* Prima: 1998

Lonsdorf, Nancy, Butler, Veronica, and Brown, Melanie. *Woman's Best Medicine, A*.Tarcher: New York, 1993

Merck Manual of Medical Information, The, Home Edition, Merck & Co.: 1997.

Mills, Simon, and Bone, Kerry, *Principles and Practice of Phytotherapy,* Churchill Livingstone: London, 2000

Mishra, Lashmi Chandra, *Scientific Basis for Ayurvedic Therapies*, CRC Press: New York, 2003

Mookerjee, Ajit, and Madhu Khanna, *The Tantric Way*, Thames and Hudson:

1977.
Mookerjee, Ajit, *Kundalini: Arousal of the Inner Energy*, Destiny: 1986.
Murray, Michael, *The Healing Power of Herbs,* Prima: 1995.
Murray, Michael, and Pizzorno, Joseph, *Encyclopedia of Natural Medicine,* Prima: 1998.
Nair, C.K.N., and Mohanan, N., *Medicinal Plants of India*
Nadkarni, AK, *Indian Materia Medica,* Popular Prakashan: Bombay, 1976
Ninivaggi, Frank John, *Elementary Textbook of Ayurveda, An*, Psychosocial Press: Madison, Connecticut, 2001
Ojha, Divakar, and Kumar, Ashok, *Panchakarma-Therapy in Ayurveda*, Chaukhamba Amarabharati Prakashan: Varanasi, 1978
Pitchford, Paul, *Healing with Whole Foods,* North Atlantic Books: Berkeley, 1993.
Radha, Swami Sivananda, *Kundalini Yoga for the West*, Timeless: 1996.
Raichur, Pratima, *Absolute Beauty,* Harper Collins: New York, 1997
Rhyner, Hans H. *Ayurveda: The Gentle Health System.* Sterling: New York, 1994
Sastry, J.L.N., *Dravyaguna Vijnana*, Chaukambha Orientalia: Varanasi, 2002
Schulz, V., Hansel, R., Tyler, V.E., *Rational Phytotherapy*, Springer: 1998
Sen, Koviraj Jayanarayan, *Pancha Karma Samgraha*, Srinabas Ayurvedic Aushadhalaya: Calcutta, no date given
Sharma, Hari. *Freedom from Disease*. Veda: Toronto. 1993
Sharma, P.V., *Cakradatta*, Chaukambha Orientalia: Varanasi, 1994
Singh, R.H., *Panca Karma Therapy*, Chowkhamba Sanskrit Series Office: Varanasi, 1992
Singhal, GD, and Patterson, TJS, *Synopsis of Ayurveda, Based on a Translation of the Susruta Samhita,* Oxford University Press: Delhi, 1993. (Susruta Samhita I.45.96.111)
Sivananda Yoga Center, The, *The Sivananda Companion to Yoga*, Gaia: 1983.
Srikantamurthym K.R., *Clinical Methods in Ayurveda*, Chaukambha Oeientalia: Varanasi, 1983
Svoboda, Robert, *Kundalini*, Brotherhood of Life: 1993.
Svoboda, Robert E., *Ayurveda: Life, Health and Longevity,* Arkana: London, 1992
Tierra, Lesley, *Healing with Chinese Herbs, The,* Crossing Press: Freedom, California, 1997
Tierra, Lesley, *Herbs of Life, The,* The Crossing Press: Freedom, California, 1992
Tierra, Michael, *Planetary Herbology,* Lotus Press, Twin Lakes, WI, 1988, www.lotuspress.com
Tillotson Alan, *One Earth Herbal Sourcebook, The*, Kensington: New York, 2001
Tirtha, Sada Shiva, Swami, *The Ayurveda Encyclopedia,* Ayurveda Holistic

Center Press: Bayville, New York, 1998

Tiwari, Maya. *Ayurveda: Secrets of Healing*. Lotus Press: Twin Lakes, WI, 1995, www.lotuspress.com

Vishnu-devananda, Swami, *The Complete Illustrated Book of Yoga*, Crown: 1960.

Vokovic, Laurel, *14-Day Herbal Cleansing,* Prentice Hall: 1998

Werbach, Melvyn, *Nutritional Influences on Illness,* Third Line Press: 1996.

Williamson, Elizabeth, *Major Herbs of Ayurveda*

Yogi Bhajan, *Teachings of Yogi Bhajan, The,* Arcline: 1977.

Yogi Bhajan, *Ancient Art of Self-Healing, The,* Silver Streak Publishers: Eugene, Oregon,1982.

RECOMMENDED READING

Bartram, Thomas, *Encyclopedia of Herbal Medicine,* Grace Publishers: Christchurch, Dorset, 1995

Bhajan, Yogi, *Ancient Art of Self-Healing, The,* Silver Streak Publishers: Eugene, Oregon, 1982.

Bhajan, Yogi, *Foods for Health & Healing, Arcline Publications: 1984*

Blumenthal, et al, *Complete German Commission E Monographs,* Integrative Medicine Communications: Austin, 1998

Brown, Susan E., *Better Bones, Better Body: A Comprehensive Self-Help Program for Preventing, Halting and Overcoming Osteoporosis*, Keats: 1996

Brown, Susan E., *Better Bones, Better Body: Beyond Estrogen and Calcium*, Contemporary Books: 2000

Erasmus, Udo, *Fats that Heal, Fats that Kill*, Alive Books: Burnaby, BC, Canada, 1986

Frawley, David, *Ayurvedic Healing,* Lotus Press: Twin Lakes, WI, 1989, www.lotuspress.com

Frawley, David, *Ayurveda and the Mind,* Lotus Press, Twin Lakes, WI, 1997, www.lotuspress.com

Frawley, David, *Yoga and Ayurveda*, Lotus Press, Twin Lakes, WI, 1999, www.lotuspress.com

Frawley, David, *Yoga for Your Type,* Lotus Press, Twin Lakes, WI, 2001, www.lotuspress.com

Gaby, Alan, *Preventing and Reversing Osteoporosis: What You Can Do About Bone Loss--A Leading Expert's Natural Approach to Increasing Bone Mass*, Prima: 1995

Gerson, Scott, *Ayurveda,* Element: 1997

Griggs, Barbara, *Green Pharmacy,* Healing Arts Press: Rochester, Vermont, 1997

Holmes, Peter, *Energetics of Western Herbs*, NatTrop: Berkeley, 1993

Johari, Harish, *Ancient Indian Massage,* Healing Arts Press: 1996

Khalsa, Karta Purkh Singh, *Body Balance*, Kensington: New York, 2004

Khalsa, Karta Purkh Singh, *Solve the Riddle of Fibromyalgia,* Natural Wellness: Montgomery, New York, 2006

Khalsa, Waheguru, *Miracle of the Healing Hands, The,* Rishi Knot Publishers:

1997

Lad, Vasant, and Frawley, David, *Yoga of Herbs, The,* Lotus Press: Twin Lakes, WI, 1986, www.lotuspress.com

Lad, Vasant, *Ayurveda: The Science of Self-Healing,* Lotus Press: Twin Lakes, WI, 1984, www.lotuspress.com

Landis, Robyn, and Khalsa, Karta Purkh Singh, *Herbal Defense*, WarnerBooks: 1997.

Lininger, Skye, et al, N*atural Pharmacy, The,* Prima: 1998

Mills, Simon, and Bone, Kerry, *Principles and Practice of Phytotherapy,* Churchill Livingstone: London, 2000

Sachs, Melanie, *Ayurvedic Beauty Care,* Lotus Press: Twin Lakes, WI, 1994, www.lotuspress.com

Svoboda, Robert E., *Ayurveda: Life, Health and Longevity,* Arkana: London, 1992

Svoboda, Robert, *Prakriti, Your Ayurvedic Constitution,* Lotus Press: Twin Lakes, WI, 1998, www.lotuspress.com

Tierra, Lesley, *Healing with Chinese Herbs,* The Crossing Press: Freedom, California, 1997

Tierra, Lesley, *Herbs of Life, The,* The Crossing Press: Freedom, California, 1992

Tierra, Lesley, *The Kid's Herb Book*, Robert D. Reid Publishers: 2000

Tierra, Michael, and Tierra, Lesley, *Chinese Traditional Herbal Medicine,* Lotus Press: Twin Lakes, WI, 1998, www.lotuspress.com

Tierra, Michael, and Tierra, Lesley, *Chinese-Planetary Herbal Diagnosis: A Primer*, Tierra: Santa Cruz, 1988

Tierra, Michael, *Planetary Herbology,* Lotus Press: Twin Lakes, WI, 1988, www.lotuspress.com

Tierra, Michael, *The Way of Herbs*, Pocket Books: 1998

Tierra, Michael, *The Way of Chinese Herbs*, Pocket Books: 1998

Tierra, Michael, *The Natural Remedy Bible*, Pocket Books: 2003

Tierra, Michael, *Treating Cancer with Herbs*, Lotus Press: Twin Lakes, WI, 2003, www.lotuspress.com

Tierra, Michael, *Biomagnetic and Herbal Therapy*, Lotus Press: Twin Lakes, WI, 1997, www.lotuspress.com

Tillotson Alan, *One Earth Herbal Sourcebook, The* Kensington: New York, 2001

Tiwari, Maya. *Ayurveda: Secrets of Healing*. Lotus: Twin Lakes, WI, 1995, www.lotuspress.com

AYURVEDA AND HERBAL RESOURCES

Planet Herbs
Internet home for Michael Tierra and the East West Herb School, East West Herb and Acupuncture Clinic, herb books and articles, online herbal forum and source for Planetary Herb Formulas including many of the traditional Ayurvedic herbs and formulas described in this book.
912 Center Street
Santa Cruz, CA 95060
(831) 429-8066
www.planetherbs.com

International Integrative Educational Institute
Karta Purkh Singh Khalsa, Founder and Course Director
Herbs & Salves Formulated by Karta Purkh Singh Khalsa
4627 Fox Hollow Road
Eugene, Oregon 97405
(541) 242-3314
www.internationalintegrative.com

The New Cleanse
Kartar S. Khalsa, DOM
P.O. Box 1515
Santa Cruz, NM 87567
(800) 563-3327
(505) 747-3323
(505) 753-6853 fax
info@thecleanse.com
www.thecleanse.com

Chrysalis Natural Medicine Clinic
Alan Keith Tillotson, PhD, AHG - Medical Herbalist
Chrysalis Natural medicine clinic specializes in herbal medicine treatments for serious or difficult to treat diseases. Phone consultations or office visits are available.

Advanced Ayurvedic training available for qualified students.
1008 Milltown Road
Wilmington, DE 19808
(302) 994-0565
http://oneearthherbs.squarespace.com/

Four Winds Natural Healing Center
Nicholas Schnell (Spirit Bear) herbalist
316 North 115th Street , Omaha, Nebraska 68154
(402) 933-6444
spiritbear4@msn.com
http://www.fourwindsnhc.com/nickcredentials.htm

Susan W. Kramer, PhD,
Herbalist - AHG, JD,
Black Belt in Bu Kyoku Kai Karate
Certified instructor of Tai Chi
1340 Woodland Hills Drive, NE
Atlanta, GA 30324
404-248-1684
swkramer@earthways.com

AYURVEDA EDUCATION

East West School of Herbalism

Michael Tierra O.M.D., L.Ac., founder of the AHG

A 36 lesson mostly distance learning herb course that includes herb studies suitable for home and professional practice, online study with supplemental lessons, articles, private student forums, weekly chat room studies directly with Michael Tierra and his staff and a yearly weeklong seminar held amidst the beautiful redwood forests in Santa Cruz Mountains where students are able to learn from a diverse number of master herbalists, including K.P. Khalsa, Lesley Tierra, David Hoffmann, Christopher Hobbs, Roy Upton and many others.

P.O. Box 275
Ben Lomond, California 95005
(831) 336-5010 (800-717-5010 (831) 336-4548 fax
www.planetherbs.com

The Ayurveda College

The Herbalists College
Karta Purkh Singh Khalsa, Course Director

The Ayurveda College offers extensive American training in Ayurveda and related fields on several campuses around the country, including courses in Ayurvedic massage, cuisine and herbalism. The college is a certified provider for massage continuing education for the National Certification Board for Therapeutic Massage and Bodywork. The faculty offers classes in a variety of aspects of Ayurveda and yoga to varied groups around America, including Bastyr University in Kenmore, Washington.

The Herbalists College provides a wide variety of education in herbal medicine on several campuses in a number of states. The flagship course is a two year training program designed to prepare for professional credentials in The American Herbalists Guild. The college offers one of the few clinical classes in herbal medicine in America.

International Integrative Educational Institute
4627 Fox Hollow
Eugene, Oregon 97405
(541) 242-3314
www.internationalintegrative.com

Evergreen Herb Garden and School

Candis Cantin, herbalist and Ayurvedic practitioner
Welcome to the Evergreen Herb Garden and the Evergreen Holistic Ministry. We provide an inspiring setting for the study of herbal medicine. Our integrative approach incorporates Western, Ayurvedic, and Chinese systems of medical treatment. Our herbal studies programs help each person find their own path to health and well-being. We are dedicated to educating people using holistic principles that honor the body, mind, and spirit. These principles empower the person with the informed awareness needed for making their own health care decisions. We welcome you to come join us, experience the wonders of natural therapies, and learn how to apply the rich healing arts of Integrative Herbology. There are over 250 different medicinal herbs growing in our gardens including many ornamentals that heal us through their beauty. At 2500 feet, our gardens provide four beautiful seasons where you can meditate and refresh your spirit. Come learn Integrative Herbology in our gardens while you experience the peace and beauty that abounds year round.
1445 Placerville, California, 95667
(530) 626-9288
www.evergreengarden.org

The National Institute of Ayurvedic Medicine

The National Institute of Ayurvedic Medicine (NIAM) is recognized as the largest and most authentic resource of information on Ayurveda in the United States. Correspondence courses events research report medicinal plants database products available with dosages and indications.
http://niam.com

FOR MORE INFORMATION

American Herbalists Guild

The American Herbalists Guild was founded in 1989 as a non-profit, educational organization to represent the goals and voices of herbalists. It is the only peer-review organization in the United States for professional herbalists specializing in the medicinal use of plants. AHG membership consists of professionals, general members (including students) and benefactors.

141 Nob Hill Road
Cheshire, CT 06410
(203) 272-6731 (203) 272-8550 fax
ahgoffice@earthlink.net
http://www.americanherbalist.com

American Association of Naturopathic Physicians

8201 Greensboro Drive, Suite 300
McLean, VA 22102
(877) 969-2267 (703) 610-9037
(703) 610-9005 fax
www.naturopathic.org

American Holistic Medical Association

4101 Lake Boone Trail, Suite 201
Raleigh, NC 27607
(919) 787-5146
www.holisticmedicine.org

National Institute of Medical Herbalists (England)

56 Longbrook Street
Exeter EX4 6AH, UK
Tel: +44 (0) 1392 426022
Fax: +44 (0) 1392 498963
nimh@ukexeter.freeuk
http://www.nimh.org.uk

National Center for Complementary and Alternative Medicine
NCCAM, National Institutes of Health
Bethesda, Maryland 20892 USA
http://nccam.nih.gov

Green Farmacy Garden
James A. (Jim) Duke, Ph.D., Botanist
8210 Murphy Road
Fulton, MD 20759
jimduke@comcast.net
(301) 498-1175
www.ars-grin.gov/duke

Kundalini Yoga
3HO Foundation
1620 Preuss Road
Los Angeles, CA 90035
(888) 346-2420
(505) 753-4988
(505) 753-1999 fax
yogainfo@3ho.org
www.3ho.org

INDEX

Agni 17, 18, 19, 20, 21, 22, 23, 25, 38, 51, 54, 56, 59, 60, 79, 95, 104, 105, 140, 167, 180, 188, 208, 212, 223, 227, 229, 251, 261, 306
Ahamkar 14
Allergy 61, 72, 121, 125, 154, 226, 227, 231, 254, 276
Ama 18, 19, 20, 46, 47, 49, 56, 65, 68, 77, 97, 99, 106, 140, 162, 170, 173, 179, 182, 184, 208, 212, 227, 229, 233, 234, 235, 240, 243, 251, 252, 289, 308
American Herbalists Guild x, xii, xiii, 331, 333
Amla 45, 67, 71, 78, 89, 90, 102, 111, 167, 174, 204, 208, 209, 214, 215, 217, 226, 233, 235, 239, 240, 244, 247, 250, 253, 254, 257, 259, 262, 264, 266, 267, 289, 302, 311
Anatomy 4, 6, 8, 17
Anupan 52, 54, 82, 83, 84, 188, 201, 202, 214, 221, 255
Asava 84, 211, 217
Baba Hari Dass x, xi, xiii, xiv, 22, 48, 49, 55, 58, 70, 71, 83, 109, 116, 156, 161, 167, 214, 221, 225, 226, 229, 242, 254
Bastyr University xiii, 88, 112, 149, 331
Bhasma 15, 85, 92, 199, 200, 201, 202, 203, 204, 213, 216, 254
Blood 13, 14, 18, 19, 21, 30, 37, 46, 47, 48, 55, 57, 58, 61, 67, 68, 69, 77, 78, 79, 83, 87, 88, 89, 90, 91, 92, 93, 94, 96, 98, 100, 102, 103, 104, 105, 106, 108, 111, 114, 115, 119, 121, 122, 123, 124, 125, 127, 129, 130, 131, 132, 134, 135, 137, 138, 139, 140, 142, 143, 144, 145, 146, 147, 148, 149, 152, 153, 154, 155, 156, 157, 158, 159, 160, 161, 162, 163, 166, 167, 168, 170, 171, 172, 173, 174, 175, 177, 178, 179, 180, 181, 182, 184, 186, 187, 188, 190, 194, 195, 198, 201, 202, 204, 205, 209, 210, 215, 220, 221, 224, 225, 234, 235, 237, 238, 244, 245, 246, 247, 248, 249, 252, 253, 261, 263, 264, 265, 267, 268, 269, 270, 271, 275, 276, 277, 282, 288, 305, 310, 311
Bowel 19, 22, 24, 30, 45, 76, 105, 108, 118, 132, 150, 168, 169, 173, 181, 192, 207, 217, 226, 234, 235, 242, 244, 249, 250, 261, 262, 279
Buddhi 15
Cancer 38, 39, 62, 101, 106, 107, 108, 122, 127, 128, 133, 134, 135, 137, 140, 145, 154, 158, 163, 164, 184, 188, 193, 194, 202, 234, 250, 266, 267, 268, 271
Castor 67, 84, 101, 116, 117, 118, 211, 235, 250, 253, 268, 279, 301, 302
Charaka Samhita 3, 55, 57, 112, 209, 216, 335

Chitta 15, 336
Chyavanprash 57, 90, 208, 209, 253, 257, 264, 266, 267, 336
Colitis 87, 89, 90, 96, 135, 152, 161, 170, 171, 173, 178, 192, 197, 244, 250, 261
constitution 12, 25, 27, 28, 29, 30, 31, 32, 33, 34, 36, 37, 43, 133, 176, 223, 273, 274, 284, 285, 287, 297, 298, 299
Detoxification 6, 39, 45, 46, 47, 49, 50, 56, 65, 115, 118, 128, 140, 210, 211, 212, 213, 215, 243, 244, 266, 278, 279, 286, 303, 304
Detoxify 26, 46, 47, 49, 58, 78, 154, 181, 208, 226, 227
Dhatu 13, 18, 19, 23, 25, 27, 80, 201
Diabetes 237, 245, 246, 247, 251, 252, 255, 304
Diagnosis xviii, 9, 11, 25, 26, 27, 36, 37, 70, 75
Diarrhea xvi, 19, 29, 34, 38, 54, 78, 89, 92, 94, 96, 100, 101, 103, 104, 105, 121, 132, 134, 144, 145, 146, 147, 148, 152, 155, 158, 160, 163, 164, 167, 170, 171, 173, 175, 176, 177, 181, 182, 188, 192, 201, 203, 204, 242, 250, 262
Diet x, xv, xvi, xvii, 7, 22, 31, 35, 41, 42, 43, 44, 45, 47, 48, 50, 51, 52, 53, 56, 57, 59, 63, 64, 65, 68, 69, 76, 77, 90, 133, 135, 138, 142, 151, 174, 185, 190, 194, 205, 217, 221, 223, 224, 225, 231, 234, 237, 239, 241, 247, 250, 252, 258, 261, 262, 268, 269, 273, 274, 276, 277, 278, 279, 283, 285, 286, 288, 297, 302
Edema 30, 37, 38, 46, 47, 76, 79, 86, 90, 93, 101, 106, 127, 129, 134, 138, 144, 147, 153, 172, 202, 203, 208, 210, 211, 238
Elements ix, 7, 8, 9, 11, 12, 13, 14, 18, 21, 22, 23, 70, 77, 78, 89, 230, 251, 276, 277, 285, 293
Enema 68, 69, 71, 209, 216, 229, 234, 302
Energetics xvii, xviii, 7, 8, 9, 42, 57, 66, 75, 79, 81, 84, 110, 112, 129, 140, 169, 170
Exercise xvii, 7, 27, 34, 35, 47, 66, 151, 223, 243, 247, 248, 258, 259, 265, 275, 281, 282, 283, 286, 299, 301, 302
Fasting 45, 47, 49, 131, 188, 234, 269, 302
Fatigue xviii, 19, 38, 39, 46, 47, 75, 79, 97, 98, 142, 166, 211, 224, 228, 248, 263, 266, 270, 285
Ghee 13, 52, 53, 54, 57, 59, 67, 71, 72, 73, 82, 83, 84, 85, 92, 94, 95, 99, 105, 111, 112, 113, 114, 115, 119, 126, 139, 153, 158, 162, 167, 172, 177, 183, 184, 187, 195, 205, 206, 209, 210, 213, 215, 216, 217, 218, 224, 234, 235, 236, 237, 239, 240, 241, 242, 243, 251, 252, 254, 257, 258, 262, 264, 268, 275, 276, 278, 279, 286, 287, 288, 289, 301, 302, 306, 307, 309, 310, 311, 312, 314
Ghrita 53, 85, 206, 240
Golden Temple xiii, 336
Gout 47, 67, 89, 114, 127, 131, 138, 139, 141, 170, 175, 178, 180, 186, 202, 208, 209, 210, 211
Greco-Roman ix
Guggul x, 78, 84, 93, 103, 139, 141, 142, 151, 161, 178, 210, 211, 216, 217, 229, 235, 237, 238, 241, 246, 248, 267, 269, 270, 302

Gunas 14, 15, 79, 80, 81
Herb Technology xiii
Honey 13, 48, 50, 51, 52, 53, 54, 61, 71, 82, 84, 88, 95, 99, 106, 118, 138, 139, 143, 147, 158, 162, 164, 168, 176, 179, 184, 186, 188, 189, 193, 195, 196, 201, 202, 204, 205, 209, 213, 214, 215, 216, 217, 224, 227, 234, 235, 237, 240, 241, 251, 252, 257, 262, 264, 265, 275, 277, 279, 286, 287, 288, 289, 301, 304, 311, 312
Hunger 13, 24, 29, 151, 288
Inflammation xvii, 8, 22, 30, 32, 38, 46, 47, 53, 67, 69, 75, 78, 88, 89, 90, 93, 100, 104, 119, 120, 127, 128, 133, 135, 148, 153, 154, 162, 163, 166, 169, 173, 175, 178, 181, 186, 191, 192, 193, 195, 203, 209, 211, 212, 219, 220, 225, 226, 227, 229, 230, 231, 232, 234, 235, 238, 241, 248, 249, 250, 251, 252, 253, 261, 263, 267, 275, 276, 277, 304
Kicharee 58, 59, 68, 194, 298, 305, 306
Kundalini xiii, 291, 293, 294, 295, 296, 334
Lifestyle x, 2, 7, 20, 31, 34, 36, 37, 38, 56, 63, 65, 95, 190, 224, 225, 253, 257, 258, 265, 273, 274, 281, 282, 283, 284, 285, 286, 297, 298, 302
Mahabhuta 8, 21
Mahad 14
Malas 23, 25, 34, 36
Manas 15, 34, 70
Massage xiii, xvi, 7, 53, 66, 67, 69, 90, 100, 115, 117, 124, 147, 161, 183, 184, 206, 209, 212, 214, 216, 230, 242, 244, 248, 254, 257, 265, 275, 276, 279, 281, 284, 289, 301, 331
Meat 35, 43, 44, 51, 55, 56, 57, 58, 71, 234, 268, 288
Medhya 15, 140, 145, 179, 201
Menthol 168, 169, 179, 248, 250, 280
Mercury 85, 134, 199, 200, 201, 202, 205
Milk 43, 44, 45, 50, 51, 52, 53, 57, 58, 60, 61, 69, 71, 73, 78, 81, 82, 83, 91, 92, 94, 97, 99, 100, 105, 106, 107, 112, 114, 115, 116, 117, 119, 123, 130, 131, 132, 133, 135, 138, 139, 149, 153, 154, 164, 167, 170, 176, 177, 183, 184, 185, 194, 195, 196, 198, 201, 202, 204, 205, 206, 208, 209, 222, 224, 234, 235, 236, 240, 241, 242, 250, 256, 257, 258, 259, 261, 264, 265, 266, 267, 269, 275, 277, 278, 279, 280, 286, 287, 288, 289, 304, 306, 310, 311, 312
Mind xii, xvii, xviii, 3, 5, 7, 8, 9, 11, 13, 14, 15, 25, 27, 28, 29, 33, 34, 39, 41, 58, 63, 65, 70, 71, 76, 78, 92, 111, 112, 113, 114, 120, 131, 144, 155, 183, 186, 189, 203, 228, 243, 253, 260, 271, 276, 277, 278, 283, 285, 286, 293, 294, 295, 297, 298, 302, 332
Mucus 13, 20, 29, 30, 32, 37, 38, 43, 47, 52, 54, 68, 72, 73, 77, 82, 91, 93, 104, 116, 122, 129, 130, 167, 184, 188, 189, 213, 214, 215, 216, 227, 230, 231, 238, 241, 244, 250, 260, 274, 275, 276, 279, 289
Mung beans x, 58, 59, 118, 275, 298, 305, 306, 314
Neti 72, 73, 114, 233, 276
Nutrition xii, 9, 42, 58, 70, 76, 108, 133, 201, 237

Obesity 38, 60, 66, 76, 79, 82, 87, 105, 141, 142, 150, 153, 162, 181, 182, 195, 202, 210, 211, 244, 270, 282
Oil 13, 44, 45, 48, 53, 62, 66, 67, 69, 71, 72, 75, 84, 86, 90, 95, 99, 100, 101, 111, 112, 113, 114, 115, 116, 117, 118, 119, 121, 122, 123, 124, 129, 133, 138, 147, 150, 158, 161, 162, 163, 164, 165, 166, 167, 168, 169, 170, 172, 177, 178, 179, 181, 182, 183, 184, 188, 189, 192, 193, 196, 209, 211, 212, 217, 218, 220, 222, 226, 230, 232, 233, 234, 235, 240, 242, 250, 253, 254, 257, 259, 262, 264, 265, 268, 269, 276, 278, 279, 280, 281, 288, 301, 302, 306, 307, 308, 309, 312, 313, 314
Oils 45, 66, 67, 77, 114, 164, 169, 189, 212, 220, 230, 232, 233, 252, 253, 254, 257, 262, 276, 277, 279, 301
Ojas 23, 78, 89, 226, 227, 287, 288
Pain 22, 23, 27, 30, 32, 33, 37, 38, 47, 49, 52, 60, 67, 91, 92, 100, 103, 110, 115, 117, 121, 122, 123, 137, 141, 150, 153, 160, 164, 168, 171, 173, 174, 177, 178, 186, 191, 192, 196, 197, 205, 208, 211, 212, 216, 219, 221, 227, 228, 229, 230, 231, 232, 242, 248, 249, 254, 255, 262, 265, 268, 276, 297, 301, 305
Panchakarma 65, 68, 69, 70, 229, 276, 287
Phlegm 14, 38, 61, 116, 136, 148, 161
Prabhava 71, 81, 179, 183, 188
Prakruti 12, 14, 27, 28, 29, 34, 42, 43, 223, 225, 228, 293
Protein xix, 48, 50, 51, 55, 56, 57, 58, 76, 78, 131, 157, 185, 205, 223, 228, 246, 258, 271, 275, 288, 303, 305
Pulse 36, 166
Purgation 69, 268
Purification 64, 65, 199
Rajas 14, 34
Rasa 18, 21, 23, 76, 77, 78, 80, 85, 159, 173, 199, 200, 202, 203, 204, 227
Rasayana 51, 63, 64, 65, 71, 97, 99, 104, 109, 111, 113, 138, 140, 141, 144, 162, 173, 202, 204, 205, 216, 217, 235, 236, 256, 285, 286
Rejuvenation 3, 59, 61, 64, 65, 69, 99, 141, 158, 209, 257, 264, 267, 284, 285, 286, 287, 288
Routine 7, 37, 45, 55, 65, 70, 217, 259, 274, 278, 279, 280, 281, 283
Salt 55, 59, 62, 69, 70, 71, 72, 73, 76, 78, 95, 147, 151, 187, 205, 210, 211, 213, 216, 233, 234, 237, 241, 242, 251, 280, 289, 302, 306, 307, 309, 310, 311, 312, 313, 314
Samskaras 15
Sattva 14, 15, 27, 34
Seasons 273, 274, 332
Semen 13, 18, 21, 24, 52, 53, 60, 67, 79, 95, 176, 235, 256, 265, 286, 287, 310
Sesame 57, 62, 67, 71, 84, 139, 161, 164, 167, 182, 183, 193, 196, 209, 212, 220, 226, 240, 254, 257, 259, 261, 264, 265, 279, 280, 281, 288, 289, 290, 301, 307, 314
Sex 52, 177, 233, 235, 256, 258, 282, 284, 285, 286, 287, 288, 289, 295

Shakti 9, 27, 293, 294, 296
Shiva 9, 105, 144, 293, 294
Sleep 30, 33, 35, 62, 79, 81, 98, 165, 166, 171, 183, 197, 228, 230, 253, 255, 257, 258, 259, 260, 261, 279, 282, 283, 285, 288, 295, 302
Sushruta Samhita 3, 4
Symptoms 1, 12, 19, 20, 21, 26, 31, 32, 34, 36, 37, 38, 39, 46, 49, 65, 66, 76, 102, 110, 133, 148, 155, 159, 167, 168, 169, 185, 211, 217, 227, 228, 230, 234, 238, 239, 243, 245, 247, 249, 250, 254, 260, 262, 264, 266
Tamas 14, 34
Tattva 8, 61, 77, 253
Temperature xvi, xvii, xviii, 8, 12, 13, 20, 29, 36, 44, 57, 66, 73, 75, 78, 79, 122, 129, 140, 162, 168, 213, 218, 228, 239, 240, 258, 261, 273, 282, 285, 289
Traditional Chinese Medicine ix, 127
Trikatu x, 139, 211, 212, 213, 214, 242, 251, 266
Triphala x, 71, 72, 73, 84, 92, 95, 113, 119, 139, 142, 202, 205, 207, 208, 210, 211, 212, 213, 214, 215, 216, 217, 218, 226, 237, 238, 239, 240, 242, 244, 251, 254, 256, 261, 262, 265, 266, 267, 270, 276, 279, 280, 281, 298, 302
Unani ix, 3, 4, 289
Urination 24, 37, 47, 78, 116, 125, 138, 145, 153, 172, 175, 204, 239
Vedas 3, 292
Vehicles 82, 84
Vikruti 12, 27, 29, 34
Vipak 23, 57, 78, 82, 145, 311, 313, 314
Vomiting 24, 47, 68, 114, 121, 123, 125, 129, 137, 144, 159, 162, 164, 167, 168, 177, 198, 204, 205, 276, 302
Yeast 46, 101, 116, 134, 159, 232
Yoga xi, xii, xiii, xiv, 3, 5, 14, 15, 17, 35, 50, 53, 56, 61, 63, 72, 142, 191, 237, 247, 248, 253, 257, 273, 280, 281, 283, 291, 293, 294, 295, 296, 297, 299, 301, 331, 334
Yogi Bhajan x, xii, xiii, xvi, 6, 7, 15, 26, 47, 48, 50, 51, 52, 56, 60, 61, 71, 72, 77, 83, 86, 87, 95, 115, 116, 118, 119, 134, 140, 162, 179, 190, 194, 199, 205, 209, 216, 217, 221, 242, 254, 256, 257, 264, 289, 291, 292, 294, 295, 297, 306, 308, 309, 311, 312, 326

(Endnotes)

1 Hoffman C, Rice D, Sung HY. Persons with chronic conditions. Their prevalence and costs. JAMA. 1996 Nov 13;276(18):1473-9.

2 Svoboda, Robert E., Ayurveda: An Alternative or Compementary Medicine? http://www.drsvoboda.com/ayurvedAlt.htm

3 Eisenberg DM, Kessler RC, Foster C, Norlock FE, Calkins DR, Delbanco TL. "Unconventional medicine in the United States: prevalence, costs, and patterns of use." N Engl J Med 1993;328:246-252.

4 Borkan J, Neher JO, Anson O, Smoker B. "Referrals for alternative therapies." J Fam Pract. 1994;39:545-550.

5 Ayurveda, Department of Ayurveda, Yoga and Naturopathy, Unani, Siddha and Homeopathy, Ministry of Health and Family Welfare, Government of India, http://indianmedicine.nic.in/html/ayurveda/ayurveda.htm

6 Ayurveda, Department of Ayurveda, Yoga and Naturopathy, Unani, Siddha and Homeopathy, Ministry of Health and Family Welfare, Government of India, http://indianmedicine.nic.in/html/ayurveda/ayurveda.htm

7 Yogi Bhajan Lecture 9/21/81

8 Yogi Bhajan Lecture (Vasant Lad guest) 1/15/94

9 Personal communication

10 Tierra, Michael, Ayurveda: The Mother of Natural Healing, Planet Herbs, http://planetherbs.com showcase/

11 Dharmananda, Subhuti, Basics of Ayurvedic Physiology, Institute of Traditional Medicine, 1997, http://www.itmonline.org/arts/ayurbasics.htm

12 Basics of Ayurveda, Nararjuna Ayurveda Group, http://www.nagarjun.com/html/n0212ayu.htm#Malas

13 Svoboda R, and Lade A, Tao and Dharma: Chinese Medicine and Ayurveda, Lotus Press, Twin Lakes, WI, 1995

14 Basic Principles of Ayurveda, India Mart, http://www.indiamart.com/ayurveda/discover-ayurveda/agni.html

15 McCaleb, Robert S., Herb Research Foundation Encyclopedia of Popular Herbs, Prima, Roseville, california, 2000.

16 Dowling RH, Veysey MJ, Pereira SP, Hussaini SH, Thomas LA, Wass JA, Murphy GM. Role of intestinal transit in the pathogenesis of gallbladder stones. Can J Gastroenterol 1997;11(1):57-64.

17 Hotz J, Plein K, [Effectiveness of plantago seed husks in comparison with wheat brain on stool frequency and manifestations of irritable colon syndrome with constipation]. *Med Klin* 1994 Dec 15;89(12):645-51

18 Blumenthal M, Busse WR, Goldberg A, et al, eds. *The Complete German Commission E Monographs: Therapeutic Guide to Herbal Medicines.* Austin: American Botanical Council and Boston: Integrative Medicine Communications, 1998, 167.

19 Yogi Bhajan Lecture 8/17/84

20 Gottlieb, Bill, New Choices in Natural Healing, All About Vatta Pitta and Kapha, http://www.mothernature.com/Library/Bookshelf/Books/21/12.cfm

21 Yogi Bhajan Lecture (Vasant Lad guest) 1/15/94

22 Rogi Pareeksha, Ayurveda, Nagarjuna Ayurveda Group, http://www.nagarjun.com/html n0400par.htm

23 Chauhan, Partap, Ayurveda Beyond Vata, Pitta and Kapha, Arogya, Jiva Ayurveda, July 17, 2002

24 Ayurveda and Ahara, Arya Vaidya Pharmacy, http://www.avpayurveda.com

25 Factors of Ayurdic Diet and Dietetics, Dr. Eddy Ayurveda School, http://www.dreddyclinic.com/online_recources/articles/ayurvedic/facts_diet.htm

26 Personal communication with Karta Purkh Singh Khalsa

27 Personal communication with Karta Purkh Singh Khalsa
28 Private Communication with Tillotson
29 Yogi Bhajan Lecture 8/17/84
30 Personal communication with Michael Tierra
31 Bhajan, Yogi, *The Ancient Art of Self Healing,* West Anandpur, Eugene, 1982, p. 60
32 Yogi Bhajan Lecture 8/17/84
33 Personal communication with Michael Tierra
34 Charaka Samhita Ci 1.3.30-31
35 Yogi Bhajan Lecture 1/8/70
36 Yogi Bhajan Lecture 1/8/70
37 Yogi Bhajan Lecture 2/21/82
38 Ten Ways to Feel Energized by Food, Maharishi Ayurveda, http://www.mapi.com/en/newsletters ayurvedic_enegy_food.html
39 Page BD Liquid chromatographic method for the determination of nine phenolic antioxidants in butter oil: collaborative study. J-AOAC-Int. 1993 Jul-Aug; 76(4): 765-79
40 Schalinske, K.L. Steele, R.D., Dietary butter protects against ultraviolet radiation-induced suppression of contact hypersensitivity in Skh:HR-1 hairless mice. J-nutr. Bethesda, Md. : American Institute of Nutrition. Mar 1996. v. 126 (3) p. 681-692.
41 Dash, Bhagwan. *Massage Therapy in Ayurveda.* Concept: New Delhi, 1992, p. 92
42 Report on butter prompts research policy changes. Nutrition-week (USA). (22 Mar 1991). v. 21(12) p. 2-3.
43 Singh RB Niaz MA Ghosh S Beegom R Rastogi V Sharma JP Dube GK Association of trans fatty acids (vegetable ghee) and clarified butter (Indian ghee) intake with higher risk of coronary artery disease in rural and urban populations with low fat consumption. Int-J-Cardiol. 1996 Oct 25; 56(3): 289-98
44 Ten Ways to Feel Energized by Food, Maharishi Ayurveda, http://www.mapi.com/en/newsletters/ayurvedic_enegy_food.html
45 Private communication. 2006.
46 Personal communication with Michael Tierra
47 August, Lynne, *Water and Salt,* Health Equations, http://healthequations.com/articles.html#
48 Midgley JP, Matthew AG, Greenwood CM, Logan AG. Effect of reduced dietary sodium on blood pressure: a metaanalysis of randomized controlled trials. JAMA 1996 May 22-29;275(20):1590-7
49 Halpern, Marc, *Journey into Ayurveda* http://www.heall.com/body/altmed/treatment/ayurveda/journey.html
50 Sadashiva Tirtha, Swami, *Ayurveda and Anemia*, Ayuveda Global Community, 2/3/2005, http://www.ayurvedahc.com/articlelive/articles/17/1/Ayurveda-&-Anemia
51 Murthy, C.S.H.N., Animal Testing in Ayurveda, *Hinduism Today,* May, 1992 http://www.hinduismtoday.com/archives/1992/05/1992-05-03.shtml
52 Personal communication with Karta Purkh Singh Khalsa
53 Sadashiva Tirtha, Swami, *Ayurveda and Anemia,* Ayuveda Global Community, 2/3/2005, http://www.ayurvedahc.com/articlelive/articles/17/1/Ayurveda-&-Anemia
54 Persona communication with Michael Tierra
55 Nagral, Kumud, (Dr. , Mrs.), Concept of Safe Motherhood in Ayurved, National Integrated Medical Association, Mumbai, http://ayurveda-foryou.com/home.html
56 Bitter Melon Monograph, Herbal Plants and Medicines, http://www.tips4betterlife.com/herbs/herb-bittermelon.html
57 Landis, Robyn, and Khalsa, Karta Purkh Singh, *Herbal Defense,* Warner Books, 1997.
58 Billing J, Sherman PW. Antimicrobial functions of spices: why some like it hot. Q Rev Biol 1998 Mar;73(1):3-49 Section of Neurobiology and Behavior, Cornell University, Ithaca, NY 14853, USA.

59 Know your onions. Food Science Central, Food Science and Technology Abstracts, April 15, 2005, http://www.foodsciencecentral.com/fsc/ixid13923

60 Murray, Michael, and Pizzorno, Joseph, Encyclopedia of Natural Medicine, Prima, Rocklin, California, 1998.

61 Yang, J; Meyers, KJ; van der Heide, J; Liu, RH (2004). Varietal differences in phenolic content and antioxidant and antiproliferative activities of onions. *Journal of Agricultural and Food Chemistry* 52 (22) 6787–6793.

62 Yogi Bhajan Lecture 2/21/82

63 Yogi Bhajan Lecture 6/21/73

64 Yogi Bhajan Lecture 6/21/73

65 Basics of Ayurveda, Nararjuna Ayurvedic Group, http://www.nagarjun.com/html/home.htm

66 Branches of Ayurveda, http://www.stayfinder.com/travelguide/india/ayurveda/ayurveda_branches.asp

67 Ayurveda, Department of Ayurveda, Yoga and Naturopathy, Unani, Siddha and Homeopathy, Ministry of Health and Family Welfare, Government of India, http://indianmedicine.nic.in/html/ayurveda/ayurveda.htm

68 Therapies and Their Uses, Arthritis Foundation http://www.arthritis.org/conditions/alttherapies/therapies_uses.asp

69 Managing Your Pain, Arthritis Foundation http://www.arthritis.org/conditions/tips_managepain.asp

70 Douillard, John, *Encyclopedia of Ayurvedic Massage,* The, North Atlantic Books, Berkeley, 2004, p. 47

71 Atreya, *Secrets of Ayurvedic Massage,* Lotus Press, Twin Lakes, WI, 2000, p. 85

72 Singh, R.H., *Pancha Karma Therapy,* Chowkhamba Sanskrit Series Office, Varanasi, 1992, p.19

73 Ojha, Divakar, and Kumar, Ashok, *Panchakarma-Therapy in Ayurveda,* Chaukhamba Amarabharati Prakashan, Varanasi, 1978, p.11

74 Sen, Koviraj Jayanarayan, *Pancha Karma Samgraha,* Srinabas Ayurvedic Aushadhalaya, Calcutta, no date given, p. 11

75 Personal Communication with Michael Tierra

76 James, Kat, *Pure decadence: becoming connoisseurs of our own inner beauty.* Better Nutrition Oct, 2002 http://www.findarticles.com/cf_0/m0FKA/10_64/91563481/print.jhtml

77 Taylor, Mikki, beauty consider this ...(Indian method proves to be effective) Essence, Nov, 2000 http://www.findarticles.com/cf_0/m1264/7_31/67263578/print.jhtml

78 deJager, Prashanti, Medhya Herbs and Therapies, *Light on Ayurveda,* IV: 3 (Spring 2005).

79 Personal commu nication with Michael Tierra

80 Charak Samhita Ci 10.25

81 Personal communication with Michael Tierra

82 Astanga Hridyam U 39.48

83 Astanga Hridyam U 40.56

84 Astanga Hridyam U 39.61

85 deJager, Prashanti, Medhya Herbs and Therapies, *Light on Ayurveda,* IV: 3 (Spring 2005).

86 Charaka Samhita Ci 1.3.30-31

87 Charaka Samhita Si 12.15

88 Boek WM, Keles N, Graamans K, Huizing EH. Physiologic and hypertonic saline solutions impair ciliary activity in vitro. Laryngoscope. 1999 Mar;109(3):396-9.

89 Herbs and Minerals, Himalaya Herbal Health Care, http://www.himalayahealthcare.com/aboutayurveda/cahs.htm

90 Personal communication with Michael Tierra

91 Chitale, P.K., *Comparative Study of Ayurveda and Treatment by Indian Drugs,* A, Sri Satguru Publications, Delhi, 1997, p.111

92 Uma Pradeep K, Geervani P, Eggum BO Common Indian spices: nutrient composition, consumption and contribution to dietary value. *Plant Foods Hum Nutr* 1993 Sep;44(2):137-48

93 Ajowan Monograph, Encyclopedia of Spices, The Epicentre, http://www.theepicentre.com/Spices/ajowan.html

94 Personal communication

95 Hamilton, Rowan. Strengths and Limitations of Aloe Vera. American Journal of Natural Medicine, December 1998, Vol. 5, No. 10, pp. 30-33.

96 Okyar A, Can A, Akev N, Baktir G, Sutlupinar N. Effect of Aloe vera leaves on blood glucose level in type I and type II diabetic rat models. Phytother Res 2001 Mar;15(2):157-61

97 Syed TA, Afzal M, Ashfaq Ahmad S, et al. Management of genital herpes in men with 0.5% Aloe vera extract in a hydrophilic cream: a placebo-controlled double-blind study. *J Dermatol Treat.* 1997;8:99–102.

98 Dash, Bhagwan. *Materia Medica of Ayurveda.* New Delhi: B. Jain Publishers. 1991. p.9

99 Dash, Bhagwan and Manfred Junius. A *Handbook of Ayurveda.* New Delhi: Concept Publishing. 1983. p.89

100 Frawley, David and Dr. Vasant Lad. *The Yoga Of Herbs: An Ayurvedic Guide to Herbal Medicine.* Lotus Press, Twin Lakes, WI, 1986. p.157

101 Nadkarni, Dr. K.M. 1976. *The Indian Materia Medica, with Ayurvedic, Unani and Home Remedies.* Revised and enlarged by A.K. Nadkarni. 1954. Reprint. Bombay: Bombay Popular Prakashan PVP. P. 482.

102 Asmawi MZ, Kankaanranta H, Moilanen E, Vapaatalo H Anti-inflammatory activities of Emblica officinalis Gaertn leaf extracts. *J Pharm Pharmacol* 1993 Jun;45(6):581-4.

103 Jose JK, Kuttan R. Hepatoprotective activity of Emblica officinalis and Chyavanaprash. *J Ethnopharmacol* 2000 Sep 1;72(1-2):135-140

104 Bhattacharya A, Chatterjee A, Ghosal S, Bhattacharya SK Antioxidant activity of active tannoid principles of Emblica officinalis (amla). *Indian J Exp Biol* 1999 Jul;37(7):676-80

105 Biswas S, Talukder G, Sharma A Protection against cytotoxic effects of arsenic by dietary supplementation with crude extract of Emblica officinalis fruit. *Phytother Res* 1999 Sep;13(6):513-6

106 Menon LG, Kuttan R, Kuttan G Effect of rasayanas in the inhibition of lung metastasis induced by B16F-10 melanoma cells. *J Exp Clin Cancer Res* 1997 Dec;16(4):365-8

107 Kumar KC S, Muller K Medicinal plants from Nepal; II. Evaluation as inhibitors of lipid peroxidation in biological membranes. *J Ethnopharmacol* 1999 Feb;64(2):135-9

108 Mathur R, Sharma A, Dixit VP, Varma M Hypolipidaemic effect of fruit juice of Emblica officinalis in cholesterolfed rabbits. *J Ethnopharmacol* 1996 Feb;50(2):61-8

109 Bhattacharya A et al. Antioxidant activity of active tannoid principles of *Emblica officinalis (amla). Indian J Exp Biol* 1999 Jul;37(7):676-80

110 Bhattacharya A et al. Antioxidant activity of active tannoid principles of *Emblica officinalis (amla). Indian J Exp Biol* 1999 Jul;37(7):676-80

111 Bhattacharya A, Kumar M, Ghosal S, Bhattacharya SK Effect of bioactive tannoid principles of Emblica officinalis on iron-induced hepatic toxicity in rats. *Phytomedicine* 2000 Apr;7(2):173-5

112 Rege NN, Thatte UM, Dahanukar SA. Adaptogenic properties of six rasayana herbs used in Ayurvedic medicine. *Phytother Res* 1999 Jun;13(4):275-91

113 Sharma N, Trikha P, Athar M, Raisuddin S. Inhibitory effect of Emblica officinalis on the in vivo clastogenicity of benzo[a]pyrene and cyclophosphamide in mice. *Hum Exp Toxicol* 2000 Jun;19(6):377-84.

114 Jeena KJ, et al. Effect of Emblica officinalis, Phyllanthus amarus and Picrorrhiza kurroa on N-nitrosodiethylamine induced hepatocarcinogenesis. *Cancer Lett.* 1999 Feb 8;136(1):11-6

115 Bandyopadhyay SK, Pakrashi SC, Pakrashi A The role of antioxidant activity of Phyllanthus emblica fruits on prevention from indomethacin induced gastric ulcer. *J Ethnopharmacol* 2000 May;70(2):171-6.

116 Biswas S, et al. Protection against cytotoxic effects of arsenic by dietary supplementation with crude extract of *Emblica officinalis* fruit. *Phytother Res.* 1999 Sep;13(6):513-6

117 Mathur Retal. Hypolipidaemic effect of fruit juice of Emblica officinalis in cholesterol-fed rabbits. *J Ethnopharmacol.* 1996 Feb;50(2):61-8.

118 Augusti KT, Arathy SL, Asha R, Ramakrishanan J, Zaira J, Lekha V, Smitha S, Vijayasree VM. A comparative study on the beneficial effects of garlic (Allium sativum Linn), amla (Emblica Officinalis Gaertn) and onion (Allium cepa Linn) on the hyperlipidemia induced by butter fat and beef fat in rats. Indian J Exp Biol 2001 Aug;39(8):760-6

119 Jacob A, et al. Effect of the Indian gooseberry (amla) on serum cholesterol levels in men aged 35-55 years. *Eur J Clin Nutr.* 1988 Nov;42(11):939-44.

120 Nadkarni, Dr. K.M. 1976. *The Indian Materia Medica, with Ayurvedic, Unani and Home Remedies.* Revised and enlarged by A.K. Nadkarni. 1954. Reprint. Bombay: Bombay Popular Prakashan PVP. p 481.

121 Kapoor, L.D. CRC *Handbook of Ayurvedic Medicinal Plants.* Boca Raton: CRC Press. 1990. p.322

122 Maharishi Ayurveda Approach to Menopause http://www.ayurveda-ayurvedic.com/natural-menopause.html

123 Kapoor LD. *Handbook of Ayurvedic Medicinal Plants.* Boca Raton, FL. CRC Press; 1990:319-320

124 Terminalia arjuna. *Altern Med Rev* 1999 Dec;4(6):436-7

125 Miller AL Botanical influences on cardiovascular disease. *Altern Med Rev* 1998 Dec;3(6):422-31

126 Shaila HP, Udupa SL, Udupa AL Hypolipidemic activity of three indigenous drugs in experimentally induced atherosclerosis. *Int J Cardiol* 1998 Dec 1;67(2):119-24

127 Ram A, Lauria P, Gupta R, Kumar P, Sharma VN Hypocholesterolaemic effects of Terminalia arjuna tree bark. *J Ethnopharmacol* 1997 Feb;55(3):165-9

128 Kumar PU, Adhikari P, Pereira P, Bhat P Safety and efficacy of Hartone in stable angina pectoris--an open comparative trial. *J Assoc Physicians India* 1999 Jul;47(7):685-9

129 Dwivedi S, Agarwal MP Antianginal and cardioprotective effects of Terminalia arjuna, an indigenous drug, in coronary artery disease. *J Assoc Physicians India* 1994 Apr;42(4):287-9

130 Bharani A, Ganguly A, Bhargava KD Salutary effect of Terminalia Arjuna in patients with severe refractory heart failure. *Int J Cardiol* 1995 May;49(3):191-9

131 Dwivedi S, Jauhari R Beneficial effects of Terminalia arjuna in coronary artery disease. *Indian Heart J* 1997 Sep- Oct;49(5):507-10

132 Seth SD, Maulik M, Katiyar CK, Maulik SK Role of Lipistat in protection against isoproterenol induced myocardial necrosis in rats: a biochemical and histopathological study. *Indian J Physiol Pharmacol* 1998 Jan;42(1):101-6

133 Kandil FE, Nassar MI A tannin anti-cancer promotor from Terminalia arjuna. *Phytochemistry* 1998 Apr;47(8):1567-8

134 Kaur S, Grover IS, Kumar S Antimutagenic potential of ellagic acid isolated from Terminalia arjuna. *Indian J Exp Biol* 1997 May;35(5):478-82

135 Pettit GR, Hoard MS, Doubek DL, Schmidt JM, Pettit RK, Tackett LP, Chapuis JC Antineoplastic agents 338. The cancer cell growth inhibitory. Constituents of Terminalia arjuna (Combretaceae). *J Ethnopharmacol* 1996 Aug;53(2):57- 63

136 Perumal Samy R, Ignacimuthu S, Sen A Screening of 34 Indian medicinal plants for antibacterial properties. *J. Ethnopharmacol* 1998 Sep;62(2):173-82

137 Kumar DS, Prabhakar YS On the ethnomedical significance of the Arjun tree, Terminalia arjuna (Roxb.) Wight & Arnot. *J Ethnopharmacol* 1987 Jul;20(2):173-90

138 Asafoetida Monograph. Encyclopedia of Spices, The Epicentre, http://www.theepicentre.com/Spices/asafetid.html

139 Dash, Bhagwan and Kashyap, Lalitesh, *Diagnosis and Treatment of Diseases in Ayurveda : Based on Ayurveda Saukhyam of Todarananda,* New Delhi, Concept, 1987, part four, page 96.

140 Chakravarthy BK, Gupta S, Gode KD. Functional beta cell regeneration in the islets of pancreas in alloxan induced diabetic rats by (-)-epicatechin. Life Sci. 1982 Dec 13;31(24):2693-7.
141 Manickam M, Ramanathan M, Jahromi MA, Chansouria JP, Ray AB. Antihyperglycemic activity of phenolics from Pterocarpus marsupium. J Nat Prod. 1997 Jun;60(6):609-10.
142 Ahmad F, Khalid P, Khan MM, Chaubey M, Rastogi AK, Kidwai JR. Hypoglycemic activity of Pterocarpus marsupium wood. J Ethnopharmacol. 1991 Oct;35(1):71-5.
143 Chakravarthy BK, Gupta S, Gambhir SS, Gode KD. Pancreatic beta-cell regeneration in rats by (-)-epicatechin. Lancet. 1981 Oct 3;2(8249):759-60.
144 Ahmad F, Khalid P, Khan MM, Rastogi AK, Kidwai JR. Insulin like activity in (-) epicatechin. Acta Diabetol Lat. 1989 Oct-Dec;26(4):291-300.
145 Rizvi SI, Abu Zaid M, Suhail M. Insulin-mimetic effect of (-) epicatechin on osmotic fragility of human erythrocytes. Indian J Exp Biol. 1995 Oct;33(10):791-2.
146 Svoboda R. 1992. Ayurveda: Life, Healthy, and Longevity. London: Arkana
147 Murray, Michael, and Pizzorno, Joseph, Encyclopedia of Natural Medicine, Prima, Rocklin, California, 1998.
148 [No authors listed] Flexible dose open trial of Vijayasar in cases of newly-diagnosed non-insulin-dependent diabetes mellitus. Indian Council of Medical Research (ICMR), Collaborating Centres, New Delhi. Indian J Med Res. 1998 Jul;108:24-9.
149 Dr. MC Pandey, Prof. PV Sharma. Hypoglycaemic effect of bark of pterocarpus marsupium roxb. The Medicine & Surgery 15 November 1975 p. 21-23.
150 Jahromi MA, Ray AB. Antihyperlipidemic effect of flavonoids from Pterocarpus marsupium. J Nat Prod. 1993 Jul;56(7):989-94.
151 Al-Hindawi, M.K., I.H. Al-Deen, M.H. Nabi, and M.H. Ismail. 1989. Anti-inflammatory activity of some Iraqi plants using intact rats. *J Ethnopharmacol.* Sep; 26(2):163-8
152 Abdel-Magied EM, Abdel-Rahman HA, Harraz FM. The effect of aqueous extracts of Cynomorium coccineum and Withania somnifera on testicular development in immature Wistar rats. *J Ethnopharmacol* 2001 Apr;75(1):1-4
153 Kuppurajan K, et al, J Res Ayu Sid, 1, 1980:247. [from: Bone K, "Withania somnifera", *Clinical Applications of Ayurvedic and Chinese Herbs,* (Queensland, Australia: Phytotherapy Press), 1996:137-41.]
154 Mishra LC, Singh BB, Dagenais S. Scientific basis for the therapeutic use of Withania somnifera (ashwagandha): a review. Altern Med Rev 2000 Aug;5(4):334-46
155 Archana R, Namasivayam A. Antistressor effect of Withania somnifera. J Ethnopharmacol 1999 Jan;64(1):91-3
156 Singh B, Saxena AK, Chandan BK, Gupta DK, Bhutani KK, Anand KK. Adaptogenic activity of a novel, withanolide-free aqueous fraction from the roots of Withania somnifera Dun. Phytother Res 2001 Jun;15(4):311-318
157 Venkatraghavan S, et al, J Res Ayu Sid, 1, 1980:370. [from: Bone K, "Withania somnifera", *Clinical Applications of Ayurvedic and Chinese Herbs,* (Queensland, Australia: Phytotherapy Press), 1996:137-41.]
158 Jain S, Shukla SD, Sharma K, Bhatnagar M. Neuroprotective Effects of Withania somnifera Dunn. in Hippocampal Sub-regions of Female Albino Rat. Phytother Res 2001 Sep;15(6):544-548
159 Dhuley JN. Adaptogenic and cardioprotective action of ashwagandha in rats and frogs. J Ethnopharmacol 2000 Apr;70(1):57-63
160 Bhattacharya SK, Bhattacharya A, Chakrabarti A. Adaptogenic activity of Siotone, a polyherbal formulation of Ayurvedic rasayanas. Indian J Exp Biol 2000 Feb;38(2):119-28
161 Bhattacharya SK, Bhattacharya A, Sairam K, Ghosal S. Anxiolytic-antidepressant activity of Withania somnifera glycowithanolides: an experimental study. Phytomedicine 2000 Dec;7(6):463-9
162 Dhuley JN. Nootropic-like effect of ashwagandha (Withania somnifera L.) in mice. Phytother Res 2001 Sep;15(6):524-528

163 Dhuley JN.Adaptogenic and cardioprotective action of ashwagandha in rats and frogs. J Ethnopharmacol 2000 Apr;70(1):57-63

164 Bhattacharya A, Ghosal S, Bhattacharya SK. Anti-oxidant effect of Withania somnifera glycowithanolides in chronic footshock stress-induced perturbations of oxidative free radical scavenging enzymes and lipid peroxidation in rat frontal cortex and striatum. J Ethnopharmacol 2001 Jan;74(1):1-6

165 Davis L, Kuttan G. Immunomodulatory activity of Withania somnifera. J Ethnopharmacol 2000 Jul;71(1-2):193-200 Amala Cancer Research Centre, Amala Nagar P.O., 630 553, Kerala, Thrissur, India.

166 Prakash J, Gupta SK, Kochupillai V, Singh N, Gupta YK, Joshi S. Chemopreventive activity of Withania somnifera in experimentally induced fibrosarcoma tumours in Swiss albino mice. Phytother Res 2001 May;15(3):240-244

167 Devi PU Withania somnifera Dunal (Ashwagandha): potential plant source of a promising drug for cancer chemotherapy and radiosensitization. Indian-J-Exp-Biol. 1996 Oct; 34(10): 927-32

168 Kanth, V.R., and P.V. Diwan. 1999. Analgesic, antiinflammatory and hypoglycaemic activities of *Sida cordifolia. Phytother Res.* Feb;13(1):75-7

169 Nadkarni, Dr. K.M. 1976. *The Indian Materia Medica, with Ayurvedic, Unani and Home Remedies.* Revised and enlarged by A.K. Nadkarni. 1954. Reprint. Bombay: Bombay Popular Prakashan PVP., p.1135.

170 Nadkarni, Dr. K.M. 1976. The Indian Materia Medica, with Ayurvedic, Unani and Home Remedies. Revised and enlarged by A.K. Nadkarni. 1954. Reprint. Bombay: Bombay Popular Prakashan PVP. P.1135.

171 Duke, James. 1999. Chemicals and their Biological Activities in: Sida rhombifolia L. (Malvaceae) Broomweed, Teaplant. Http://www.ars-grin.gov/cgi-bin/duke/farmacy2.pl. Agricultural Research Service (ARS), United States Department of Agriculture.

172 Nadkarni, Dr. K.M. 1976. The Indian Materia Medica, with Ayurvedic, Unani and Home Remedies. Revised and enlarged by A.K. Nadkarni. 1954. Reprint. Bombay: Bombay Popular Prakashan PVP. P.1137.

173 Nadkarni, Dr. K.M. 1976. The Indian Materia Medica, with Ayurvedic, Unani and Home Remedies. Revised and enlarged by A.K. Nadkarni. 1954. Reprint. Bombay: Bombay Popular Prakashan PVP. P.1137.

174 Varrier, P.S. 1996. I*ndian Medicinal Plants: A Compendium of 500 species.* Edited by PK Warrier, VPK Nambiar and C Ramankutty. vol 5. Hyderabad: Orient Longman. P. 135.

175 Nadkarni, Dr. K.M. 1976. The Indian Materia Medica, with Ayurvedic, Unani and Home Remedies. Revised and enlarged by A.K. Nadkarni. 1954. Reprint. Bombay: Bombay Popular Prakashan PVP. P.1137.

176 Berberine. *Altern Med Rev* 2000 Apr;5(2):175-7

177 Iizuka N, Miyamoto K, Okita K, Tangoku A, Hayashi H, Yosino S, Abe T, Morioka T, Hazama S, Oka M Inhibitory effect of Coptidis Rhizoma and berberine on the proliferation of human esophageal cancer cell lines. *Cancer Lett* 2000 Jan 1;148(1):19-25

178 Lin JG, Chung JG, Wu LT, Chen GW, Chang HL, Wang TF Effects of berberine on arylamine N-acetyltransferase activity in human colon tumor cells. *Am J Chin Med* 1999;27(2):265-75

179 Grippa E, Valla R, Battinelli L, Mazzanti G, Saso L, Silvestrini B Inhibition of Candida rugosa lipase by berberine and structurally related alkaloids, evaluated by high-performance liquid chromatography. *Biosci Biotechnol Biochem* 1999 Sep;63(9):1557-62

180 Halder RK, Neogi NC, Rathor RS. Pharmacological investigations on Berberine hydrochloride. Ind. J. Pharmacol. 1970; 2:26.

181 Bhide, M. B. and Dutta, N. K. The antagonist action of berberine hydrochloride against certain biogenic substances, Ind. J. Physiol. Pharmacol., 12: 19-22, 1968

182 Nadkarni, Dr. K.M. 1976. The Indian Materia Medica, with Ayurvedic, Unani and Home Remedies. Revised and enlarged by A.K. Nadkarni. 1954. Reprint. Bombay: Bombay Popular Prakashan PVP. p. 947-8.

183 Thyagarajan SP, Subramanian S, Thirunalasundar Total Effect of Phyllanthus amarus on chronic carriers of hepatitis B virus. Lancet 1988: ii: pp.764–6
184 Kapoor LD. *Handbook of Ayurvedic Medicinal Plants.* Boca Raton, FL. CRC Press; 1990
185 Anand KK, Singh B, Saxena AK, Chandan BK, Gupta VN, Bhardwaj V3,4,5-Trihydroxy benzoic acid (gallic acid), the hepatoprotective principle in the fruits of Terminalia belerica-bioassay guided activity. *Pharmacol Res* 1997 Oct;36(4):315-21
186 Shaila HP, Udupa AL, Udupa SL Preventive actions of Terminalia belerica in experimentally induced atherosclerosis. *Int J Cardiol* 1995 Apr;49(2):101-6
187 Aegle marmelos Monograph, Himalaya Healthcare, http://www.himalayahealthcare.com/herbfinder/h_aegle.htm
188 Singh A Rao AR Evaluation of the modulatory influence of black pepper (Piper nigrum, L.) on the hepatic detoxication system. Cancer-Lett. 1993 Aug 16; 72(1-2): 5-9
189 Kaoul I and A Kapil. *Evaluation of the liver protective potential of piperine, an active principal of black and long peppers.*Planta Medica 1993. 59: 413-417.
190 Shanmugasundaram KR et al, *Amritabindu for depletion of antioxidants. Journal of Ethnopharmacology.* 1994. 42(2): 83-93.
191 Liao S; Hiipakka RA Selective inhibition of steroid 5 alpha-reductase isozymes by tea epicatechin-3-gallate and epigallocatechin-3-gallate. Biochem Biophys Res Commun, 1995 Sep 25, 214:3, 833-8
192 Gupta S, Ahmad N, Mohan RR, Husain MM, Mukhtar H Prostate cancer chemoprevention by green tea: in vitro and in vivo inhibition of testosterone-mediated induction of ornithine decarboxylase. *Cancer Res* 1999 May1;59(9):2115-20
193 *Mayo Clin Health Lett* 1999 Apr;17(4):4 Ingredient in green tea kills prostate cancer cells, study finds.
194 Masami Suganuma, Sachiko Okabe, Yasuko Kai, Naoko Sueoka, Eisaburo Sueoka, and Hirota Fujiki Synergistic Effects of (-)-Epigallocatechin Gallate with (-)-Epicatechin, Sulindac, or Tamoxifen on Cancer-preventive Activity in the Human Lung Cancer Cell Line PC-9 CANCER RESEARCH 59, 44-47, January 1, 1999]
195 Rasheed A, Haider M Antibacterial activity of Camellia sinensis extracts against dental caries. *Arch Pharm Res* 1998 Jun;21(3):348-52
196 Otake S, Makimura M, Kuroki T, Nishihara Y, Hirasawa M Anticaries effects of polyphenolic compounds from Japanese green tea. *Caries Res* 1991;25(6):438-43
197 Rasheed A, Haider M Antibacterial activity of Camellia sinensis extracts against dental caries. *Arch Pharm Res* 1998 Jun;21(3):348-52
198 Van Het Hof KH, Wiseman SA, Yang CS, Tijburg LB Plasma and lipoprotein levels of tea catechins following repeated tea consumption. *Proc Soc Exp Biol Med* 1999 Apr;220(4):203-9
199 Stensvold I, Tverdal A, Solvoll K, Foss OP. Tea consumption. relationship to cholesterol, blood pressure, and coronary and total mortality. Prev Med 1992 Jul;21(4):546-53
200 Han LK, Takaku T, Li J, Kimura Y, Okuda H Anti-obesity action of oolong tea. *Int J Obes Relat Metab Disord* 1999 Jan;23(1):98-105
201 Dulloo AG, Duret C, Rohrer D, Girardier L, Mensi N, Fathi M, Chantre P, Vandermander J. Efficacy of a green tea extract rich in catechin polyphenols and caffeine in increasing 24-h energy expenditure and fat oxidation in humans. Am J Clin Nutr 1999 Dec;70(6):1040-5
202 Kono S, Shinchi K, Ikeda N, Yanai F, Imanishi K. Green tea consumption and serum lipid profiles: a cross-sectional study in northern Kyushu, Japan. Prev Med 1992 Jul;21(4):526-31
203 Hu, Z. (1992) Mitogenic activity of (-) epigallocatechin gallate on B-cells and investigation of structure-function relationship. *Int. J. Immunopharmacol.* 14 : 1399-1407.
204 Ryu, E. (1982) Prophylactic effect of tea on pathogenic microorganism infection to animals and humans. *Int. J. Zoonoses.* 9 : 126-131.
205 Clark KJ, Grant PG, Sarr AB, Belakere JR, Swaggerty CL, Phillips TD, Woode GN An in vitro study of theaflavins extracted from black tea to neutralize bovine rotavirus and bovine coronavirus infections. *Vet Microbiol* 1998 Oct;63(2-4):147-57

206 Nakane, H. and Ono,K. (1989) Differential inhibition of HIV-reverse transcriptase and various DNA and RNA polymerases by some catechin derivatives. Nucleic Acids Research, Symposium series 21, 115.

207 TS Yam, JM Hamilton-Miller, S Shah, The effect of a component of tea (Camellia sinensis) on methicillin resistance, PBP2' synthesis, and beta-lactamase production in Staphylococcus aureus. J. Antimicrob. Chemother. 1998 42: 211-216

208 Shetty, M. et al 1994 Antibacterial activity of tea (*Camellia sinensis*) and coffee (Coffee arabica) with specialreference to *Salmonella typhimurium. J. Commun. Dis.* 26: 147-150.

209 Conney, A.H., et al. "Inhibitory effect of green tea on tumorigenesis by chemicals and ultraviolet light," Prev Med, 21(3): 361-69, May 1992.

210 Sohn OS; Surace A; Fiala ES; Richie JP Jr; Colosimo S; Zang E; Weisburger JH Effects of green and black tea on hepatic xenobiotic metabolizing systems in the male F344 rat. Xenobiotica 1994 Feb; 24 (2): 119-27

211 Liao S; Hiipakka RA Selective inhibition of steroid 5 alpha-reductase isozymes by tea epicatechin-3-gallate and epigallocatechin-3-gallate. Biochem Biophys Res Commun, 1995 Sep 25, 214:3, 833-8

212 Sadakata, S. Et al. (1995). Mortality among female practitioners of Chanyou (Japanese tea ceremony). *Tohoku J. Exp. Med.* 166:475-477.

213 Rai D, Bhatia G, Palit G, Pal R, Singh S, Singh HK. Adaptogenic effect of Bacopa monniera (Brahmi). Pharmacol Biochem Behav. 2003 Jul; 75(4): 823-30.

214 Chowdhuri DK, Parmar D, Kakkar P, Shukla R, Seth PK, Srimal RC. Antistress effects of bacosides of Bacopa monnieri: modulation of Hsp70 expression, superoxide dismutase and cytochrome P450 activity in rat brain. Phytother Res. 2002 Nov; 16(7): 639-45.

215 Kidd PM.A review of nutrients and botanicals in the integrative management of cognitive dysfunction. Altern Med Rev 1999 Jun;4(3):144-61

216 Roodenrys S, Booth D, Bulzomi S, Phipps A, Micallef C, Smoker J. Chronic effects of Brahmi (Bacopa monnieri) on human memory. Neuropsychopharmacology. 2002 Aug; 27(2): 279-81.

217 Singh, R.H. and Singh, L.(1980). Studies on the anti-anxiety effect of the Medhya Rasayana drug Brahmi *(Bacopa monniera Wet.)- Part 1. J. Res. Ayurveda and Siddha* 1:133-148

218 Ashok D.B. Vaidya, The Status And Scope Of Indian Medicinal Plants Acting On Central Nervous System Indian J Pharmacol 1997; 29: S340-S343

219 Quadri A.A., Mentat (BR-16A) in mentally retarded children with behavioural problems. *Current Medical Practice* 1993; (37): 121-125

220 Agrawal, A., Gupta, U., Dixit, S.P., Dubey, G.P. (1993) Management of mental deficiency by an indigenous drug Brahmi. Pharmacopsychoecologia, Vol 6(1) 1-5.

221 Quadri A.A., Mentat (BR-16A) in mentally retarded children with behavioural problems. *Current Medical Practice* 1993; (37): 121-125

222 Sharma R, Chaturvedi C, Tewari PV. Efficacy of Bacopa monniera in revitalizing intellectual functions in children. J Res Edu Ind Med 1987:1-12.

223 Negi, K.S. et al. (2000) Indian Journal of Psychiatry, Vol 42 April, Supplement, http://www.ijponline.org/indIJP-%20PsychoPharmacology.html

224 Mukherjee, GD and Dey, CD (1968) Comparative study on the antiepileptic action of some common phytoproducts. Journal of Experimental Medical Sciences.11(4):82-85

225 Vohora D, Pal SN, Pillai KK.Protection from phenytoin-induced cognitive deficit by Bacopa monniera, a reputed Indian nootropic plant. J Ethnopharmacol 2000 Aug;71(3):383-90

226 Tripathi YB Chaurasia S Tripathi E Upadhyay A Dubey GP Bacopa monniera Linn. as an antioxidant: mechanism of action. Indian-J-Exp-Biol. 1996 Jun; 34(6): 523-6 1996

227 Russo A, Izzo AA, Borrelli F, Renis M, Vanella A. Free radical scavenging capacity and protective effect of Bacopa monniera L. on DNA damage. Phytother Res. 2003 Sep; 17(8): 870-5.

228 Nadkarni, Dr. K.M. 1976. *The Indian Materia Medica, with Ayurvedic, Unani and Home Remedies.* Revised and enlarged by A.K. Nadkarni. 1954. Reprint. Bombay: Bombay Popular Prakashan PVP. p. 469
229 Saxena, A.K. et al. 1993. Hepatoprotective effects of Eclipta alba on subcellular levels in rats. J Ethnopharmacol. Dec;40(3):155-61
230 Singh B, Saxena AK, Chandan BK, Agarwal SG, Anand KK. In vivo hepatoprotective activity of active fraction from ethanolic extract of Eclipta alba leaves. Indian J Physiol Pharmacol. 2001 Oct;45(4):435-41.
231 Frawley, David and Vasant Lad. 1986. *The Yoga Of Herbs: An Ayurvedic Guide to Herbal Medicine.* Twin Lakes, WI: Lotus Press. P. 163.
232 Dash, Bhagwan. *Materia Medica of Ayurveda.* New Delhi: B. Jain Publishers. 1991. p.82
233 Eclipta Monograph, Himalaya Herbal Healthcare, http://www.himalayahealthcare.com/herbfinder/h_eclipt.htm
234 Kumari CS, Govindasamy S, Sukumar E. Lipid lowering activity of Eclipta prostrata in experimental hyperlipidemia. J Ethnopharmacol. 2006 Jan 4; [Epub ahead of print]
235 Charaka Samhita Ci 10.27
236 Srikantha Murthy, K.R. *Vagbhata's Astanga Hrdayam.* vol. 3. Varanasi: Krishnadas Academy. 1995. p. 387
237 Personal interview
238 Weiss, Rudolf. 1988. *Herbal Medicine.* Translated by A.R. Meuss. Beaconsfield, England: Beaconsfield Publishers.
239 Menon M.K. and P.C. Dandiya. 1967. The mechanism of the tranquillizing action of asarone from Acorus calamus Linn. J Pharm Pharmacol. Mar;19(3):170-5
240 Miller, Richard Alan. 1993. *The Magical and Ritual use of Herbs.* Rochester, Vermont: Destiny Books. P. 58.
241 deJager, Prashanti, Medhya Herbs and Therapies, *Light on Ayurveda,* IV: 3 (Spring 2005).
242 deJager, Prashanti, Medhya Herbs and Therapies, *Light on Ayurveda,* IV: 3 (Spring 2005).
243 Personal communication with Michael Tierra
244 Personal Communication with Karta Purkh Singh Khalsa
245 Al-Zuhair H, el-Sayeh B, Ameen HA, al-Shoora H Pharmacological studies of cardamom oil in animals. *Pharmacol Res* 1996 Jul-Aug;34(1-2):79-82
246 Black Cardamom Monograph, Gernot Kinzer's Spice Pages, http://www.kfunigraz.ac.at/~katzer/engl/Amom_sub.html
247 Kapoor, L. D., CRC *Handbook of Ayurvedic Medicinal Plants*
248 Tierra, Michael and Lesley, *Overview: Planetary Herbology* www.planetherbs.com
249 Tierra, Michael and Lesley, *Overview Planetary Herbology* http://www.planetherbs.com/articles/introduction_to_planetary_herbol.htm
250 Johari, Harish. *Ayurvedic Massage.* Healing Arts. Rochester, 1996.
251 Alternative Medicine Online http://library.thinkquest.org/24206/ayurvedamedicine. html?tqskip1=1&tqtime=0529#common
252 Lad, Vasant, *The Complete Book of Ayurvedic Home Remedies,* Harmony Books, New York, 1998, p.202
253 Frawley, David. Ayurvedic Healing, Lotus Press: Twin Lakes, WI
254 Yogi Bhajan Lecture 8/13/76
255 Bensky, Dan, and Gamble, Andrew, *Chinese Materia Medica,* Eastland Press, Seattle, 1986.
256 Hu CQ Chen K Shi Q Kilkuskie RE Cheng YC Lee KH Anti-AIDS agents, 10. Acacetin-7-O-beta-Dgalactopyranoside, an anti-HIV principle from Chrysanthemum morifolium and a structure-activity correlation with some related flavonoids. J-Nat-Prod. 1994 Jan; 57(1): 42-51
257 Wang HK, Xia Y, Yang ZY, Natschke SL, Lee KH Recent advances in the discovery and development of flavonoids and their analogues as antitumor and anti-HIV agents. *Adv Exp Med Biol* 1998;439:191-225

258 Dhuley JN Anti-oxidant effects of cinnamon (Cinnamomum verum) bark and greater cardamom (Amomum subulatum) seeds in rats fed high fat diet. *Indian J Exp Biol* 1999 Mar;37(3):238-42
259 Mancini-Filho J, Van-Koiij A, Mancini DA, Cozzolino FF, Torres RP Antioxidant activity of cinnamon (Cinnamomum Zeylanicum, Breyne) extracts. *Boll Chim Farm* 1998 Dec;137(11):443-7
260 Kurokawa M, Kumeda CA, Yamamura J, Kamiyama T, Shiraki K Antipyretic activity of cinnamyl derivatives and related compounds in influenza virus-infected mice. *Eur J Pharmacol* 1998 May 1;348(1):45-51
261 Jennifer Wurges, Cinnamon bark, Gale Encyclopedia of Alternative Medicine, http://www.findarticles.com/cf_0/g2603/0000/2603000034/p1/article.jhtml
262 Eugene Zampieron, ND, Cinnamon.(therapeutic uses) Healthy & Natural Journal Dec, 2000 http://www.findarticles.com/cf_0/m0HKL/6_7/76471212/p1/article.jhtml
263 Monograph- Cinnamon, Bastyr University Department of Botanical Medicine
264 Peter Landau, *Cinnamon Found to Kill Deadly E.coli Bacteria.* Chemical Market Reporter, August 23, 1999 http://www.findarticles.com/cf_0/m0FVP/8_256/55549452/p1/article.jhtml
265 Inouye S, Yamaguchi H, Takizawa T., Screening of the antibacterial effects of a variety of essential oils on respiratory tract pathogens, using a modified dilution assay method. J Infect Chemother 2001 Dec;7(4):251-4
266 Chang ST, Chen PF, Chang SC. Antibacterial activity of leaf essential oils and their constituents from Cinnamomum osmophloeum. J Ethnopharmacol 2001 Sep;77(1):123-7Department of Forestry, National Taiwan University, No 1
267 Judy Mcbride, Cinnamon Extracts Boost Insulin Sensitivity. (Agricultural Research Service) July, 2000 http://www.findarticles.com/cf_0/m3741/7_48/63986959/p1/article.jhtml
268 Lee Scheier, *Salicylic acid: One more reason to eat your fruits and vegetables.* (For Your Information). Journal of the American Dietetic Association Dec, 2001 http://www.findarticles.com/cf_0/m0822/12_101/80949235/p1/article.jhtml
269 Patti Woods-Lavoie Heating Things Up (in the Kitchen), Better Nutrition, Feb, 2001, http://www.findarticles.com/cf_0/m0FKA/2_63/78476721/print.jhtml
270 http://www.medsupport.org/brainscents.htm
271 Personal communication from Yogi Bhajan with Karta Purkh Singh Khalsa
272 Arai I, Amagaya S, Komatsu Y, Okada M, Hayashi T, Kasai M, Arisawa M, Momose Y Improving effects of the extracts from Eugenia uniflora on hyperglycemia and hypertriglyceridemia in mice. *J Ethnopharmacol* 1999 Dec 15;68(1-3):307-14
273 Coleus Monograph, DiagnoseMe, http://www.diagnose-me.com/treat/T390160.html
274 Seamon, K.B., and Daly, J.W. Forkskolin: A unique diterpene activator of cAMP-generating systems. J. Cyclic Nucleotide Research 7 (1981): 201-24
275 Coleus Monograph, GrowGreen Bio Sciences, http://www.growgreen.in/medicinal-herbs.html
276 Badmaev, Vladimir, Majeed, Muhammed, Ayurvedic herb Coleus forskohlii shows promise in enhancing lean body mass, Health Supplement Retailer, http://www.hsrmagazine.com/articles/071feat3.html
277 Han LK, Morimoto C, Yu RH, Okuda H. Effects of Coleus forskohlii on fat storage in ovariectomized rats. Yakugaku Zasshi. 2005 May;125(5):449-53.
278 Chithra V, Leelamma S Coriandrum sativum changes the levels of lipid peroxides and activity of antioxidant enzymes in experimental animals. *Indian J Biochem Biophys* 1999 Feb;36(1):59-61
279 Cumin Monograph, Encyclopedia of Spices, The Epicentre, http://www.theepicentre.com/Spices/cumin.html
280 Nadkarni, AK, Indian Materia Medica, Popular Prakashan, Bombay, 1976, p.1195.
281 Murray, Michael, and Pizzorno, Joseph, Encyclopedia of Natural Medicine, Prima, Rocklin, California, 1998.
282 Baba K et al. Antitumor activity of hot water extract of dandelion, *Taraxacum officinale*-correlation between antitumor activity and timing of administration. *Yagugaku Zasshi* 1981; 101: 583-43.

283 McDaniel, Douglas, "Traditional Chinese Specific Condition Review: Mastitis," *Protocol Journal of Botanical Medicine,* Spring, 1996, p.76.

284 Bensky, Dan, and Gamble, Andrew, *Chinese Materia Medica,* Eastland Press, Seattle, 1986, p.129.

285 Baba K et al. Antitumor activity of hot water extract of dandelion, *Taraxacum officinale*-correlation between antitumor activity and timing of administration. Yagugaku Zasshi 1981; 101: 583-43.

286 Yu Tiao-zhong, "Herba Taraxaci Mongolici Cum Radice (Pu Gong Ying) as the Main Treatment in Gynecological Recalcitrant, Difficult Conditions", Xin Zhong Yi *(New Chinese Medicine),* #5, 1996, p.46

287 Stansbury, Jill, "Botanical Therapies for Fibrocystic Breast Disease," Medical Herbalism, Summer 1997, p.1.

288 Stansbury, Jill, "Botanical Therapies for Fibrocystic Breast Disease," Medical Herbalism, Summer 1997, p.1.

289 Abdul Ghani AS Amin R The vascular action of aqueous extracts of Foeniculum vulgare leaves. JEthnopharmacol. 1988 Dec; 24(2-3): 213-8

290 Tanira MOM, Shah AH, Mohsin A, et al. Pharmacological and toxicological investigations on *Foeniculum vulgare* dried fruit extract in experimental animals. *Phytother Res* 1996;10:33-6.

291 Vasudevan K, Vembar S, Veeraraghavan K, Haranath PS Influence of intragastric perfusion of aqueous spice extracts on acid secretion in anesthetized albino rats. *Indian J Gastroenterol* 2000 Apr-Jun;19(2):53-6

292 Falcao, Ronnie, LM, MS, Breastfeeding, http://www.gentlebirth.org/archives/bestfeed.html

293 Organic Mother's Milk, Traditional Medicinals, http://www.traditionalmedicinals.com/?id=30&pid=14 294 Zia T, Hasnain SN, Hasan SK. Evaluation of the oral hypoglycaemic effect of Trigonella foenum-graecum L. (methi) in normal mice. J Ethnopharmacol 2001 May;75(2-3):191-195

295 Platel K, Srinivasan K. Influence of dietary spices and their active principles on pancreatic digestive enzymes in albino rats. Nahrung 2000 Feb;44(1):42-46

296 Balabanov P, Karamanos AP. Central effects of AC-1 and TFG-1. Folia Med (Plovdiv) 1998;40(3BSuppl 3):110-113

297 Taylor WG, Elder JL, Chang PR, Richards KW. Microdetermination of diosgenin from fenugreek (Trigonella foenum-graecum) seeds. J Agric Food Chem 2000 Nov;48(11):5206-5210

298 Murakami T, Kishi A, Matsuda H, Yoshikawa M. Medicinal foodstuffs. XVII. Fenugreek seed. (3): structures of new furostanol-type steroid saponins, trigoneosides Xa, Xb, XIb, XIIa, XIIb, and XIIIa, from the seeds of Egyptian Trigonellafoenum-graecum L. Chem Pharm Bull (Tokyo) 2000 Jul;48(7):994-1000

299 Sharma RD, Sarkar A, Hazra DK, et al. Use of fenugreek seed powder in the management of non-insulin dependent diabetes mellitus. *Nutr Res.* 1996;16:1331–1339.

300 Madar Z, Abel R, Samish S, Arad J. Glucose-lowering effect of fenugreek in non-insulin dependent diabetics. Eur J Clin Nutr 1988 Jan;42(1):51-54

301 Sharma RD, Raghuram TC, Rao NS. Effect of fenugreek seeds on blood glucose and serum lipids in type I diabetes. Eur J Clin Nutr 1990 Apr;44(4):301-306

302 Broca C, Manteghetti M, Gross R, Baissac Y, Jacob M, Petit P, Sauvaire Y, Ribes G. 4-Hydroxyisoleucine: effects of synthetic and natural analogues on insulin secretion. Eur J Pharmacol 2000 Mar 3;390(3):339-345 303 Broca C, Gross R, Petit P, Sauvaire Y, Manteghetti M, Tournier M, Masiello P, Gomis R, Ribes G. 4- Hydroxyisoleucine: experimental evidence of its insulinotropic and antidiabetic properties. Am J Physiol 1999 Oct;277(4 Pt 1):E617-E623

304 Sauvaire Y, Petit P, Broca C, Manteghetti M, Baissac Y, Fernandez-Alvarez J, Gross R, Roye M, Leconte A, Gomis R, Ribes G. 4-Hydroxyisoleucine: a novel amino acid potentiator of insulin secretion. Diabetes 1998 Feb;47(2):206-210

305 Sharma RD, et al. Hypolipidaemic effect of fenugreek seeds: a chronic study in non-insulin dependent diabetic patients. Phytother Res 1996;10:332-4.
306 Ravikumar P, Anuradha CV. Effect of fenugreek seeds on blood lipid peroxidation and antioxidants in diabetic rats. Phytother Res 1999 May;13(3):197-201
307 Sowmya P, Rajyalakshmi P. Hypocholesterolemic effect of germinated fenugreek seeds in human subjects. Plant Foods Hum Nutr 1999;53(4):359-365
308 Evans AJ, Hood RL, Oakenfull DG, Sidhu GS. Relationship between structure and function of dietary fibre: a comparative study of the effects of three galactomannans on cholesterol metabolism in the rat. Br J Nutr 1992 Jul;68(1):217-229
309 Fenugreek, The Natural Pharmacist, http://www.tnp.com/encyclopedia/substance/45
310 Choudhary D, Chandra D, Choudhary S, Kale RK. Modulation of glyoxalase, glutathione S-transferase and antioxidant enzymes in the liver, spleen and erythrocytes of mice by dietary administration of fenugreek seeds. Food Chem Toxicol 2001 Oct;39(10):989-997
311 Sur P, Das M, Gomes A, Vedasiromoni JR, Sahu NP, Banerjee S, Sharma RM, Ganguly DK. Trigonella foenum graecum (fenugreek) seed extract as an antineoplastic agent. Phytother Res 2001 May;15(3):257-259
312 Schmidt, Michael A., *Smart Fats,* North Atlantic Books, Berkeley, California, 1997
313 Silagy CA, Neil HA. A meta-analysis of the effect of garlic on blood pressure. J Hypertens 1994 Apr;12(4):463-8
314 Auer W, Eiber A, Hertkorn E, Hoehfeld E, Koehrle U, Lorenz A, Mader F, Merx W, Otto G, Schmid-Otto B, et al. Hypertension and hyperlipidaemia: garlic helps in mild cases. Br J Clin Pract Suppl 1990 Aug;69:3-6
315 Steiner M, Khan AH, Holbert D, Lin RI. A double-blind crossover study in moderately hypercholesterolemic men that compared the effect of aged garlic extract and placebo administration on blood lipids. Am J Clin Nutr 1996 Dec;64(6):866-70
316 Jonkers D, van den Broek E, van Dooren I, Thijs C, Dorant E, Hageman G, Stobberingh E Antibacterial effect of garlic and omeprazole on Helicobacter pylori. *J Antimicrob Chemother* 1999 Jun;43(6):837-9
317 Kasuga S, Ushijima M, Morihara N, Itakura Y, Nakata Y [Effect of aged garlic extract (AGE) on hyperglycemia induced by immobilization stress in mice]. *Nippon Yakurigaku Zasshi* 1999 Sep;114(3):191-7
318 Kumar GR, Reddy KP Reduced nociceptive responses in mice with alloxan induced hyperglycemia after garlic (Allium sativum Linn.) treatment. *Indian J Exp Biol* 1999 Jul;37(7):662-6
319 Arora DS, Kaur J Antimicrobial activity of spices. *Int J Antimicrob Agents* 1999 Aug;12(3):257-62.
320 Deshpande RG, Khan MB, Bhat DA, Navalkar RG Inhibition of Mycobacterium avium complex isolates from AIDS patients by garlic (Allium sativum). *J Antimicrob Chemother* 1993 Oct;32(4):623-6
321 Abdullah TH In vitro efficacy of a compound derived from garlic against Pneumocystis carinii. *J Natl Med Assoc* 1996 Nov;88(11):694, 704
322 Lee JH, Kang HS, Roh J Protective effects of garlic juice against embryotoxicity of methylmercuric chloride administered to pregnant Fischer 344 rats. *Yonsei Med* J 1999 Oct;40(5):483-9.
323 Helen A, Rajasree CR, Krishnakumar K, Augusti KT, Vijayammal PL Antioxidant role of oils isolated from garlic (Allium sativum Linn) and onion (Allium cepa Linn) on nicotine-induced lipid peroxidation. *Vet Hum Toxicol* 1999 Oct;41(5):316-9
324 Balasenthil S, Arivazhagan S, Ramachandran CR, Nagini S Effects of garlic on 7,12-Dimethylbenz[a]anthraceneinduced hamster buccal pouch carcinogenesis. *Cancer Detect Prev* 1999;23(6):534-8.

325 Chung JG Effects of garlic components diallyl sulfide and diallyl disulfide on arylamine N-acetyltransferase activity in human bladder tumor cells. *Drug Chem Toxicol* 1999 May;22(2):343-58.
326 Denisov LN, Andrianova IV, Timofeeva SS [Garlic effectiveness in rheumatoid arthritis]. *Ter Arkh* 1999;71(8):55-8
327 Yogi Bhajan Lecture 4/11/83
328 Zhao C, Shichi H Prevention of acetaminophen-induced cataract by a combination of diallyl disulfide and Nacetylcysteine. *J Ocul Pharmacol Ther* 1998 Aug;14(4):345-55
329 Marz RW, Ismail C, Popp MA [Profile and effectiveness of a phytogenic combination preparation for treatment of sinusitis]. *Wien Med Wochenschr* 1999;149(8-10):202-8
330 Frawley, David, and Lad, Vasant, *The Yoga of Herbs,* Lotus Press, Twin Lakes, WI, 1986.
331 Ahmed RS Sharma SB Biochemical studies on combined effects of garlic (Allium sativum Linn) and ginger (Zingiber officinale Rosc) in albino rats. *Indian J Exp Biol.* 1997 Aug; 35(8): 841-3
332 Ernst E, Pittler MH. Efficacy of ginger for nausea and vomiting: a systematic review of randomized clinical trials. Br J Anaesth 2000 Mar;84(3):367-71.
333 McCaleb, Robert S., Herb Research Foundation Encyclopedia of Popular Herbs, Prima, Roseville, California, 2000.
334 M, Busse WR, Goldberg A, et al, eds. *The Complete German Commission E Monographs: Therapeutic Guide to Herbal Medicines.* Austin: American Botanical Council and Boston: Integrative Medicine Communications, 1998, 167.
335 Gupta YK, Sharma M. Reversal of pyrogallol-induced delay in gastric emptying in rats by ginger (Zingiber officinale).Methods Find Exp Clin Pharmacol 2001 Nov;23(9):501-3.
336 Vutyavanich T, Kraisarin T, Ruangsri RA. Ginger for nausea and vomiting in pregnancy: randomized, doublemasked, placebo-controlled trial. Obstet Gynecol., 2001; 97:577-82.
337 Keating A, Chez R. Ginger syrup as an anti emetic in early pregnancy, *Altern Ther Health Med* 2002;8:89-91.
338 Ginger. The Chopra Center, http://www.chopra.com/article.asp?program=general&id=25
339 Fuhrman B, Rosenblat M, Hayek T, Coleman R, Aviram M Ginger extract consumption reduces plasma cholesterol, inhibits LDL oxidation and attenuates development of atherosclerosis in atherosclerotic, apolipoprotein E-deficient mice. *J Nutr* 2000 May;130(5):1124-31.
340 Bhandari U, Sharma JN, Zafar R The protective action of ethanolic ginger (Zingiber officinale) extract in cholesterol fed rabbits. *J Ethnopharmacol* 1998 Jun;61(2):167-7.
341 Bordia A, Verma SK, Srivastava KC Effect of ginger (Zingiber officinale Rosc.) and fenugreek (Trigonella foenumgraecum L.) on blood lipids, blood sugar and platelet aggregation in patients with coronary artery disease. *Prostaglandins Leukot Essent Fatty Acids* 1997 May;56(5):379-84
342 Thomson M, Al-Qattan KK, Al-Sawan SM, Alnaqeeb MA, Khan I, Ali M. The use of ginger (Zingiber officinale Rosc.) as a potential anti-inflammatory and antithrombotic agent. Prostaglandins Leukot Essent Fatty Acids 2002 Dec;67(6):475-8.
343 Vimala S, Norhanom AW, Yadav M Anti-tumour promoter activity in Malaysian ginger rhizobia used in traditional medicine. *Br J Cancer* 1999 Apr;80(1-2):110-6
344 Lee E, Park KK, Lee JM, Chun KS, Kang JY, Lee SS, Surh YJ Suppression of mouse skin tumor promotion and induction of apoptosis in HL-60 cells by Alpinia oxyphylla Miquel (Zingiberaceae). *Carcinogenesis* 1998 Aug;19(8):1377-81
345 Park KK, Chun KS, Lee JM, Lee SS, Surh YJ Inhibitory effects of [6]-gingerol, a major pungent principle of ginger, on phorbol ester-induced inflammation, epidermal ornithine decarboxylase activity and skin tumor promotion in ICR mice. *Cancer Lett* 1998 Jul 17;129(2):139-44
346 Sharma JN, Srivastava KC, Gan EK Suppressive effects of eugenol and ginger oil on arthritic rats. *Pharmacology* 1994 Nov;49(5):314-8.
347 Srivastava KC, Mustafa T Ginger (Zingiber officinale) and rheumatic disorders. *Med Hypotheses* 1989 May;29(1):25- 8

348 Weinberg, Norma Pasekoff, *Natural and Herbal Remedies for Carpal Tunnel Syndrome* (Storey Books, Pownal Vermont, 2000)
349 Mustafa T, Srivastava KC. Ginger (Zingiber officinale) in migraine headache. J Ethnopharmacol 1990 Jul;29(3):267- 73.
350 Joanna Piatek, *Cooking with Ginger,* Digs Magazine.com http://www.digsmagazine.com/nourish/nourish_farmerjoginger. htm
351 http://www.culinarycafe.com/Spices_Herbs/Ginger.html
352 McCormick Spice Usage http://www.mccormick.com/content.cfm?id=10092
353 Uma Pradeep K, Geervani P, Eggum BO. Common Indian spices: nutrient composition, consumption and contribution to dietary value. Plant Foods Hum Nutr 1993 Sep;44(2):137-48
354 Phillips OA, Mathew KT, Oriowo MA. Antihypertensive and vasodilator effects of methanolic and aqueous extracts of Tribulus terrestris in rats. J Ethnopharmacol. 2006 Apr 6;104(3):351-5. Epub 2005 Nov 9.
355 1-TOP Capsules http://www.impotence-herbal.com/action.htm
356 Gauthaman K, Ganesan AP, Prasad RN. Sexual effects of puncturevine (Tribulus terrestris) extract (protodioscin): an evaluation using a rat model. J Altern Complement Med. 2003 Apr;9(2):257-65.
357 Vedavathy S, Rao KN. 1991. Antipyretic activity of six indigenous medicinal plants of Tirumala Hills, Andhra Pradesh, India. *Journal of Ethnopharmacology* 33(1-2): p 193-196.
358 Prince PS. Menon VP. Gunasekaran G. 1999. Hypolipidemic action of Tinospora cordifolia roots in alloxan diabetic rats. *Journal of Ethnopharmacology* 64(1): p 53-57.
359 Rao EV, Rao MV. 1981. Studies on the polysaccharide preparation (Guduchisatwa) derived from Tinospora cordifolia. *Indian Journal of Pharmaceutical Sciences* 43(May-Jun):103-106.
360 Nadkarni K. M. 1908. Indian Materia Medica Plants. Popular Prakashan Private Ltd., Bombay, India. 1908
361 Verma SK, Bordia A. Effect of Commiphora mukul (gum guggulu) in patients of hyperlipidemia with special reference to HDL-cholesterol. Indian J Med Res 1988 Apr;87:356-60
362 Satyavati GV. Gum guggul (Commiphora mukul)--the success story of an ancient insight leading to a modern discovery. Indian J Med Res 1988 Apr;87:327-35
363 Tripathi YB, Malhotra OP, Tripathi SN. Thyroid stimulating action of Z-guggulsterone obtained from Commiphora mukul. Planta Med 1984 Feb;(1):78-80
364 Satyavati GV, Dwarakanath C, Tripathi SN. Experimental studies on the hypocholesterolemic effect of Commiphora mukul. Engl. (Guggul). Indian J Med Res 1969 Oct;57(10):1950-62
365 Paranjpe P, Patki P, Patwardhan B. Ayurvedic treatment of obesity: a randomised double-blind, placebo-controlled clinical trial. J Ethnopharmacol 1990 Apr;29(1):1-11
366 Antonio J, Colker CM, Torina GC, et al. Effects of a standardized guggulsterone phosphate supplement on body composition in overweight adults: A pilot study. *Curr Ther Res* 1999;60:220-7.
367 Shanmugasundaram KR, Panneerselvam C, Sumudram P, Shanmugasundaram ERB. Insulinotropic activity of G. sylvestre, R.Br. and Indian medicinal herb used in controlling diabetes mellitus. Pharmacol Res Commun 1981;13:475–86.
368 Bishayee A, Chatterjee M. Hypolipidemic and antiatherosclerotic effects of oral Gymnema sylvestre R.Br. leaf extract in albino rats fed on a high fat diet. Phytother Res 1994;8:118–20.
369 The National Institute of Ayurvedic Medicine http://www.niam.com/
370 Baskaran K, Ahmath BK, Shanmugasundaram KR, Shanmugasundaram ERB. Antidiabetic effect of a leaf extract from Gymnema sylvestre in non-insulin-dependent diabetes mellitus patients. J Ethnopharmacol 1990;30:295–305.
371 Shanmugasundaram ER, Rajeswari G, Baskaran K, Rajesh Kumar BR, Radha Shanmugasundaram K, Kizar Ahmath B. Use of Gymnema sylvestre leaf extract in the control of blood glucose in insulin-dependent diabetes mellitus. J Ethnopharmacol. 1990 Oct;30(3):281-94.

372 Baskaran K, Kizar Ahamath B, Radha Shanmugasundaram K, Shanmugasundaram ER. Antidiabetic effect of a leaf extract from Gymnema sylvestre in non-insulin-dependent diabetes mellitus patients. J Ethnopharmacol. 1990 Oct;30(3):295-300.
373 Prakash AO, Mather S, Mather R. Effect of feeding Gymnema sylvestre leaves on blood glucose in beryllium nitrate treated rats. J Ethnopharmacol 1986;18:143-146.
374 Shanmugasundaram ER, Gopinath KL. Shanmugasundaram KR, Rojendran VM. Possible regeneration of the islets of Langerhans in streptozotocin-diabetic rats given Gymnema sylvestre leaf extracts. J Ethnopharmacol 1990;30:265-279.
375 Kapoor LD. *Handbook of Ayurvedic Medicinal Plants.* Boca Raton, FL. CRC Press; 1990:322
376 Jagtap AG, Karkera SG. Potential of the aqueous extract of Terminalia chebula as an anticaries agent. *J Ethnopharmacol.* 1999 Dec 15;68(1-3):299-306
377 Saleem A, Husheem M, Harkonen P, Pihlaja K. Inhibition of cancer cell growth by crude extract and the phenolics of Terminalia chebula retz. fruit. J Ethnopharmacol 2002 Aug;81(3):327-36
378 Suguna L, Singh S, Sivakumar P, Sampath P, Chandrakasan G. Influence of Terminalia chebula on dermal wound healing in rats. Phytother Res 2002 May;16(3):227-31
379 Odigie IP, Ettarh RR, Adigun SA. Chronic administration of aqueous extract of Hibiscus sabdariffa attenuates hypertension and reverses cardiac hypertrophy in 2K-1C hypertensive rats. J Ethnopharmacol. 2003 Jun;86(2-3):181-5.
380 Herrera-Arellano A, Flores-Romero S, Chavez-Soto MA, Tortoriello J. Effectiveness and tolerability of a standardized extract from Hibiscus sabdariffa in patients with mild to moderate hypertension: a controlled and randomized clinical trial. Phytomedicine. 2004 Jul;11(5):375-82.
381 Ali BH, Al Wabel N, Blunden G. Phytochemical, pharmacological and toxicological aspects of Hibiscus sabdariffa L.: a review. Phytother Res. 2005 May;19(5):369-75.
382 Jambolan Monograph, The New Crop Resource Online Program, Pudue University, http://www.hort.purdue.edu/newcrop/morton/jambolan.html
383 Smith, Ed, Single Herb Extracts, http://www.herbaled.org/THM/Singles/jambul.html
384 Chakravarti, Sree, A Healer's Journey, Rudra Press, 1993
385 Jambul Mongraph, Ayurveda Marketplace, http://www.ayurveda-herbal-remedy.com/indian herbs/syzygiumcumini.html
386 Jones SM, Zhong Z, Enomoto N, Schemmer P, Thurman RG Dietary juniper berry oil minimizes hepatic reperfusion injury in the rat. *Hepatology,* 1998 Oct;28(4):1042-50
387 Caceres DD, Hancke JL, Burgos RA, Sandberg F, Wikman GK Use of visual analogue scale measurements (VAS) to asses the effectiveness of standardized Andrographis paniculata extract SHA-10 in reducing the symptoms of common cold. A randomized double blind-placebo study. *Phytomedicine,* 1999 Oct;6(4):217-23
388 Thom, E. Wollan, T. A controlled clinical study of Kanjang mixture in the treatment of uncomplicated upper respiratory tract infections PTR,-Phytother-res. Sussex : John Wiley & Sons. May 1997. v. 11 (3) p. 207-210. 1997 0951-418X
389 Chang RS, Ding L, Chen GQ, Pan QC, Zhao ZL, Smith KM Dehydroandrographolide succinic acid monoester as an inhibitor against the human immunodeficiency virus. *Proc Soc Exp Biol* Med 1991 May;197(1):59-66
390 Calabrese C, Berman SH, Babish JG, Ma X, Shinto L, Dorr M, Wells K, Wenner CA, Standish LJ A phase I trial of andrographolide in HIV positive patients and normal volunteers. *Phytother Res* 2000 Aug;14(5):333-8
391 Kokam Mon ograph, India Agro Industry, http://www.agriculture-industry-india.com/spices/ kokam.html
392 Journal of the Canadian Association of Herbal Practitioners, (Winter 1996).
393 Holarrhena antidysenterica Monograph, Siris Impex, http://www.sirisimpex.com/holarrhena.htm
394 Holarrhena antidysenterica Monograph, Himalaya Herbal Healthcare, http://www.himalayahealthcare.com/herbfinder/h_holarr.htm

395 Kavitha D, Shilpa PN, Devaraj SN. Antibacterial and antidiarrhoeal effects of alkaloids of Holarrhena antidysenterica
WALL. Indian J Exp Biol. 2004 Jun;42(6):589-94.
396 Chakraborty A, Brantner AH. Antibacterial steroid alkaloids from the stem bark of Holarrhena pubescens. J Ethnopharmacol, 1999 Dec 15;68(1-3):339-44.
397 Joy KL, Kuttan R. Anti-diabetic activity of Picrorrhiza kurroa extract. J Ethnopharmacol, 1999 Nov 1;67(2):143-8.
398 British Journal of Dermatology, 1994; 130:488-93.
399 Yokozawa T, Liu ZW, Chen CP Protective effects of Glycyrrhizae radix extract and its compounds in a renal hypoxia (ischemia)-reoxygenation (reperfusion) model, *Phytomedicine* 2000 Jan;6(6):439-45
400 Yamashiki M, Nishimura A, Huang XX, Nobori T, Sakaguchi S, Suzuki H Effects of the Japanese herbal medicine "Sho-saiko-to" (TJ-9) on interleukin-12 production in patients with HCV-positive liver cirrhosis. *Dev Immunol* 1999;7(1):17-22
401 Vaidya, Ashok D.B. The Status And Scope Of Indian Medicinal Plants Acting On Central Nervous System. Indian J Pharmacol 1997; 29: S340-S343
402 Shulka, Bharat, *Benefits of Brahmi,* Ayurvedic Global Community, http://ayurvedahc.com/index.htm
403 Nalini K, et al. Effect of Centella asiatica fresh leaf aqueous extract on learning and memory and biogenic amine turnover in albino rats. Fitoterapia 1992; 63(3): 232-7
404 Mook-Jung I, Shin JE, Yun SH, Huh K, Koh JY, Park HK, Jew SS, Jung MW. Protective effects of asiaticoside derivatives against beta-amyloid neurotoxicity. *J Neurosci Res* 1999; Nov 1;58(3):417-25
405 Veerendra Kumar MH, Gupta YK. Effect of Centella asiatica on cognition and oxidative stress in an intracerebroventricular streptozotocin model of Alzheimer's disease in rats. Clin Exp Pharmacol Physiol. 2003 May- Jun;30(5-6):336-42.
406 Chen, Y.J., Y.S. Dai, B.F. Chen, A. Chang, H.C. Chen, Y.C. Lin, K.H. Chang, Y.L. Lai , C.H. Chung CH and Y.J. Lai. 1999. The effect of tetrandrine and extracts of *Centella asiatica* on acute radiation dermatitis in rats. *Biol Pharm Bull.* Jul; 22(7):703-6
407 Shukla, A., A.M. Rasik, G.K. Jain, R. Shankar. D.K. Kulshrestha, and B.N. Dhawan. 1999a. In vitro and in vivo wound healing activity of asiaticoside isolated from *Centella asiatica. J Ethnopharmacol* Apr; 65(1):1-11.
408 Chatterjee, T.K., A. Chakraborty, M. Pathak, and G.C. Sengupta. 1992. Effects of plant extract Centella asiatica (Linn.) on cold restraint stress ulcer in rats. *Indian J Exp Biol.* Oct; 30(10):889-91
409 Manduk Parni Monograph, Jiva Ayurveda, http://www.ayurvedic.org/ayubasics/mandukparni.asp?nm=Common%20Herbs&nm2=Manduk%20Parni
410 Rubia cordifolia Monopgraph, Himalaya Herbal Healthcare, http://www.himalayahealthcare.com/aboutayurveda/cahr.htm
411 Personal Communication with Michael Tierra
412 Dolara P, Luceri C, Ghelardini C, Monserrat C, Aiolli S, Luceri F, Lodovici M, Menichetti S, Romanelli MN Analgesic effects of myrrh. *Nature* 1996 Jan 4;379(6560):29
413 Neem Monograph, Jiva Ayurveda, Ayubasics, http://www.ayurvedic.org/ayubasics/neem.asp?nm=Common%20Herbs&nm2=Neem
414 Yogi Bhajan Lecture 5/3/74
415 Nutmeg, Gernot Katzer's Spice pages http://wwwang. kfunigraz.ac.at/~katzer/engl/generic_frame.html?Curc_dom.html
416 Lad, Vasant, an5/3/74 d Frawley, David, *The Yoga of Herbs,* Lotus Press, Twin Lakes, 1986, p. 133
417 Nair, C.K.N., *Medicinal Plants of India,* Shri Surendra Partap, Delhi, 1998, p. 304
418 Kapoor, L.D., *Handbook of Ayurvedic Medicinal Plants.* Boca Raton, FL. CRC Press; 1990, p. 238
419 Lad, Vasant, and Frawley, David, *The Yoga of Herbs,* Lotus Press, Twin Lakes, 1986, p. 133
420 Dash, Bhagwan, *Diagnosis and Treatment of Diseases in Ayurveda,* Concept, New Delhi, 1982,

part four, p. 268

421 Bensky, Dan, and Gamble, Andrew, *Chinese Materia Medica,* Eastland Press, Seattle, 1986, p. 548.

422 The Pharmacology of Nutmeg, *The Lawrence Review of NaturalProducts,* April 1984, vol.5, number 3

423 Bensky, Dan, and Gamble, Andrew, *Chinese Materia Medica,* Eastland Press, Seattle, 1986, p. 549.

424 Stein U, Greyer H, Hentschel H. Nutmeg (myristicin) poisoning--report on a fatal case and a series of cases recorded by a poison information centre. Forensic Sci Int. 2001 Apr 15;118(1):87-90.

425 Sangalli BC, Chiang W. Toxicology of nutmeg abuse. J Toxicol Clin Toxicol. 2000;38(6):671-8.

426 Hallstrom H, Thuvander A. Toxicological evaluation of myristicin. Nat Toxins. 1997;5(5):186-92.

427 Zheng GQ, Kenney PM, Zhang J, Lam LK. Inhibition of benzo[a]pyrene-induced tumorigenesis by myristicin, a volatile aroma constituent of parsley leaf oil. Carcinogenesis. 1992 Oct;13(10):1921-3.

428 Leung, Albert Y., *Encyclopedia of Common Natural Ingredients,* Wiley Interscience, New York, 1980, p.243

429 Weil, Andrew, The use of nutmeg as a psychotropic agent, United Nations Office on Drugs and Crime, 1966 http://www.unodc.org/unodc/bulletin/bulletin_1966-01-01_4_page003.html#s001

430 Nadkarni, Dr. K.M. 1976. *The Indian Materia Medica, with Ayurvedic, Unani and Home Remedies.* Revised and enlarged by A.K. Nadkarni. 1954. Reprint. Bombay: Bombay Popular Prakashan PVP, p. 830

431 Kapoor, L.D., *Handbook of Ayurvedic Medicinal Plants.* Boca Raton, FL. CRC Press; 1990, p. 238

432 Nutmeg, Gernot Katzer's Spice pages http://wwwang. kfunigraz.ac.at/~katzer/engl/generic_frame.html?Curc_dom.html

433 Nutmeg and derivatives, Food and Agriculture Organization of The United States, Rome, September, 1994 http://www.fao.org/docrep/v4084e/v4084e04.htm

434 Van Gils C, Cox PA. Ethnobotany of nutmeg in the Spice Islands. J Ethnopharmacol. 1994 Apr;42(2):117-24.

435 Schultes, Richard Evans and Hofmann, Albert. The Botany and Chemistry of Hallucinogens, Charles C. Thomas Publishers, p. 121

436 Sangalli BC, Chiang W. Toxicology of nutmeg abuse. J Toxicol Clin Toxicol. 2000;38(6):671-8.

437 The Pharmacology of Nutmeg, *The Lawrence Review of Natural Products,* April 1984, vol.5, number 3

438 Hallstrom H, Thuvander A. Toxicological evaluation of myristicin. Nat Toxins. 1997;5(5):186-92.

439 Grover JK, Khandkar S, Vats V, Dhunnoo Y, Das D. Pharmacological studies on Myristica fragrans--antidiarrheal, hypnotic, analgesic and hemodynamic (blood pressure) parameters. Methods Find Exp Clin Pharmacol. 2002 Dec;24(10):675-80.

440 Sherry CJ, Burnett RE. Enhancement of ethanol-induced sleep by whole oil of nutmeg. Experientia. 1978 Apr 15;34(4):492-3.

441 Lansdorf, Nancy, Maharishi Ayurveda for Common Disorders: Insomnia http://www.ayurvedaayurvedic.com/recommendations/asgb-68.html

442 Bhajan, Yogi, *The Ancient Art of Self Healing,* West Anandpur, Eugene, 1982, p. 57

443 Grover JK, Khandkar S, Vats V, Dhunnoo Y, Das D. Pharmacological studies on Myristica fragrans--antidiarrheal, hypnotic, analgesic and hemodynamic (blood pressure) parameters. Methods Find Exp Clin Pharmacol. 2002 Dec;24(10):675-80.

444 Bhajan, Yogi, *The Ancient Art of Self Healing,* West Anandpur, Eugene, 1982, p. 10

445 Dash, Bhagwan, *Five Specialized Therapies of Ayurveda,* Concept, New Delhi,1992, p.223

446 Jain, S.K., and DeFillips, Robert A., *Medicinal Plants of India,* Reference Publications, Algonac, Michigan, 1991, p.441

447 Herbal Monograph, Nutmeg, Himalaya Herbal Healthcare http://www.himalayahealthcare.com/

herbfinder/h_myrist.htm
448 Bhajan, Yogi, *The Ancient Art of Self Healing,* West Anandpur, Eugene, 1982, p. 10
449 1-TOP Capsules http://www.impotence-herbal.com/action.htm
450 Lad, Vasant, and Frawley, David, *The Yoga of Herbs,* Lotus Press, Twin Lakes, WI, 1986, p. 133
451 Grover JK, Khandkar S, Vats V, Dhunnoo Y, Das D. Pharmacological studies on Myristica fragrans--antidiarrheal, hypnotic, analgesic and hemodynamic (blood pressure) parameters. Methods Find Exp Clin Pharmacol. 2002 Dec;24(10):675-80.
452 Dastur, J.F., *Everybody's Guide to Ayurvedic Medicine,* Tarepoevala, Bombay, 1978,p. 59
453 Myristica- Nutmeg, King's American Dispensatory http://www.ibiblio.org/herbmed/eclectic/kings/myristica.html
454 Lad, Vasant, *Complete Book of Ayurvedic Home remedies, The,* Harmony Books, New York, 1998, p. 163
455 Kumar, Abhimanyu, Primary Care of Atisar (Diarrhea), Ayurveda News, Chakrapani Ayurveda Clinic http://chakrapaniayurveda.com/
456 Nadkarni, Dr. K.M. 1976. *The Indian Materia Medica, with Ayurvedic, Unani and Home Remedies.* Revised and enlarged by A.K. Nadkarni. 1954. Reprint. Bombay: Bombay Popular Prakashan PVP, p. 832
457 Personal communication with Michael Tierra
458 Nadkarni, Dr. K.M. 1976. *The Indian Materia Medica, with Ayurvedic, Unani and Home Remedies.* Revised and enlarged by A.K. Nadkarni. 1954. Reprint. Bombay: Bombay Popular Prakashan PVP, p. 832
459 Murthy, K.R., translator, *Sarngadhar-Samhita,* Chaukamba Orientalia, Delhi, 1995, p. 92
460 Dash, Bhagwan, *Diagnosis and Treatment of Diseases in Ayurveda,* Concept, New Delhi, 1982, part four, p. 217
461 Nutmeg, http://sivasakti.com/
462 Pruthi, J.S., *Spices and Condiments,* National Book Trust, New Delhi, 1976, p.171
463 Morita T, Jinno K, Kawagishi H, Arimoto Y, Suganuma H, Inakuma T, Sugiyama K. Hepatoprotective Effect of Myristicin from Nutmeg (Myristica fragrans) on Lipopolysaccharide/d-Galactosamine-Induced Liver Injury. J Agric Food Chem. 2003 Mar 12;51(6):1560-5.
464 Dash, Bhagwan, *Diagnosis and Treatment of Diseases in Ayurveda, Concept,* New Delhi, 1982, part six, p. 29
465 Webb, Ginger, *Traditional Uses of Nutmeg in Spice Islands,* Herbalgram no. 38, p. 14
466 Palau Pinang, Nutmeg Balm http://www.penangherbs.com/nutmegbalm.html
467 Tibetan Nutmeg Lotion http://www1.ivenue.com/diamondwayayurveda/item8000.ctlg
468 1-TOP Capsules http://www.impotence-herbal.com/action.htm
469 Yogi Bhajan, private communication.
470 Liu JH, Chen GH, Yeh HZ, Huang CK, Poon SK Enteric-coated peppermint-oil capsules in the treatment of irritable bowel syndrome: a prospective, randomized trial. *J Gastroenterol* 1997 Dec;32(6):765-8
471 Freise J, Kohler S [Peppermint oil-caraway oil fixed combination in non-ulcer dyspepsia--comparison of the effects of enteric preparations]. *Pharmazie* 1999 Mar;54(3):210-5
472 Micklefield GH, Greving I, May B Effects of peppermint oil and caraway oil on gastroduodenal motility. *Phytother Res* 2000 Feb;14(1):20-3
473 Felter, Harvey Wickes, M.D., *The Eclectic Materia Medica, Pharmacology and Therapeutics*
474 Felter, Harvey Wickes, M.D., and Lloyd, John Uri, Phr. M., Ph. D., *King's American Dispensatory*
475 The Columbia Electronic Encyclopedia, Columbia University Press
476 The Natural Standard www.naturalstandard.com
477 Blumenthal, Mark, *The Complete Commission E Monographs,* The American Botanical Council, Austin, Texas, 1998
478 Gobel H, Schmidt G, Soyka D. Effect of peppermint and eucalyptus oil preparations on neurophysiological and experimental algesimetric headache parameters. Cephalalgia. 1994

Jun;14(3):228-34

479 Schattner P, Randerson D. Tiger Balm as a treatment of tension headache. A clinical trial in general practice. Aust Fam Physician. 1996 Feb;25(2):216, 218, 220 passim.

480 Shoba G, Joy D, Joseph T, Majeed M, Rajendran R, Srinivas PS, Influence of piperine on the pharmacokinetics of curcumin in animals and human volunteers. Planta Med 1998 May;64(4):353-356

481 Seeram NP, Adams LS, Henning SM, Niu Y, Zhang Y, Nair MG, Heber D. In vitro antiproliferative, apoptotic and antioxidant activities of punicalagin, ellagic acid and a total pomegranate tannin extract are enhanced in combination with other polyphenols as found in pomegranate juice. J Nutr Biochem. 2005 Jun;16(6):360-7.

482 Fil MI, et al. Antioxidant activity of pomegranate juice and its relationship with phenolic composition and processing. J Agric Food Chem 2000;48:4581-9.

483 Rosenblat M, Volkova N, Coleman R, Aviram M. Pomegranate byproduct administration to apolipoprotein edeficient mice attenuates atherosclerosis development as a result of decreased macrophage oxidative stress and reduced cellular uptake of oxidized low-density lipoprotein. J Agric Food Chem, 2006 Mar 8;54(5):1928-35.

484 Opium Poppy- traditional medicine, Plant Cultures, Royal Botanic Gardens, Kew, http://www.plantcultures.org.uk/index.html

485 Hotz J, Plein K[Effectiveness of plantago seed husks in comparison with wheat brain on stool frequency and manifestations of irritable colon syndrome with constipation]. *Med Klin* 1994 Dec 15;89(12):645-51

486 Prior A, Whorwell PJ Double blind study of ispaghula in irritable bowel syndrome. *Gut* 1987 Nov;28(11):1510-3

487 Kumar A, Kumar N, Vij JC, Sarin SK, Anand BS Optimum dosage of ispaghula husk in patients with irritable bowel syndrome: correlation of symptom relief with whole gut transit time and stool weight. *Gut* 1987 Feb;28(2):150-5

488 Rauwolfia serpentina Monograph, Himalaya Herbal Healthcare, http://www.himalayahealthcare.com/herbfinder/h_rauwolfia.htm

489 Sushruta Samhita U.60.47

490 Asparagus adscendens Monograph, Himalaya Herbal Healthcare, http://www.himalayahealthcare.com/herbfinder/h_asparagus.htm

491 Tandon, M., Shukla, Y.N. and Thakur, R.S. 1990. Steroid glycosides from Asparagus adscendens. Phytochemistry 29: 2957-2959.

492 Nandan Musli, http://www.nandanmusli.com/safeaphrodisiac.htm

493 Safed Musli Monograph, Grow Green Bio-Sciences, http://www.growgreen.in/medicinal-herbs.html

494 Nadkarni, K.M., *Indian Materia Medica,* Popular Prakashan, Bombay, 1976, p. 151

495 Milot, Brenda, Historical Evidence Supports Medicinal Use of Saffron, *HerbalGram.* 2005;68:32-33

496 Nadkarni, Dr. K.M. 1976. The Indian Materia Medica, with Ayurvedic, Unani and Home Remedies. Revised and enlarged by A.K. Nadkarni. 1954. Reprint. Bombay: Bombay Popular Prakashan PVP. p. 1101

497 Murray, Michael, and Pizzorno, Joseph, Encyclopedia of Natural Medicine, Prima, Rocklin, California, 1998.

498 Chen T, Li J, Cao J, Xu Q, Komatsu K, Namba T A new flavanone isolated from rhizoma smilacis glabrae and the structural requirements of its derivatives for preventing immunological hepatocyte damage. *Planta Med* 1999 Feb;65(1):56-9

499 Bernardo RR, Pinto AV, Parente JP Steroidal saponins from Smilax officinalis. *Phytochemistry* 1996 Sep;43(2):465-9

500 Ju Y, Jia Z, Sun X Steroidal saponins from Smilax menispermoidea and S. lebrunii. *Phytochemistry* 1994 Nov;37(5):1433-6

501 *New England Journal of Medicine,* 1942; 227: 128-33

502 Franz G. The senna drug and its chemistry. Pharmacology 1993 Oct;47 Suppl 1:2-6
503 Krumbiegel G, Schulz HU. Rhein and aloe-emodin kinetics from senna laxatives in man. Pharmacology 1993 Oct;47 Suppl 1:120-4
504 Astanga Hridyam U.39.47
505 Bhattacharya SK, Bhattacharya A, Chakrabarti A. Adaptogenic activity of Siotone, a polyherbal formulation of Ayurvedic rasayanas. Indian J Exp Biol 2000 Feb;38(2):119-28
506 Asparagus Monograph, Himalaya Herbal Healthcare, http://www.himalayahealthcare.com/herbfinder/h_asparagus1.htm
507 Dalvi SS Nadkarni PM Gupta KC Effect of Asparagus racemosus (Shatavari) on gastric emptying time in normal healthy volunteers. J-Postgrad-Med. 1990 Apr; 36(2): 91-4
508 Horseradish Tree. http://www.livingdesert.org/plants/horseradish_tree.asp
509 Fritz M. A common tree with rare power. Los Angeles Times 2000 Mar 27;partA:1.
510 The Moringa Tree. http://www.treesforlife.org/project/moringa/default.en.asp
511 Freiberger CE, et al. Nutrient content of the edible leaves of seven wild plants from Niger. Plant Foods Hum Nutr 1998;53(1):57-69.
512 Babal, Ken, C.N.. Shelf Stockers for 2001, Nutrition Science News, January, 2001, http://www.newhope.com/nutritionsciencenews/NSN_backs/Jan_01/shelfstockers.cfm
513 Fritz M. A common tree with rare power. Los Angeles Times 2000 Mar 27;partA:1.
514 Pankaja N, Prakash J. Availability of calcium from kilkeerai (Amaranthus tricolor) and drumstick (Moringa oleifera) greens in weanling rats. Nahrung. 1994;38(2):199-203.
515 Moringa, Hope Seeds, http://hopeseeds.org/garden/moringa.htm
516 The Moringa Tree. http://www.islamonline.net/english/science/2003/02/article06.shtml#*
517 The Australian New Crops Newsletter, 19.2 Moringa, January, 1998. http://www.newcrops.uq.edu.au/newslett/ncnl9192.htm
518 Ayurveda Dictionary. http://www.ayurveda.com.au/Ayursite1/html/herbsdic.html#M
519 Moringa oleifera. http://www.ayurveda-herbal-remedy.com/indian-herbs/moringa-oleifera.html
520 Faizi S, et al. Hypotensive constituents from the pods of Moringa oleifera. Planta Med 1998 Apr;64(3):225-8.
521 Eilert U, et al. The antibiotic principle of seeds of Moringa oleifera and Moringa stenopetala. Planta Res 1981;42:55-61.
522 Moringa Monograph. http://www.himalayahealthcare.com/herbfinder/h_moring.htm
523 deJager, Prashanti, Sri Tulsiji: Queen of Herbs, LOAJ, I:2 (Fall 2002) 4-9.
524 deJager, Prashanti, Sri Tulsiji: Queen of Herbs, LOAJ, I:2 (Fall 2002) 4-9.
525 Nadkarni, K.M., Indian Materia Medica, Popular Prakashan, Bombay, 1976, p.863.
526 Kapoor, L.D., The CRC Handbook of Ayurvedic Medicinal Plants, CRC Press, Baton Rouge, 1990, p. 249.
527 deJager, Prashanti, Sri Tulsiji: Queen of Herbs, LOAJ, I:2 > (Fall 2002) 4-9.
528 National Institute of Ayurvedic Medicine, 584 Milltown Road Brewster, New York 10509 USA http://www.niam.com/
529 Sarkar A, Lavania SC, Pandey DN, Pant MC Changes in the blood lipid profile after administration of Ocimum sanctum (Tulsi) leaves in the normal albino rabbits. Indian J Physiol Pharmacol 1994 Oct;38(4):311-2
530 Rai V, Iyer U, Mani UV Effect of Tulasi (Ocimum sanctum) leaf powder supplementation on blood sugar levels, serum lipids and tissue lipids in diabetic rats. Plant Foods Hum Nutr 1997;50(1):9-16
531 Singh, N. *Ann. Nat. Acad. Ind. Med.,* 1986, 2(1):14-26.
532 Agrawal P, Rai V, Singh RB Randomized placebo-controlled, single blind trial of holy basil leaves in patients with noninsulin-dependent diabetes mellitus. Int J Clin Pharmacol Ther 1996 Sep;34(9):406-9
533 Karthikeyan K, Ravichandran P, Govindasamy S, Chemopreventive effect of Ocimum sanctum on DMBA-induced hamster buccal pouch carcinogenesis. Oral Oncol 1999 Jan;35(1):112-9
534 Uma Devi P, Ganasoundari A, Rao BS, Srinivasan KK In vivo radioprotection by ocimum

flavonoids: survival of mice. Radiat Res 1999 Jan;151(1):74-8
535 Devi PU, Bisht KS, Vinitha M A comparative study of radioprotection by Ocimum flavonoids and synthetic aminothiol protectors in the mouse. Br J Radiol 1998 Jul;71(847):782-4
536 Phadke SA, Kulkarni SD Screening of in vitro antibacterial activity of Terminalia chebula, Eclapta alba and Ocimum sanctum. Indian J Med Sci 1989 May;43(5):113-7
537 Godhwani S, Godhwani JL, Vyas DS Ocimum sanctum- a preliminary study evaluating its immunoregulatory profile in albino rats. J Ethnopharmacol 1988 Dec;24(2-3):193-8
538 Mandal S, Das DN, De K, Ray K, Roy G, Chaudhuri SB, Sahana CC, Chowdhuri MK Ocimum sanctum Linn--a study on gastric ulceration and gastric secretion in rats. Indian J Physiol Pharmacol 1993 Jan;37(1):91-2
539 Singh S, Majumdar DK Evaluation of antiinflammatory activityof fatty acids of Ocimum sanctum fixed oil. Indian J Exp Biol 1997 Apr;35(4):380-3
540 Sembulingam K, Sembulingam P, Namasivayam A Effect of Ocimumsanctum Linn on noise induced changes in plasma corticosterone level. Indian J Physiol Pharmacol 1997 Apr;41(2):139-43
541 deJager, Prashanti, Sri Tulsiji: Queen of Herbs, LOAJ, I:2 (Fall 2002) 4-9.
542 Maulik G, Maulik N, Bhandari V, Kagan VE, Pakrashi S, Das DK Evaluation of antioxidant effectiveness of a few herbal plants. Free Radic Res 1997 Aug;27(2):221-8
543 Werbach M and Murray M. 1994. Botanical Influences on Illness. Tarzana, California: Third Line Press
544 Michael T. Murray, N.D., The Healing Power of Herbs, Prima, Rocklin, California, 1995.
545 Murray, Michael, and Pizzorno, Joseph, Encyclopedia of Natural Medicine, Prima, Rocklin, California, 1998.
546 Patacchini R, Maggi CA, Meli A. Capsaicin-like activity of some natural pungent substances on peripheral endings of visceral primary afferents. Naunyn Schmiedebergs Arch Pharmacol 1990 Jul;342(1):72-7
547 Ramsewak RS, DeWitt DL, Nair MG Cytotoxicity, antioxidant and anti-inflammatory activities of curcumins I-III from Curcuma longa. *Phytomedicine* 2000 Jul;7(4):303-8
548 Ammon HP, Wahl MA. Pharmacology of Curcuma longa. Planta Med 1991 Feb;57(1):1-7.
549 Thamlikitkul V, Bunyapraphatsara N, Dechatiwongse T, et al. Randomized double blind study of *Curcuma domestica Val. for dyspepsia. J Med Assoc Thai.* 1989;72:613–620.
550 World Health Organization, *WHO Monographs on Selected Medicinal Plants, Geneva,* 1999.
551 deJager, Prashanti, Turmeric: Ayurvedic Spice of Life, Part I, LOAJ, I:3 (Spring 2003) 12-16, Part II, LOAJ, I: 4 (Summer 2003) 23-27.
552 deJager, Prashanti, Turmeric: Ayurvedic Spice of Life, Part I, LOAJ, I:3 (Spring 2003) 12-16, Part II, LOAJ, I: 4 (Summer 2003) 23-27.
553 Srinivas L, Shalini VK, Shylaja M. Turmerin: a water soluble antioxidant peptide from turmeric [Curcuma longa] Arch Biochem Biophys 1992 Feb 1;292(2):617-23
554 S Awasthi, SK Srivatava, JT Piper, SS Singhal, M Chaubey, and YC Awasthi Am J Clin Nutr 1996;64:761-766.
555 Aggarwal BB, Kumar A, Bharti AC. Anticancer potential of curcumin: preclinical and clinical studies. Anticancer Res 2003 Jan-Feb;23(1A):363-98
556 Nagabhushan M, Amonkar AJ, Bhide SV. In vitro antimutagenicity of curcumin against environmental mutagens. Food Chem Toxicol 1987 Jul;25(7):545-7
557 Lin SC, Lin CC, Lin YH, Supriyatna S, Teng CW. Protective and therapeutic effects of Curcuma xanthorrhiza on hepatotoxin-induced liver damage. Am J Chin Med 1995;23(3-4):243-54
558 Deshpande UR, Gadre SG, Raste AS, Pillai D, Bhide SV, Samuel AM. Protective effect of turmeric (Curcuma longa L.) extract on carbon tetrachloride-induced liver damage in rats. Indian J Exp Biol 1998 Jun;36(6):573-7
559 Yogi Bhajan Lecture 2/12/92
560 Mazumder A, Raghavan K, Weinstein J, Kohn KW, Pommier Y. Inhibition of human immunode-

ficiency virus type-1 integrase by curcumin. Biochem Pharmacol 1995 Apr 18;49(8):1165-70
561 Lad, Vasant, and Frawley, David, *The Yoga of Herbs,* Lotus Press, Twin Lakes, WI 1986
562 Houghton PJ The scientific basis for the reputed activity of Valerian *J Pharm Pharmacol* 1999 May;51(5):505-12.
563 Bourin M, Bougerol T, Guitton B, Broutin E A combination of plant extracts in the treatment of outpatients with adjustment disorder with anxious mood: controlled study versus placebo. *Fundam Clin Pharmacol* 1997;11(2):127-32
564 Leathwood PD, Chauffard F, Heck E, Munoz-Box R Aqueous extract of valerian root (Valeriana officinalis L.) improves sleep quality in man. *Pharmacol Biochem Behav* 1982 Jul;17(1):65-71
565 Mercury, The Wonder Substance, Jiva Ayurveda, http://www.ayurvedic.org/ayurveda/arogya_topics.asp?nm1=Newsletter%20%3E%20Arogya%20Archive#Mercury
566 Yogi Bhajan Lecture 9/17-18/92
567 Personal communication with Karta Purkh Singh Khalsa
568 Shilajatu Monograph, Healthepic, http://www.healthepic.com/ayurveda/rasayana/shilajatu.htm
569 Shilajatu Monograph, Healthepic, http://www.healthepic.com/ayurveda/rasayana/shilajatu.htm
570 Ayurveda Pharmacopoeia, Department of Ayurveda, Yoga and Naturopathy, Unani, Siddha and Homeopathy, Ministry of Health and Family Welfare, Government of India, http://indianmedicine.nic.in/html/ayurveda/ayurveda.htm
571 Dharmananda, Subhuti, Chyawanprash, The Premier Rasayana of Ayurveda, Institute for Traditional Medicine, http://www.itmonline.org/
572 Yogi Bhajan Lecture 9/5/81
573 Frawley, David, *Ayurvedic Healing,* Lotus Press: Twin Lakes, WI
574 Chyavanprasha Monograph, Healthepic, http://www.healthepic.com/ayurveda/rasayana/chyavanaprasha.htm
575 Tillotson, Alan, Khalsa, Karta Purkh Singh, Caldecott, Todd, *Triphala,* Canadian Journal of Herbalism, Vol. XXII, 2001.
576 Jose JK, Kuttan R. Hepatoprotective activity of Emblica officinalis and Chyavanaprash. J Ethnopharmacol 2000 Sep;72(1-2):135-40
577 Manjunatha S, Jaryal AK, Bijlani RL, Sachdeva U, Gupta SK. Effect of Chyawanprash and vitamin C on glucose tolerance and lipoprotein profile. Indian J Physiol Pharmacol 2001 Jan;45(1):71-9
578 Tierra, Michael, Asafoetida: For Digestive Waekness, Food Allergies and Candida, http://www.planetherbs.com/articles/asafoetida.html
579 Ayurveda Pharmacopoeia, Department of Ayurveda, Yoga and Naturopathy, Unani, Siddha and Homeopathy, Ministry of Health and Family Welfare, Government of India, http://indianmedicine.nic.in/html/ayurveda/ayurveda.htm
580 Frawley, David. *Ayurvedic Healing,* Lotus Press: Twin Lakes, WI
581 Ayurveda Pharmacopoeia, Department of Ayurveda, Yoga and Naturopathy, Unani, Siddha and Homeopathy, Ministry of Health and Family Welfare, Government of India, http://indianmedicine.nic.in/html/ayurveda/ayurveda.htm
582 India. Ministry of Health and Family Planning. *The Ayurvedic Formulary of India.* Part 1. 1st ed. Delhi. 1978. p. 226.
583 Sharma KR, Bhatia RP, Kumar V Role of the indigenous drug saptamrita lauha in hemorrhagic retinopathies. *Ann Ophthalmol* 1992 Jan;24(1):5-8
584 Personal communication with Michael Tierra
585 Srikantha Murthy, K.R. Sarnagadhar-Samhita: A Treatise on Ayurveda. Chaukhambha Varanasi: Orientalia; 1984. p.85
586 India. Ministry of Health and Family Planning. The Ayurvedic Formulary of India. Part 1. 1st ed. Delhi. 1978. p. 89
587 Srikantha Murthy, K.R. *Sarnagadhar-Samhita: A Treatise on Ayurveda.* Chaukhambha Varanasi: Orientalia; 1984. p.85
588 India. Ministry of Health and Family Planning. *The Ayurvedic Formulary of India.* Part 1. 1st ed.

Delhi. 1978. p. 85
589 Lad, V., and Frawley, D. *Yoga of Herbs,* The. Lotus Press, Twin Lakes, WI, 1986
590 Vaidya Mana Bajracharya, Robert Abel, and Alan Tillotson, 1997, Self-published
591 Sharma, R.K. and Bhagwan Dash. *Agnivesa's Caraka Samhita (Text with English Translation and Critical Exposition based on Cakrapani Datta's Ayurveda Dipika)* vol. 3. Varanasi: Chaukhambha Orientalia; 1988.
592 Sharma, R.K. and Bhagwan Dash. *Agnivesa's Caraka Samhita (Text with English Translation and Critical Exposition based on Cakrapani Datta's Ayurveda Dipika)* vol. 3. Varanasi: Chaukhambha Orientalia; 1988, p 49.
593 Srikantha Murthy, K.R. *Vagbhata's Astanga Hrdayam. vol. 3.* Varanasi: Krishnadas Academy. 1995. p. 387
594 Sharma, PV. *Cakradatta* (Text with English Translation): *A Treatise on the Principles and Practices of Ayurvedic Medicine.* Varanasi: Chaukhambha Orientalia. 1994. p. 166.
595 Vaidya Mana Bajra Bajracharya. Personal communication (with Alan Tillotson). 1976.
596 Sharma, PV. *Cakradatta* (Text with English Translation): *A Treatise on the Principles and Practices of Ayurvedic Medicine.* Varanasi: Chaukhambha Orientalia. 1994. p. 17.
597 Sharma, PV. *Cakradatta* (Text with English Translation): *A Treatise on the Principles and Practices of Ayurvedic Medicine.* Varanasi: Chaukhambha Orientalia. 1994. p. 241.
598 Nadkarni, Dr. K.M. *The Indian Materia Medica, with Ayurvedic, Unani and Home Remedies.* Revised and enlarged by A.K. Nadkarni. 1954. Reprint. Bombay: Bombay Popular Prakashan PVP. 1976. P. 1204
599 Personal communication
600 Yogi Bhajan. Personal communication (with K.P.S. Khalsa). 1975.
601 Sharma, PV. *Cakradatta* (Text with English Translation): *A Treatise on the Principles and Practices of Ayurvedic Medicine.* Varanasi: Chaukhambha Orientalia. 1994. p. 410.
602 Sharma, PV. *Cakradatta* (Text with English Translation): *A Treatise on the Principles and Practices of Ayurvedic Medicine.* Varanasi: Chaukhambha Orientalia. 1994. p. 424.
603 Dash, Bhagwan. *Ayurvedic Cures for Common Diseases.* Hind Pocket: Delhi. 1995
604 Dash, Bhagwan. *Ayurvedic Cures for Common Diseases.* Hind Pocket: Delhi. 1995, p. 84
605 Dash, Bhagwan. High Blood Pressure and Sleeplessness. Jain: New Delhi, 1993
606 Paranjpe P, Patki P, Patwardhan B Ayurvedic treatment of obesity: a randomised double-blind, placebo-controlled clinical trial. *J Ethnopharmacol* 1990 Apr;29(1):1-11
607 Thakur CP, Thakur B, Singh S, Sinha PK, Sinha SK. The Ayurvedic medicines Haritaki, Amala and Bahira reduce cholesterol-induced atherosclerosis in rabbits. *Int J Cardiol.* 1988 Nov;21(2):167-75.
608 Yogi Bhajan Lecture 2/21/82
609 Yogi Bhajan Lecture 7/10/80
610 Blumenthal, Mark, *The Complete German Commission E Monographs,* American Botanical Council, Austin, 1998
611 Sarrell EM, Mandelberg A, Cohen HA. Efficacy of naturopathic extracts in the management of ear pain associated with acute otitis media. Arch Pediatr Adolesc Med 2001 Jul;155(7):796-9
612 Willow Bark Monograph, European Scientific Cooperative on Phytotherapy Monographs, Exeter, UK, 1997
613 Willow Bark Monograph, American Herbal Pharmacopoeia, Santa Cruz, California, 1999.
614 McCaleb, Robert S., Herb Research Foundation Encyclopedia of Popular Herbs, Prima, Roseville, california, 2000.
615 Personal communication with Michael Tierra
616 Yogi Bhajan Lectire 2/12/92
617 Personal communication
618 Prakriti, Your Ayurvedic Constitution, Lotus Press: Twin Lakes, WI
619 The Yoga of Herbs Lotus, 1986
620 Bhattacharya SK, Bhattacharya A, Chakrabarti A. Adaptogenic activity of Siotone, a polyherbal

formulation of Ayurvedic rasayanas. Indian J Exp Biol 2000 Feb;38(2):119-28
621 Müller K, Ziereis K, Gawlik I. The antipsoriatic Mahonia aquifolium and its active constituents; II. Antiproliferative activity against cell growth of human keratinocytes. Planta Med. 1995 Feb;61(1):74-5.
622 Personal communication with Michael Tierra
623 Bunyapraphatsara N, Jirakulchaiwong S, Thirawarapan S, et al. The efficacy of Aloe vera cream in the treatment of first, second, and third degree burns in mice. *Phytomedicine* 1996; 2(3): 247-251.
624 Mint Monograph. Jiva Ayurveda, http://www.ayurvedic.org/ayubasics/mint.asp?nm=Common%20Herbs&nm2=Mint
625 Personal communication wih Michael Tierra
626 Mihalic, Rhonda, A Joint Effort, Health Supplement Retailer, August 2001, p. 26 http://www.hsrmagazine.com/articles/181feat3.html
627 Study shows sleep disruption to be chief complaint. Arthritis Foundation http://www.arthritis.org/resources/news/news_sleep.asp
628 Mihalic, Rhonda, A Joint Effort, Health Supplement Retailer, August 2001, p. 26 http://www.hsrmagazine.com/articles/181feat3.html
629 Felson DT. Weight and osteoarthritis. Am J Clin Nutr 1996 Mar;63(3 Suppl):430S-432S
630 National Institute of Arthritis and Musculoskeletal and Skin Diseases http://www.nih.gov/niams/healthinfo/arthexfs.htm
631 Bland JH. The reversibility of osteoarthritis: a review. Am J Med 1983 Jun 14;74(6A):16-26
632 Marcus Adam Top Complaint Among Arthritics Isn't Pain http://www.healthscout.com/template.asp?page=newsDetail&ap=1&id=91385
633 Study shows sleep disruption to be chief complaint Arthritis Foundation http://www.arthritis.org/resources/news/news_sleep.asp
634 Babal, Ken, Shelf Stockers for 2001,Nutrition Science News, January, 2001, www.healthwellexchange.com/nutritionsciencenews/NSN_backs/Jan_01/shelfstockers.cfm
635 Duke James The Most Important MEDICINE You'll Ever GROW. Mother Earth News Jan, 2001 www.findarticles.com/cf_0/m1279/2001_Jan/66961755/print.jhtml
636 Ammon HP, Safayhi H, Mack T, Sabieraj J Mechanism of antiinflammatory actions of curcumine and boswellic acids. *J Ethnopharmacol* 1993 Mar;38(2-3):113-9
637 Ammon HP, Mack T, Singh GB, Safayhi H Inhibition of leukotriene B4 formation in rat peritoneal neutrophils by an ethanolic extract of the gum resin exudate of Boswellia serrata. *Planta Med* 1991 Jun;57(3):203-7
638 Singh GB, Atal CK. Pharmacology of an extract of salai guggal ex-Boswellia serrata, a new non-steroidal antiinflammatory agent. Agents Actions 1986 Jun;18(3-4):407-12.
639 Arora RB, Kapoor V, Basu N, Jain AP Anti-inflammatory studies on Curcuma longa (turmeric). *Indian J Med Res* 1971 Aug;59(8):1289-95
640 Yegnanarayan R, Saraf AP, Balwani JH Comparison of anti-inflammatory activity of various extracts of Curcuma longa (Linn). *Indian J Med Res* 1976 Apr;64(4):601-8
641 Srimal RC, Dhawan BN Pharmacology of diferuloyl methane (curcumin), a non-steroidal anti-inflammatory agent. *J Pharm Pharmacol* 1973 Jun;25(6):447-52
642 Mukhopadhyay A, Basu N, Ghatak N, Gujral PK Anti-inflammatory and irritant activities of curcumin analogues in rats. *Agents Actions* 1982 Oct;12(4):508-15
643 Ghatak N, Basu N Sodium curcuminate as an effective anti-inflammatory agent. *Indian J Exp Biol* 1972 May;10(3):235-6
644 Murray, Michael, and Pizzorno, Joseph, *Encyclopedia of Natural Medicine,* Prima, Rocklin, California, 1998.
645 Sidhu GS, Singh AK, Thaloor D, Banaudha KK, Patnaik GK, Srimal RC, Maheshwari RK Enhancement of wound healing by curcumin in animals. *Wound Repair Regen* 1998 Mar-

Apr;6(2):167-77

646 Patacchini R, Maggi CA, Meli A Capsaicin-like activity of some natural pungent substances on peripheral endings of visceral primary afferents. *Naunyn Schmiedebergs Arch Pharmacol* 1990 Jul;342(1):72-7

647 Ramsewak RS, DeWitt DL, Nair MG Cytotoxicity, antioxidant and anti-inflammatory activities of curcumins I-III from Curcuma longa. *Phytomedicine* 2000 Jul;7(4):303-8

648 Kulkarni RR, Patki PS, Jog VP, Gandage SG, Patwardhan B Treatment of osteoarthritis with a herbomineral formulation: a double-blind, placebo-controlled, cross-over study. *J Ethnopharmacol* 1991 May-Jun;33(1-2):91-5

649 Willow Bark Monograph, European Scientific Cooperative on Phytotherapy Monographs, Exeter, UK, 1997

650 Schmid B, Ludtke R, Selbmann HK, Kotter I, Tschirdewahn B, Schaffner W, Heide L. Efficacy and tolerability of a standardized willow bark extract in patients with osteoarthritis: randomized placebo-controlled, double blind clinical trial. Phytother Res 2001 Jun;15(4):344-50

651 Mills SY, Jacoby RK, Chacksfield M, Willoughby M. Effect of a proprietary herbal medicine on the relief of chronic arthritic pain: a double-blind study. Br J Rheumatol 1996 Sep;35(9):874-8

652 Begum VH, Sadique J Long term effect of herbal drug Withania somnifera on adjuvant induced arthritis in rats. *Indian J Exp Biol* 1988 Nov;26(11):877-82

653 Lakshmi-Chandra Mishra Alternative Medicine Review. Scientific Basis for the Therapeutic Use of Withania somnifera (Ashwagandha): A Review. 2000;5(4) 334-346.

654 Kulkarni RR, Patki PS, Jog VP, et al. Treatment of osteoarthritis with a herbomineral formulation: a double-blind, placebo-controlled, cross-over study. J Ethnopharmacol 1991;33:91-95.

655 Personal communication with Michael Tierra

656 Personal communication with Michael Tierra

657 Asthma Prevalence, Health Care Use and Mortality, 2000-200, National Center for Health Statistics http://www.cdc.gov/nchs/products/pubs/pubd/hestats/asthma/asthma.htm

658 U.S. asthma rates on the rise, CDC says, 2/27/2004 http://www.usatoday.com/news/health/2004-02-27-asthmacdc_x.htm

659 David Wolfson, ND Solving Sinusitis, Nutrition Science News, April 2000, http://www.healthwellexchange.com/nutritionsciencenews/NSN_backs/Apr_00/sinusitis.cfm

660 Poole MD. A focus on acute sinusitis in adults: changes in disease management. Am J Med 1999 May 3;106(5A):38S-47S

661 National Institute of Ayurvedic Medicine, http://www.niam.com

662 Murray, Michael, and Pizzorno, Joseph, Encyclopedia of Natural Medicine, Prima, Rocklin, California, 1998.

663 Yaegaki K, Coil JM Examination, classification, and treatment of halitosis; clinical perspectives. *J Can Dent Assoc* 2000 May;66(5):257-61

664 Abstracts, American Society for Microbiology General Meeting, Washington, D.C., May 18-22, 2003. News release, University of Illinois, Chicago.

665 Suri, Savitha, Preventing Benign Prostatic Hypertrophy through Ayurveda, May 22, 2005, http://www.boloji.com/ayurveda/av041.htm

666 *Prostate Protection System,* Your Ayurvedic Guide to Self-Care, http://www.mapi.com/catalog/indexprostate. html?session_id=741243_8872956_1058394939&affil=&prod_page=catalog/index-prostate.html

667 Dash, Bhagwan and Kashyap, Lalitesh, *Diagnosis and Treatment of Diseases in Ayurveda: Based on Ayurveda Saukhyam of Todarananda,* New Delhi, Concept, 1987, part four, page 89.

668 McCarty MF. Up-regulation of hepatic IGFBP-1 production as a strategy for preventing benign prostatic hyperplasia. Med Hypotheses. 2001 Jan;56(1):1-4.

669 Koskimaki J, Hakama M, Huhtala H, Tammela TL. Association of dietary elements and lower

urinary tract symptoms. Scand J Urol Nephrol. 2000 Feb;34(1):46-50.

670 American Dietetic Association; Dietitians of Canada. Position of the American Dietetic Association and Dietitians of Canada: vegetarian diets. Can J Diet Pract Res. 2003 Summer;64(2):62-81.

671 Deneo-Pellegrini, H., et al. *Foods, nutrients and prostate cancer: a case- control study in Uruguay.* British Journal of Cancer, Vol. 80, No. 3/4, May 1999, pp. 591-97

672 Dash, Bhagwan and Kashyap, Lalitesh, *Diagnosis and Treatment of Diseases in Ayurveda: Based on Ayurveda Saukhyam of Todarananda,* New Delhi, Concept, 1987, part four, page 96.

673 *Prostate Health- Focus on Prevention,* Ayurvedic News, Health and Wholeness, http://www.yourayurvedastore.com/newsletter/articles/a-prostatehealth.html

674 Ayurveda Pharmacopoeia, Department of Ayurveda, Yoga and Naturopathy, Unani, Siddha and Homeopathy, Ministry of Health and Family Welfare, Government of India, http://indianmedicine.nic.in/html/ayurveda/ayurveda.htm

675 Bhajan, Yogi, *Ancient Art of Self Healing,* West Anandpur (publisher), Eugene, Oregon, 1982., p. 86

676 Wright, Jonathan V., Fifty years of canker sore misery and the simple treatment that ended them. Health News and Review, Summer 1994, v4, n3, p2 (1).

677 Linda B. White, M.D. *Pathway To A Healthy Heart* http://www.healthwell.com/delicious-online/D_Backs/Feb_97/heart.cfm?path=hw

678 Jill Stansbury, N.D., *Change of Heart,* http://www.healthwell.com/hnbreakthroughs/may99/changeofheart.cfm?path=hw&cond=25&mcat=58

679 Berger, Fran, *Eat Your Heart Out,* Health Scout, www.healthscout.com/cgibin/ WebObjects/Af.woa/wa/article?ap=1&id=103368

680 Kapoor LD. *Handbook of Ayurvedic Medicinal Plants.* Boca Raton, FL. CRC Press; 1990:319-320

681 Bharani A, Ganguly A, Bhargava KD Salutary effect of Terminalia Arjuna in patients with severe refractory heart failure. *Int J Cardiol* 1995 May;49(3):191-9

682 Dwivedi S, Jauhari R Beneficial effects of Terminalia arjuna in coronary artery disease. *Indian Heart J* 1997 Sep- Oct;49(5):507-10

683 Seth SD, Maulik M, Katiyar CK, Maulik SK Role of Lipistat in protection against isoproterenol induced myocardial necrosis in rats: a biochemical and histopathological study. *Indian J Physiol Pharmacol* 1998 Jan;42(1):101-6

684 Silagy CA, Neil HA. A meta-analysis of the effect of garlic on blood pressure. J Hypertens 1994 Apr;12(4):463-8

685 Auer W, Eiber A, Hertkorn E, Hoehfeld E, Koehrle U, Lorenz A, Mader F, Merx W, Otto G, Schmid-Otto B, et al. Hypertension and hyperlipidaemia: garlic helps in mild cases. Br J Clin Pract Suppl 1990 Aug;69:3-6

686 Steiner M, Khan AH, Holbert D, Lin RI. A double-blind crossover study in moderately hypercholesterolemic men that compared the effect of aged garlic extract and placebo administration on blood lipids. Am J Clin Nutr 1996 Dec;64(6):866-70

687 Verma SK, Bordia A. Effect of Commiphora mukul (gum guggulu) in patients of hyperlipidemia with special reference to HDL-cholesterol. Indian J Med Res 1988 Apr;87:356-60

688 Satyavati GV. Gum guggul (Commiphora mukul)--the success story of an ancient insight leading to a modern discovery. Indian J Med Res 1988 Apr;87:327-35

689 Tripathi YB, Malhotra OP, Tripathi SN. Thyroid stimulating action of Z-guggulsterone obtained from Commiphora mukul. Planta Med 1984 Feb;(1):78-80

690 Satyavati GV, Dwarakanath C, Tripathi SN. Experimental studies on the hypocholesterolemic effect of Commiphora mukul. Engl. (Guggul). Indian J Med Res 1969 Oct;57(10):1950-62

691 Antonio J, Colker CM, Torina GC, et al. Effects of a standardized guggulsterone phosphate supplement on body composition in overweight adults: A pilot study. *Curr Ther Res*

1999;60:220-7.
692 American Academy of Ophthalmology (2001). Cataract in the Adult Eye (Preferred Practice Pattern). San Francisco: American Academy of Ophthalmology. http://my.webmd.com/hw/health_guide_atoz/hw35464.asp?navbar=hw36827#hw35464-Bib
693 Dash, Bhagwan. *Fundamentals of Ayurvedic Medicine.* Bansal: Delhi, 1980, p.25
694 Devaraj, T.L. Speaking of Ayurvedic Remedies for Common Diseases. Sterling: New Delhi, 1985, p.120
695 Dash, Bhagwan. *Ayurvedic Cures for Common Diseases.* Hind Pocket: Delhi. 1995, p.84
696 Lad, V., and Frawley, D. *Yoga of Herbs, The.* LotusPress, Twin Lakes, WI, 1986, p.158
697 Frawley, David. *Ayurvedic Healing,* Lotus Press: Twin Lakes, WI
698 S Awasthi, SK Srivatava, JT Piper, SS Singhal, M Chaubey, and YC Awasthi Am J Clin Nutr 1996;64:761-766.
699 Heyn, Birgit. *Ayurvedic Medicine.* Thorsons: Wellingborough, 1987, p.112
700 Frawley, David. *Ayurvedic Healing,* Lotus Press: Twin Lakes, WI, p.245
701 Hameed, H. Abdul. *Complete Book of Home Remedies, The.* Orient: Delhi, 1982, p.54
702 Dash, Bhagwan. *Ayurvedic Cures for Common Diseases.* Hind Pocket: Delhi. 1995, p.84
703 Dash, Bhagwan. *High Blood Pressure and Sleeplessness.* Jain: New Delhi, 1993, p.57
704 Devaraj, T.L. Speaking of Ayurvedic Remedies for Common Diseases. Sterling: New Delhi, 1985, p.121
705 Kapoor, L.D. CRC *Handbook of Ayurvedic Medicinal Plants.* CRC Press: New York, 1989, p.234
706 Frawley, David. *Ayurvedic Healing,* Lotus Press: Twin Lakes, WI p.245
707 Tiwari, Maya. *Ayurveda: Secrets of Healing.* LotusPress, Twin Lakes, WI, 1995, p.136
708 Dash, Bhagwan. *Massage Therapy in Ayurveda.* Concept: New Delhi, 1992, p.68
709 Welihinda, J., et al. Effect of Momordica charantia on the glucose tolerance in maturity onset diabetes. J. Ethopharmacol 17 (1986): 277-82
710 Shanmugrasundram, E.R.B., et al. *Use of Gymnema sylvestre leaf extract in the control of blood glucose in insulindependent diabetes mellitus.* J. Ethnopharmacol 30 (1990): 281-94
711 Dash, Bhagwan, and Kashyap, Lalitesh. *Materia Medica of Ayurveda.* Concept: New Delhi, 1979, p.4
712 Tavani A, Negri E, La Vecchia C. Food and nutrient intake and risk of cataract. Ann Epidemiol. 1996 Jan;6(1):41-6.
713 Jacques PF, Chylack LT Jr. Epidemiologic evidence of a role for the antioxidant vitamins and carotenoids in cataract prevention. Am J Clin Nutr. 1991 Jan;53(1 Suppl):352S-355S.
714 Hankinson SE, Stampfer MJ, Seddon JM, Colditz GA, Rosner B, Speizer FE, Willett WC. Nutrient intake and cataract extraction in women: a prospective study. BMJ. 1992 Aug 8;305(6849):335-9.
715 Frawley, David, and Lad, Vasant, The Yoga of Herbs, LotusPress, Twin Lakes, WI, 1986.
716 Jain, S.K., and DeFillips, Robert A., Medicinal Plants of India, Reference Publications, Algonac, Michigan, 1991, p.372.
717 Nadkarni, K.M., Indian Materia Medica, Popular Prakashan, Bombay, 1976, p.863.
718 Kapoor, L.D., The CRC Handbook of Ayurvedic Medicinal Plants, CRC Press, Baton Rouge, 1990, p. 249.
719 Phadke SA, Kulkarni SD Screening of in vitro antibacterial activity of Terminalia chebula, Eclapta alba and Ocimum sanctum. Indian J Med Sci 1989 May;43(5):113-7
720 Godhwani S, Godhwani JL, Vyas DS Ocimum sanctum-a preliminary study evaluating its immunoregulatory profile in albino rats. J Ethnopharmacol 1988 Dec;24(2-3):193-8
721 Hotz J, Plein K[Effectiveness of plantago seed husks in comparison with wheat brain on stool frequency and manifestations of irritable colon syndrome with constipation]. *Med Klin* 1994 Dec 15;89(12):645-51
722 Prior A, Whorwell PJ Double blind study of ispaghula in irritable bowel syndrome. *Gut* 1987

Nov;28(11):1510-3

723 Kumar A, Kumar N, Vij JC, Sarin SK, Anand BS Optimum dosage of ispaghula husk in patients with irritable bowel syndrome: correlation of symptom relief with whole gut transit time and stool weight. *Gut* 1987 Feb;28(2):150-5

724 Personal communication with Michael Tierra

725 Depression Health Center. WebMD Health, http://my.webmd.com/medical_information/condition_centers/depression/default.htm

726 Berger, Fran, Exercise Those Aging Brains, January 23, 2001, Health Scout, www.healthscout.com/cgibin/ WebObjects/Af.woa/wa/article?ap=1&id=107423

727 Wiener Medizinische Wocheschrift, 1975; 1223:705-9

728 Chakravarti, Sree, A Healer's Journey, Rudra Press, 1993

729 Keitel W, Frerick H, Kuhn U, Schmidt U, Kuhlmann M, Bredehorst A. Capsicum pain plaster in chronic nonspecific low back pain. Arzneimittelforschung 2001 Nov;51(11):896-903

730 Srimal RC, Dhawan BN. Pharmacology of diferuloyl methane (curcumin), a non-steroidal anti-inflammatory agent. J Pharm Pharmac 1973;25:447-52.

731 Halpern, Marc, Ayurveda And The Treatment of Digestive Disease, California College of Ayurveda, www.ayurvedacollege.com

732 Rasyid A, Lelo A. The effect of curcumin and placebo on human gall-bladder function: an ultrasound study. *Aliment Pharmacol Ther.* 1999;13:245–249.

733 Ammon HP, Wahl MA. Pharmacology of Curcuma longa. *Planta Med.* 1991;57:1–7.

734 Thamlikitkul V, Bunyapraphatsara N, Dechatiwongse T, et al. Randomized double blind study of *Curcuma domestica Val. for dyspepsia. J Med Assoc Thai.* 1989;72:613–620.

735 World Health Organization, WHO Monographs on Selected Medicinal Plants, Geneva, 1999.

736 Blumenthal M, Busse WR, Goldberg A, et al, eds. *The Complete German Commission E Monographs: Therapeutic Guide to Herbal Medicines.* Austin: American Botanical Council and Boston: Integrative Medicine Communications, 1998, 167.

737 McCaleb, Robert S., Herb Research Foundation Encyclopedia of Popular Herbs, Prima, Roseville, california, 2000.

738 Seamon, K.B., and Daly, J.W. Forkskolin: A unique diterpene activator of cAMP-generating systems. J. Cyclic Nucleotide Research 7 (1981): 201-24

739 Caprioli, J., and Sears, M. Forskolin lowers intraocular pressure in rabbits, monkeys, and man. Lancet i (1983): 958- 60

740 Mengi, S.A., and Desphande, S. G. Comparative evaluation of Butea frondosa and flurbiprofen for ocular antiinflammatory activity in rabbits. J. Pharm. Pharmacol. 47 (1995): 997-1001

741 Indian Tinospora Shows Positive Results in Treating Allergic Rhinitis, *HerbalGram.* 2006;69:27

742 Yogi Bhajan. Personal communication (with K.P.S. Khalsa). 1975.

743 Badar VA, Thawani VR, Wakode PT, Shrivastava MP, Gharpure KJ, Hingorani LL, Khiyani RM. Efficacy of Tinospora cordifolia in allergic rhinitis. J Ethnopharmacol. 2005 Jan 15;96(3):445-9. Epub 2004 Nov 23

744 Riehemann K Behnke B Schulze Osthoff K Plant extracts from stinging nettle (Urtica dioica), an antirheumatic remedy, inhibit the proinflammatory transcription factor NF-kappaB. FEBS-Lett. 1999 Jan 8; 442(1): 89-94 1999

745 Mittman P Randomized, double-blind study of freeze-dried Urtica dioica in the treatment of allergic rhinitis. Planta- Med. 1990 Feb; 56(1): 44-7 1990

746 Obertreis B Giller K Teucher T Behnke B Schmitz H Anti-inflammatory effect of Urtica dioica folia extract in comparison to caffeic malic acid Arzneimittelforschung. 1996 Jan; 46(1): 52-6 1996

747 Chrubasik S Enderlein W Bauer R Grabner W Evidence for antirheumatic effectiveness of Herba Urtica dioica in acute arthritis: a pilot study. Phytomedicine 1997; 4:105-8.

748 Ayurveda Pharmacopoeia, Department of Ayurveda, Yoga and Naturopathy, Unani, Siddha and Homeopathy, Ministry of Health and Family Welfare, Government of India, http://

indianmedicine.nic.in/html/ayurveda/ayurveda.htm

749 Personal communication with Michael Tierra

750 Dinsmoor, Robert Scott, *Impotence,* Gale Encyclopedia of Medicine, www.gale.com

751 Yogi Bhajan Lecture 8/13/76

752 Bhajan, Yogi, *Ancient Art of Self Healing,* West Anandpur (publisher), Eugene, Oregon, 1982., p. 15.

753 Nandan Musli, http://www.nandanmusli.com/safeaphrodisiac.htm

754 Nadkarni, K.M., *Indian Materia Medica,* Popular Prakashan, Bombay, 1976, p. 151

755 Abdel-Magied EM, Abdel-Rahman HA, Harraz FM. The effect of aqueous extracts of Cynomorium coccineum and Withania somnifera on testicular development in immature Wistar rats. J Ethnopharmacol 2001 Apr;75(1):1-4

756 Dhuley JN.Adaptogenic and cardioprotective action of ashwagandha in rats and frogs. J Ethnopharmacol 2000 Apr;70(1):57-63

757 Jose JK, Kuttan R. Hepatoprotective activity of Emblica officinalis and Chyavanaprash. J Ethnopharmacol 2000 Sep;72(1-2):135-40

758 Manjunatha S, Jaryal AK, Bijlani RL, Sachdeva U, Gupta SK. Effect of Chyawanprash and vitamin C on glucose tolerance and lipoprotein profile. Indian J Physiol Pharmacol 2001 Jan;45(1):71-9

759 Lad, Vasant, and Frawley, David, The *Yoga of Herbs,* Lotus Press, Twin Lakes, 1986, p. 142

760 Nadkarni, Dr. K.M. 1976. *The Indian Materia Medica, with Ayurvedic, Unani and Home Remedies.* Revised and enlarged by A.K. Nadkarni. 1954. Reprint. Bombay: Bombay Popular Prakashan PVP., p.1135.

761 Baidyanath Ayurveda http://www.baidyanath.com/messageoil.htm

762 Tierra, Michael, *Ayurveda and Insomina,* http://planetherbs.com

763 Houghton PJ The scientific basis for the reputed activity of Valerian *J Pharm Pharmacol* 1999 May;51(5):505-12.

764 Bourin M, Bougerol T, Guitton B, Broutin E A combination of plant extracts in the treatment of outpatients with adjustment disorder with anxious mood: controlled study versus placebo. *Fundam Clin Pharmacol* 1997;11(2):127-32

765 Leathwood PD, Chauffard F, Heck E, Munoz-Box R Aqueous extract of valerian root (Valeriana officinalis L.) improves sleep quality in man. *Pharmacol Biochem Behav* 1982 Jul;17(1):65-71

766 Lansdorf, Nancy, Maharishi Ayurveda for Common Disorders: Insomnia http://www. ayurvedaayurvedic. com/recommendations/asgb-68.html

767 Liu JH, Chen GH, Yeh HZ, Huang CK, Poon SK Enteric-coated peppermint-oil capsules in the treatment of irritable bowel syndrome: a prospective, randomized trial. *J Gastroenterol* 1997 Dec;32(6):765-8

768 Freise J, Kohler S [Peppermint oil-caraway oil fixed combination in non-ulcer dyspepsia--comparison of the effects of enteric preparations]. *Pharmazie* 1999 Mar;54(3):210-5

769 Micklefield GH, Greving I, May B Effects of peppermint oil and caraway oil on gastroduodenal motility. *Phytother Res* 2000 Feb;14(1):20-3

770 Hotz J, Plein K[Effectiveness of plantago seed husks in comparison with wheat bran on stool frequency and manifestations of irritable colon syndrome with constipation]. *Med Klin* 1994 Dec 15;89(12):645-51

771 Prior A, Whorwell PJ Double blind study of ispaghula in irritable bowel syndrome. *Gut* 1987 Nov;28(11):1510-3

772 Kumar A, Kumar N, Vij JC, Sarin SK, Anand BS Optimum dosage of ispaghula husk in patients with irritable bowel syndrome: correlation of symptom relief with whole gut transit time and stool weight. *Gut* 1987 Feb;28(2):150-5

773 Sharma KR, Bhatia RP, Kumar V. Role of the indigenous drug saptamrita lauha in hemorrhagic retinopathies. Ann Ophthalmol. 1992 Jan;24(1):5-8.

774 Nalini K, et al. Effect of Centella asiatica fresh leaf aqueous extract on learning and memory and

biogenic amine urnover in albino rats. Fitoterapia 1992; 63(3): 232-7
775 Mook-Jung I, Shin JE, Yun SH, Huh K, Koh JY, Park HK, Jew SS, Jung MW.Protective effects of asiaticoside derivatives against beta-amyloid neurotoxicity. J Neurosci Res 1999 Nov 1;58(3):417-25.
776 Vohora D, Pal SN, Pillai KK.Protection from phenytoin-induced cognitive deficit by Bacopa monniera, a reputed Indian nootropic plant. J Ethnopharmacol 2000 Aug;71(3):383-90.
777 Bhattacharya SK, Bhattacharya A, Chakrabarti A. Adaptogenic activity of Siotone, a polyherbal formulation of Ayurvedic rasayanas. Indian J Exp Biol 2000 Feb;38(2):119-28
778 Okyar A, Can A, Akev N, Baktir G, Sutlupinar N. Effect of Aloe vera leaves on blood glucose level in type I and type II diabetic rat models. Phytother Res 2001 Mar;15(2):157-61
779 Yogi Bhajan Lecture 8/13/76
780 Yogi Bhajan Lecture 8/13/76
781 Lad, Vasant, and Frawley, David, *The Yoga of Herbs,* Lotus Press, Twin Lakes, WI, 1986, p. 133
782 Nandan Musli, http://www.nandanmusli.com/safeaphrodisiac.htm
783 Nadkarni, K.M., *Indian Materia Medica,* Popular Prakashan, Bombay, 1976, p. 151
784 Modi, Ramesh, *Aamla, An Important Ayurvedic Medicine,* Ayurved Centre, Toronto, Canada, http://www.ayurvedtoronto.netfirms.com/aamla.htm
785 Bhajan, Yogi, *Ancient Art of Self Healing,* West Anandpur (publisher), Eugene, Oregon, 1982., p. 15.
786 Oi, Y., T. Kawada, K. Iwai, et al. Garlic supplementation enhances norepinephrine secretion, growth of brown adipose tissue, and triglyceride catabolism inrats. J Nutr Biochem, 1995; 6: 250-5
787 Ryttig KR, Tellnes G, Haegh L, Boe E, Fagerthun H. A dietary fibre supplement and weight maintenance after weight reduction: a randomized, double-blind, placebo-controlled long-term trial. Int J Obes 1989;13(2):165-71
788 Turnbull WH, Thomas HG. The effect of a Plantago ovata seed containing preparation on appetite variables, nutrient and energy intake. Int J Obes Relat Metab Disord 1995 May;19(5):338-42
789 Verma SK, Bordia A. Effect of Commiphora mukul (gum guggulu) in patients of hyperlipidemia with special reference to HDL-cholesterol. Indian J Med Res 1988 Apr;87:356-60
790 Satyavati GV. Gum guggul (Commiphora mukul)--the success story of an ancient insight leading to a modern discovery. Indian J Med Res 1988 Apr;87:327-35
791 Tripathi YB, Malhotra OP, Tripathi SN. Thyroid stimulating action of Z-guggulsterone obtained from Commiphora mukul. Planta Med 1984 Feb;(1):78-80
792 Satyavati GV, Dwarakanath C, Tripathi SN. Experimental studies on the hypocholesterolemic effect of Commiphora mukul. Engl. (Guggul). Indian J Med Res 1969 Oct;57(10):1950-62
793 Antonio J, Colker CM, Torina GC, et al. Effects of a standardized guggulsterone phosphate supplement on body composition in overweight adults: A pilot study. *Curr Ther Res* 1999;60:220-7.
794 Paranjpe P, Patki P, Patwardhan B. Ayurvedic treatment of obesity: a randomised double-blind, placebo-controlled clinical trial. J Ethnopharmacol 1990 Apr;29(1):1-11
795 *Phytotherapy Research,* 1994; 8: 118-20
796 Personal communication, referencing a quote from Christopher Hobbs, L.Ac.
797 Private communication with Alan Tillotson
798 Sastry, J.L.N., Dravyaguna Vijnana, Chaukambha Orientalia, Varanasi, 2002, p.228
799 Sharma, Ram, and Dash, Bhagwan, *Caraka Samhita,* Chowkhamba, Varanasi, 1992
800 Anselmo, Peter, with Brooks, James, *Ayurvedic Secrets to Longevity and Total Health,* Prentice Hall, Englewood Cliffs, 1996
801 Lad, Vasant, *Ayurveda Today,* Spring, 1995, p.3
802 Ranade, Subash, *Natural Healing through Ayurveda,* Passage Press, Salt Lake City, 1993
803 Yogi Bhajan, *The Ancient Art of Self Healing,* West Anandpur, 1982
804 Frawley, David, *Yoga International,* January/February 1996

805 Svoboda, Robert, Ritual Success, www.drsvoboda.com
806 Satcakra-nirupana, v. 3
807 Svoboda, Robert, Cultivating Prana, www.drsvoboda.com
808 Yogi Bhajan Lecture 9/17-18/92
809 Chauhan, Partap, The Real Ayurveda, Jiva Ayurveda, http://www.ayurvedic.org/
810 Personal communication with Karta Purkh Singh Khalsa
811 Yogi Bhajan Lecture 2/12/92
812 Yogi Bhajan Lecture, Man to Man number 2

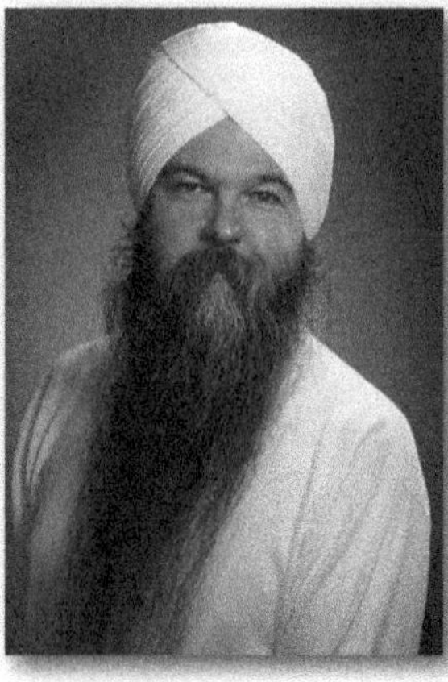

Karta Purkh Singh Khalsa, D.N.-C., A.H.G., R.C., is an herbalist, nutritionist, yoga teacher and educator who has been making natural healing approaches palatable to the modern mind for over thirty five years. He was the herbal apprentice of an Ayurvedic master, Yogi Bhajan for thirty-two years, and is the only American to hold the title "Yogaraj" in Ayurvedic herbalism.

Khalsa was the founder of Seattle's first multidisciplinary holistic clinic. He is the author or editor of over 30 books, and, with over 1,300 articles in publication, is a frequent contributor to mainstream and professional publications. He served two terms on the governing council of the American Herbalists Guild. He is on the faculty in the botanical medicine department of Bastyr University, a top naturopathic medical school.

Karta Purkh Singh and his wife, Jagdish Kaur Khalsa, also a long time close student of Yogi Bhajan, live in Eugene, Oregon, where they share a home with their teenage daughter.

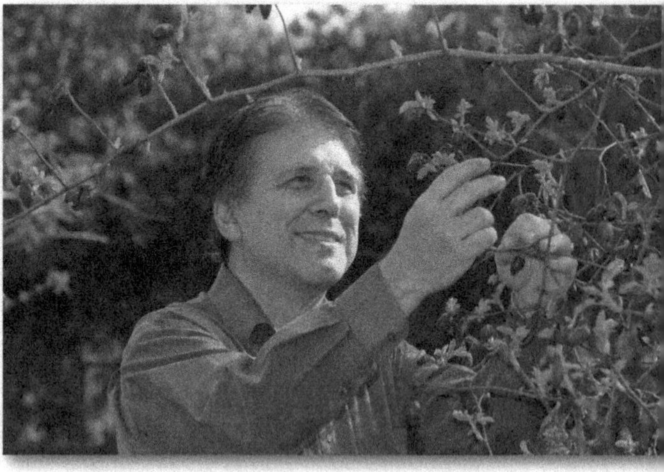

Michael Tierra, L.Ac., O.M.D., A.H.G., is one of the founders of the North American natural health movement, and was one of the first acupuncturists to be licensed in the United States. He began his herbal studies in 1968, when he learned the wild forest plants and healing ways of the Karok and Yurok Indians.

Starting in 1970, Michael apprenticed with a variety of natural healing experts. In particular, he studied Ayurvedic medicine and yoga with Baba Hari Dass.

Later he authored many the nationally acclaimed herbal books, including the first two books of this trilogy, The Way of Herbs and The Way of Chinese Herbs. His East West Correspondence Courses in Herbology has educated a generation of herbalists.

In 1989, Michael Tierra founded the American Herbalists Guild, with the goal of establishing standards for the professional practice of clinical herbal medicine in the United States.

Tierra lectures throughout the world. Each year, in the spring, Michael and his wife, Lesley, travel abroad to teach at the East West College.

BIOMAGNETIC
and Herbal Therapy

Dr. Michael Tierra

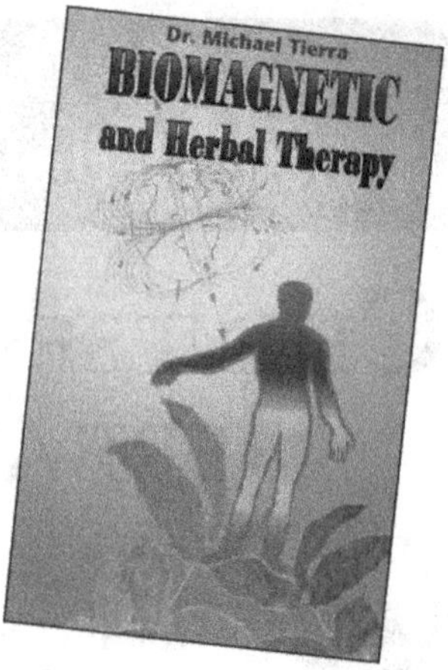

Trade Paper
ISBN 978-0-9149-5533-7
108 pp $10.95

Magnetic energy is the structural force of the universe. In this book the respected herbalist and healer, Dr. Michael Tierra, enlightens us on the healing influence of commercially available magnets for many conditions and describes the sometimes miraculous relief from such problems as joint pain, skin diseases, acidity, blood pressure, tumors, kidney, liver and thyroid problems, and more. Magnetizing herbs, teas, water and their usage in conjunction with direct placement of magnets for synergistic effectiveness is presented in a systematic, succinct and practical manner for the benefit of the professional and lay person alike. Replete with diagrams and appendices, this is a "how to do" practical handbook for augmenting health and obtaining relief from pain.

The paradigm of health in the future is based on energy flow. This paradigm reaches back to the ancient healing arts of the traditional Chinese, the Ayurvedic and the Native American cultures. It is connected to the work of Hippocrates, the "father" of Western medicine, in ancient Greek culture, and found its way through the herbal and homeopathic science that has flourished in Europe over the last few hundred years.

Dr. Tierra is the author of the all-time best selling herbal *The Way of Herbs* as well as the synthesizing work *Planetary Herbology.* He is a practicing herbalist and educator in the field with a background of studies spanning the Chinese and Ayurvedic, the Native American and the European herbal traditions.

Available at bookstores and natural food stores nationwide or order your copy directly by sending $10.95 plus $2.50 shipping/handling ($.75 s/h for each additional copy ordered at the same time) to:

Lotus Press, PO Box 325, Dept. TCH, Twin Lakes, WI 53181 USA
toll free order line: 800 824 6396 office phone: 262 889 8561
office fax: 262 889 2461 email: lotuspress@lotuspress.com
web site: www.lotuspress.com

Lotus Press is the publisher of a wide range of books and software in the field of alternative health, including Ayurveda, Chinese medicine, herbology, aromatherapy, Reiki and energetic healing modalities. Request our free book catalog.

Planetary Herbology

by Dr. Michael Tierra

A major work integrating the herbal traditions of the East with those of the West by the bestselling author of "The Way of Herbs". This practical handbook and reference guide is a landmark publication in this field. For unprecedented usefulness in practical applications, the author provides a comprehensive listing of the more than 400 medicinal herbs available in the west, classified according to their chemical constituents, properties and actions, indicated uses and suggested dosages.

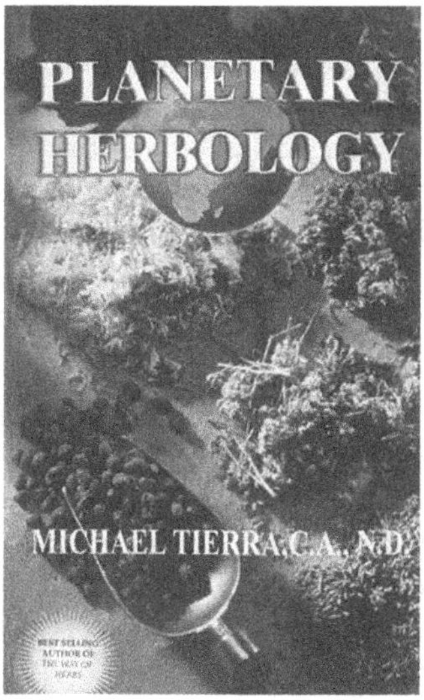

Trade Paper Book ISBN: 978-0-9415-2427-8 490 pp pb $19.95

Available at bookstores and natural food stores nationwide or order your copy directly by sending $17.95 plus $2.50 shipping/handling ($.75 s/h for each additional copy ordered at the same time) to:

Lotus Press, PO Box 325, Dept. NW, Twin Lakes, WI 53181 USA
toll free order line: 800 824 6396 office phone: 262 889 8561
office fax: 262 889 2461 email: lotuspress@lotuspress.com
web site: www.lotuspress.com

Lotus Press is the publisher of a wide range of books and software in the field of alternative health, including Ayurveda, Chinese medicine, herbology, aromatherapy, Reiki and energetic healing modalities. Request our free book catalog.